CLINICAL SKILLS

FOR

SPEECH-LANGUAGE PATHOLOGISTS

D1532657

CLINICAL SKILLS

FOR
SPEECH-LANGUAGE PATHOLOGISTS

Stanley A. Goldberg, Ph.D.
San Francisco State University

SINGULAR PUBLISHING GROUP
SAN DIEGO · LONDON

Singular Publishing Group, Inc.
401 West A Street, Suite 325
San Diego, California 92101-7904

19 Compton Terrace
London N1 2UN, UK

e-mail: singpub©mail.cerfnet.com
Website: http://www.singpub.com

© 1997 by Singular Publishing Group, Inc.
Second Singular Printing June 1998

Typeset in 10/12 New Century Schoolbook by So Cal Graphics
Printed in the United States of America by BookCrafters

Library of Congress Cataloging-in-Publication Data

Goldberg, Stanley, A.
    Clinical skills for speech-language clinicians / Stanley A.
Goldberg.
      p.   cm.
    Includes bibliographical references and index.
    ISBN 1-56593-686-8
    1. Speech therapy.   I. Title.
    [DNLM: 1. Speech-Language Pathology—methods. 2. Speech
Disorders—therapy.
    3. Language Disorders—therapy.   WL 340.2
G618c 1996]
RC423.G633   1996
616.85'506—dc20
DNLM/DLC
for Library of Congress
                   96-33065
                   CIP

Contents

Acknowledgments

I would like to acknowledge and thank Dr. Noma Anderson for her review of the entire text. Dr. Jean Van Keulen, Dr. Addison Watanabe, and Ms. Rhonda Friedlander for their review and helpful suggestions on Chapter 3. The Confederated Salish and Kootenai Tribes of the Flathead Indian Reservation and Ms. Rhonda Friedlander and her family for giving of their time and sharing of their culture. To the United States Office of Special Education and Rehabilitation for their support in my efforts to improve the quality of therapy provided to children receiving services in the nation's public schools (Grant Number H029820261-93).

Dedicated to

The many students and clinicians who have been
gracious enough to allow me to observe, dissect, and
comment on their therapy. Without your graciousness,
this book would never have been possible.

Those clinicians who have currently, and will continue,
to provide the best possible therapy for their clients,
often in the face of overwhelming economic and
political pressures.

Section I

INTRODUCTION TO THERAPY

CHAPTER

1

Introduction

*C*linicians in helping professions occupy a very special place in all societies. Clients and their families entrust them with at least one aspect of their lives. It may be to cure a physical illness, to understand an emotional problem, or to learn a new communicative behavior. In order to help the person, they are given permission to suggest changes, restructure interactions, and modify behaviors which often will affect core features of the person's identity. The enormity of the power they are willingly given is overshadowed only by the amount of responsibility it demands. In the hands and words of clinicians comes the power to unalterably affect peoples lives. Nothing they do in therapy should be haphazard or casual. Not only do clients and their families have the right to expect competent, efficient, ethical, and caring interactions, but speech-language clinicians are ethically obligated to provide it.

Providing services of the highest quality involves a multidimensional process which often is as complicated as the disorder being treated. This process takes the form of skills which are both technical and process oriented. Both types of skills transcend many fields and become the means by which the knowledge and compassion of clinicians are transformed into helping behaviors. The purpose of this text is to describe these skills, provide empirical evidence for their value, and explain in detail how they should be used with individuals who have communicative disorders.

A MAP OF THE BOOK

A new technology called Global Positioning System (GPS) navigation uses the position of satellites to tell you within 5 feet where you are anywhere in the world. With a small hand-held receiver you can plot a course, record, and save location positions that can be used as future reference points. Final destinations can be established and the best route determined before the journey begins. Whether the journey is on land or water, knowing where you are going allows you to plan more efficiently, prepare for what you will encounter on the way, and, by knowing the route and destination, derive more out of the experience. The same principles apply to this text. By understanding what the text is intended to do and knowing what will be encountered on the journey, you will be able to derive more benefits from the text than if a road map was not provided.

Text Structure

If a helping profession calls itself a clinical science, it needs to answer the following questions regarding all forms of intervention. *What* should be done to effect positive change in clients? *Why* should it be done? And *How* should it be accomplished? Together, the answers to these three questions constitute the backbone of any scientific approach in the clinical sciences. The absence of the first leads to a state of ignorance. Without answers to the second question, there is no justifiable basis for intervention. Not being able to answer the third question causes professional helplessness. These three questions are posed and answered for all skills in this text.

What. "What" refers to general principles or maxims that are skills to be used by clinicians. They are written in specific behavioral terms such as "develop rapport" or "reinforce correct responses." For each skill there will be a definition and a description. When possible, two examples will be provided, one that uses everyday experiences as a reference point and another based on at least one communicative disorder. This will allow both inexperienced and experienced clinicians to see the rationale for the skill's use. If the skill has specific behavioral components, as most do, each will be delineated and their sequence described.

Why. "Why" questions refer to the justification for a skill's use. Answers to these questions can range from very weak to very strong. The weakest and least justifiable relies on a personal conviction or theoretical position, where no references are made to objective data. The position is held on the basis of faith, intuition, or the need to be theoretically consistent. When reality conflicts with the belief or theory, reality is often ignored with this type of justification. A second type of justification is based on

clinical experience with similar cases. The assumption is that, since a significant number of past cases bear enough similarities with a present case, an inductive leap of faith can be made. Although stronger than the first form of justification, the use of clinical experiences may be flawed by the lack of a wide range of experiences. Given the infinite variety of people, differences between a present case and past cases may be too great to draw any inferences. The next form of justification, and one of the strongest, is based on experimental studies that are well controlled and generalizable to a wide range of clinical situations. Although the study may not have directly involved the area of communicative disorders, the principles and conditions of the study are transferable to a specific communication disorder. For example, the importance of establishing trust when working with drug-dependent clients is probably no different than its importance when working with a vocal abusing client. The last, and strongest, form of justification are clinical studies occurring within the field of communicative disorders. With this form of justification, no inferences need be made. The skills have been studied directly in the treatment of communicatively disordered individuals.

Although the last form of justification is the strongest, it is the one least available in our field. A 20-year review of the literature in speech-language pathology reveals that few studies have objectively examined the effect specific clinical skills have on communicatively disabled clients. The closest researchers in our field came to studying clinical skills was the examination of supervisory practices. Interest in this area began in the late 1970s and abated considerably by the late 1980s (Oratio & Hood, 1977; Stackhouse & Furnham, 1983; Dowling, 1986; Shapiro & Anderson, 1988). During these 10 years of intense research, the primary focus was not on the identification of critical skills, but rather on (1) the creation of acceptable clinical evaluation formats; (2) analysis of supervisor-supervisee interaction patterns; and (3) methods for determining the degree of acceptability of supervision styles. These studies, although important for the development of supervisory practice in speech-language pathology, focused on how to evaluate clinical skills rather than determining what skills should be evaluated. Few data-based clinical studies in the area of speech-language pathology have attempted to substantiate not only what a skill looks like within a clinical context, but also its importance in terms of affecting the outcome of therapy. Most justifications therefore will need to involve one of the remaining three types. Of the three, the strongest would be using research generated in other areas.

Fortunately, a substantial amount of applicable research has been conducted in fields other than speech-language therapy. These include physician training, psychoanalysis, psychology, physical therapy, occupational therapy, counseling, social work, business, nursing, and instructional technology. The results of studies in these areas, although not necessarily pertaining directly to communicative disorders, contain elements of clinical interactions and change that are applicable to our clients. For a very few clinical skills, experimental studies were not located. For those, the justification becomes based on 25 years of clinical experience. Hopefully, with future research, these also will have an experimental justification.

HOW. "How" involves the application of the skill. It is the step between knowledge about the disorders and its transfer into helping behaviors. For example, it is one thing to know that clients who are leaving off the final phoneme of words need to be taught to produce that phoneme. It is another to know how to emphasize certain components in the stimulus configuration that will facilitate its production and result in the retention of the behavior.

There are certain ways in which one can learn the "how" skills in any field, whether that field involves the amelioration of communication problems or more manual skills such as plumbing. The most common approach involves a course of study followed by supervised practice. Just as student clinicians are supervised by clinical supervisors, the work of journey-person plumbers is closely watched by their supervising master plumbers. The purpose of the supervised clinical practice for both student speech-language clinicians and journey-person plumbers is to develop the skills necessary for the practice of their profession. One of these professions has a long history of successful training. The other has for the past 50 years been less successful. Unfortunately for us, the profession of speech-language pathology has been the less successful one. With little interest in the identification of critical clinical skills, there was even less concern with how to teach them to student clinicians. The assumptions of supervision researchers and the underlying basis of their studies was that, by understanding the dynamics of the supervisory process, the clinical competence of students would be enhanced. And by setting high academic standards for students, many of the problems found in poor clinical practice would be eliminated. Unfortunately, this educational strategy has not resulted in its intended goals. Upon graduating from training programs many clinicians find that they are ill-prepared to meet many of the needs of their clients and are forced to gain knowledge of skills on a trial-and-error basis. Although many of the skills are eventually acquired, others are not. They are ones clinicians know are necessary, but do not have the knowledge required to develop them. And that knowledge cannot be acquired just through experience. For example, unless one knows the research on stimulus configuration, the probability that the stimulus best suited for retention will be used is rather small. Without either experimental knowledge or clinical experience, justifications are often based on faith.

To facilitate the learning process in this text, forms, sample dialogues, and check sheets are provided. Some are designed merely to give an example of how something should be done. Others present formats for evaluating client behaviors, still others are constructed so that clinicians can evaluate their own behaviors. The design of these supplemental materials allows for the full spectrum of clinical experience, from neophytes to clinicians with advanced skills. Clinicians with more experience may choose to ignore sample dialogues and concentrate on the self-analysis forms. Newer clinicians will benefit from using all of the material.

Terminology

Five terms should be understood before beginning this book. These are *foundational, transitional, complex, technical,* and *process-oriented*. The first three refer to the level of sophistication needed to acquire skills, and the last two refer to types of skills.

Levels of Sophistication. Skills can be placed on a continuum of complexity, ranging from foundational to complex. Foundational skills are those that form a base on which more advanced skills rest. Transitional skills utilize components of the foundational skills and apply them in more sophisticated ways. Complex skills involve a considerable amount of inductive reasoning. Inductive reasoning refers to the process where an individual encounters a situation which does not match one he or she has previously learned or encountered. In order to adequately deal with it, a new set of principles or practices must be constructed.

Types of Skills. The skills in this book are divided into those that are primarily technical and those which are primarily process-oriented. A technical skill is defined by a precise condition and specific interaction steps. For example, "reinforcing correct responses" would be a technical skill because it has a precise condition (occurs when a response is identical to what is requested) and specific interaction steps (after a correct response is provided, an appropriate reinforcer is administered). A process-oriented skill is less precise, and involves structuring responses or statements that are likely to result in the client developing a desired perception. An example would be "can develop rapport," because it involves using a set of clinician verbal and nonverbal behaviors that can result in the client perceiving something personal and positive about the clinician.

Qualifications to the Classification System. Categorizing skills in terms of sophistication and type is a heuristic exercise. In other words, the categorization is done for ease of organization and use. There is nothing absolute or impermeable about the system. Yet, the system makes intuitive sense. Anyone who has used a wide variety of skills can attest to the ease in using some and the tremendous difficulty in using others. Twenty-five years of experience and clinical judgments were used in categorizing the skills. Although some skills have been identified as being purely technical and others purely interpersonal, there is disagreement on others (Goldberg, 1990). Alternative grouping of skills is possible. Regardless of where skills are placed, the integrity of their justification and methods for use remains valid.

Major Sections

Section I is a basic introduction to the investigation of clinical skills. In Sections II, III, and IV, 295 techniques and clinical behaviors are addressed. They are grouped into larger skill categories such as *advance organizing statements* and *rapport*. This will allow the reader who is using the text as a clinical reference manual to quickly find the information that is of interest.

SECTION 1: Introduction to Therapy.

Three chapters are contained in the Introduction to Therapy section. The first chapter is the one you are reading and essentially provides a map of the book. The second chapter involves a presentation of the principles of change. In that chapter some of the most basic considerations for therapy are addressed. These involve concepts about change, its importance, factors of resistance, and methods for enhancing its development. The third chapter provides the reader with a very broad view of culture, which looks at cultural sensitivity as something that has many dimensions and something that can be learned.

SECTION 2: Foundational Skills.

In the second section, foundational skills and clinical behaviors are presented. Although the notion of *foundational* may imply that these are skills associated only with beginning training, even experienced clinicians may find them novel. Although some of these skills are routinely taught to beginning graduate students in speech-language pathology, others are not. And even if they are considered as part of the beginning arsenal of clinical skills for student clinicians, they often lack the "why" and "how" necessary for their effective practice. A list of all foundational skills appears in Table 1–1. In Chapter 4, the foundational technical skills are grouped into 8 categories containing 50 behaviors and techniques. These range from very precise behaviors such as "incorporating flexibility into the design of materials" to more general behaviors such as "using methods for developing consistency." In Chapter 5, 58 process-oriented behaviors and techniques are grouped into 11 categories.

SECTION 3: Transitional Skills.

Transitional skills are skills that require more sophistication and experience to develop than those in the foundational section. They lie between the foundational skills and complex skills in terms of their learning requirements. Although the transitional skills appear after foundational skills in this text, this does not necessarily reflect the order of their appearance in therapy. The same is true of complex skills. For example, *group therapy* skills are classified as complex skills, yet they are immediately important from the beginning of most sessions in school settings. Knowing how to terminate clients is identified as a transitional skill, yet the need for this skill occurs only at the end of therapy. Transitional skills are summarized in Table 1–2. In Chapter 6, 43 behaviors and techniques are listed under 5 technical skills. Chapter 7 contains 39 behaviors and techniques in eight process-oriented categories.

SECTION 4: Complex Skills.

Complex skills are skills that require the most significant amount of sophistication and experience. How often have you observed someone doing outstanding therapy, or better still, noted your own excellent therapy and marveled at how everything "clicked"? How you or the person observed seemed to do everything right, how you or they maximized the client's communicative ability, accomplishing a nonreligious equivalent of a "laying on of hands"? Usually, people walk away from the event, holding the person in awe, and not quite understanding how the changes were accomplished. Although the master clinician possesses the same foundational and transitional skills as most other clinicians, their mastery of complex skills differentiates them from other colleagues in their field. Complex skills are summarized in Table 1–3. In Chapter 8, 62 technical behaviors and techniques are presented in 7 categories. In Chapter 9 there are 43 process-oriented behaviors and techniques in 6 skill categories.

TABLE 1–1
Foundational Skills Classification

TECHNICAL (47 techniques and behaviors)	PROCESS-ORIENTED (58 techniques and behaviors)
Materials and Activities ➢ Age Appropriate ➢ Interesting ➢ Safe ➢ Generalizability	**Rapport** Methods ➢ Personal Warmth ➢ Commonality of Interests ➢ Genuine Concern
Advance Organizing Statements ➢ Purpose of Activity ➢ Conduct of Activity ➢ Justification for Activities ➢ Consequences of Behaviors	**Empathy and Compassion** Types ➢ Emotional ➢ Cognitive Uses ➢ Style of Communicating
Operant Techniques Positive Reinforcement ➢ Intrinsic Reinforcement ➢ Extrinsic Reinforcement ➢ Extraneous Reinforcement ➢ Criteria for Advancement Punishment ➢ Aversive Stimuli ➢ Response Cost Reinforcement Schedules ➢ Ratio Schedule of Reinforcement ➢ Interval Schedule of Reinforcement ➢ Mixed Schedule of Reinforcement	**Speech Characteristics** Intonation Patterns ➢ Age Factors ➢ Intensity and Amplitude ➢ Intonation for Effect ➢ Ending Intonation Patterns Paralanguage ➢ Identifiers ➢ Characterizers
Planning Activities Time ➢ Immediate ➢ Intermediate ➢ Long Range Organization ➢ Categorical ➢ Sequential Materials/Activities ➢ Safety ➢ Expense Stimulus Configurations ➢ Simplification ➢ Rate of Presentation ➢ Variations ➢ Visualness ➢ Redundancy ➢ Task Complexity	**Communicating at Client's Level** Communication Style ➢ Professional Jargon ➢ Profanity ➢ Age Considerations

TECHNICAL (47 techniques and behaviors)	PROCESS-ORIENTED (58 techniques and behaviors)
Planning Activities *(Continued)* ➢ Figure-Ground ➢ Context ➢ Categorization	**Communicating for Comprehension** ➢ Preceding Statements ➢ Asking Questions ➢ Simplification ➢ Visual and Graphic Instructions ➢ Confirmation Through Demonstration
Objectives ➢ Gaining Information ➢ Redirecting Attitudes ➢ Learning Strategies ➢ Teaching Specific Behaviors	**Respect** Cultural Values ➢ Acceptable/Unacceptable Activities ➢ Goals Personal Needs ➢ Effects of the Disorder ➢ Acceptance of Activities Caring Interaction Style ➢ Conveying Painful Information
Modeling ➢ Presentation of the Model ➢ Types of Models ➢ Sequence of Presenting and Withdrawing	**Maximizing Response Opportunities** Response Time ➢ Complexity, Age, Practice ➢ Interpretations Response Cuing ➢ Types of Cues ➢ Cue Fading
Consistency Areas of Importance ➢ Interaction Style ➢ Skills ➢ Consequences Effects ➢ Presence of Consistency ➢ Absence of Consistency	**Being Attentive** Conversational Follow-Through ➢ Importance of Statements ➢ Relevance Asking Relevant Questions ➢ Going Beyond Listening ➢ Expanding Areas of Interest
Professional Terminology and Style Terminology ➢ Descriptions of Behaviors and Events Justification ➢ Immediate ➢ Delayed	**Flexibility** Areas of Flexibility ➢ Cultural Differences ➢ Age Components ➢ Freedom Within Parameters ➢ Shifts in Clinical Focus *(continued)*

TABLE 1–1 *(continued)*

TECHNICAL (47 techniques and behaviors)	PROCESS-ORIENTED (58 techniques and behaviors)
	Client Decision Making
	Models for Involvement ➢ Simple ➢ Sophisticated
	Determining Goals ➢ Children ➢ Adolescents ➢ Adults
	Selecting Methods and Techniques ➢ Children ➢ Adolescents ➢ Adults
	Selecting Extraneous Reinforcers ➢ Children
	Nonverbal Behaviors
	Clients ➢ Face ➢ Arms/Hands ➢ Legs/Feet ➢ Posture
	Clinicians ➢ Face ➢ Arms/Hands ➢ Legs/Feet ➢ Posture
	Functions of Nonverbal Behaviors ➢ Amplification ➢ Contradiction ➢ Qualification ➢ Unrelated Message

TABLE 1–2
Transitional Skills Classification

TECHNICAL (44 techniques and behaviors)	PROCESS-ORIENTED (34 techniques and behaviors)
Control Verbal Interactions ➢ Children ➢ Adolescents ➢ Adults Material and Activity Design ➢ Sequentially Ordered Activities ➢ Structured Activities Contingencies ➢ Consequences for Actions ➢ Representing Contingencies	**Acknowledgment** Verbal ➢ Conversational Follow-Through ➢ Asking Relevant Questions ➢ Paraphrasing/Simple Rephrasing ➢ Client-Centered Therapy Techniques Vocal ➢ Prosody or Intonation ➢ Paralanguage Nonverbal ➢ Intentional Messages ➢ Unintentional Messages
Response Differentiation Successive Approximations ➢ Selecting End Behaviors ➢ Approximation Steps ➢ Step Components Multiple Cuing ➢ Hierarchy of Abstractness ➢ Types of Cues ➢ Number of Cues ➢ Modality of Cues ➢ Combining Successive Approximations with Multiple Cuing	**Acceptance** Withholding Judgments ➢ Effects of Prior Judgments ➢ Developing Trust Providing Judgments ➢ Behaviors ➢ Attitudes and Intonation Patterns
Parental Involvement Consultation ➢ Increasing Parent-Clinician Interactions ➢ Problem Identification and Monitoring ➢ Sharing Relevant Information ➢ Understanding Behaviors ➢ Supporting Parents ➢ Examining Overlapping Roles ➢ Training General Considerations ➢ Use of Strategies ➢ Comprehensiveness Procedures ➢ Goal Section ➢ Written Instructions ➢ Wording ➢ Observations ➢ Exact Words	**Self-Disclosure** Cultural Considerations ➢ Caucasians ➢ African Americans and Hispanics ➢ Native Americans ➢ Asian Americans/Pacific Islanders

(continued)

TABLE 1-2 *(continued)*

TECHNICAL (44 techniques and behaviors)	PROCESS-ORIENTED (34 techniques and behaviors)
Parental Involvement *(Continued)* ➤ Joint Therapy ➤ Solo Therapy ➤ Home Therapy	**Preparing For Termination** Clinician ➤ Prognosis ➤ Utilization of Strategies ➤ Generalization of Behaviors Client ➤ Responsibility for Change ➤ Ongoing Analysis of Behaviors and Goals ➤ Phasing Out of Direct Contact
Process of Learning Stages of Learning ➤ Apprehending ➤ Acquisition ➤ Retention ➤ Retrieval Levels ➤ Signal ➤ Stimulus-Response ➤ Chaining ➤ Verbal Association ➤ Discrimination ➤ Concept ➤ Rule ➤ Problem Solving	**Effective Use of Time** Minimizing Extraneous Activities ➤ Child/Adolescent ➤ Adult Maximizing Responses ➤ Efficient Structuring of Activities ➤ Requiring Multiple Responses
	Matching Activities to Learning Styles Individual Cognitive Styles ➤ Reflective Learning Style ➤ Active Learning Style Cultural Learning Styles ➤ Ethnic ➤ Religious ➤ Geographic/Regional ➤ Socioeconomic ➤ Disability ➤ Age
	Rephrasing Positive Effects ➤ Indicating Clinician Attention ➤ Restructuring ➤ Summation Methods ➤ Personalization

TABLE 1–3
Complex Skills Classification

TECHNICAL (62 techniques and behaviors)	PROCESS-ORIENTED (44 techniques and behaviors)
Changing Attitudes Discussion ➤ Client-Centered ➤ Logical Structuring ➤ Demonstration	**Confrontation** Effectiveness Methods ➤ Enlisting Client Input ➤ Structuring Confrontations Problems ➤ Losing Face ➤ Cultural Considerations ➤ Aftermath ➤ Clients' Deference to Clinicians
Monitoring Degrees ➤ Binary ➤ Gradations Types ➤ Interval Contingent ➤ Signal Contingent ➤ Event Contingent Clinician Monitoring ➤ Modality ➤ Shifting From Clinician to Client Client ➤ Nonverbal Signal ➤ Verbal Signal	**Group Therapy** Basic Considerations ➤ Preparation ➤ Group Composition ➤ General Competency ➤ Settings ➤ Cultural Considerations ➤ Clinical Orientation Interpersonal Issues ➤ Gender Leadership ➤ Ethnic Leadership ➤ Role Relationships ➤ Member-to-Member Feedback ➤ Group Interactive Styles ➤ Active Involvement Management ➤ Control ➤ Efficiency Functions ➤ Teaching New Behaviors ➤ Generalization of Behaviors ➤ Gathering Data ➤ Discussion
Using Strategies General Considerations ➤ Criteria for Selecting Strategies ➤ Behavior vs. Strategy ➤ Strategies and Intelligence ➤ Source of Strategies ➤ Internal vs. External *(continued)*	*(continued)*

TABLE 1–3 *(continued)*

TECHNICAL (62 techniques and behaviors)	PROCESS-ORIENTED (44 techniques and behaviors)
Using Strategies *(Continued)* ➤ Training Requirements for Effectiveness ➤ Practice vs. Strategies ➤ Classifying Clients by Strategy Use ➤ Strategies and Performance Speed ➤ Strategy Examples ➤ Effort, Strategy Selection, and Usage General Strategies ➤ Major Life Transitions ➤ Categorization ➤ Visualization ➤ Stress Reduction ➤ Post Organizers ➤ Elaboration ➤ Active Involvement ➤ Visual Cues ➤ Summary Skills ➤ Problem-Solving Applications ➤ Methodology ➤ Combining Strategies ➤ Combining Strategies with Monitoring ➤ Strategies and Feedback ➤ Strategies Within Comprehensive Approaches ➤ Contrasting Strategies Areas for Strategy Usage ➤ Detailed Information and Behaviors ➤ Central Ideas or Concepts	**Feedback** Client to Clinician ➤ Requests Clinician to Client ➤ Timing ➤ Specificity ➤ Levels of Acceptability Types ➤ Levels of Sophistication ➤ Positive and Instructional Feedback ➤ Semantics of Positive and Negative Words
Generalization Timing ➤ A Stage of Therapy ➤ An Integrated Part of Therapy Stimulus Generalization ➤ Configurations ➤ Training Sequence ➤ Rationale Response Generalization ➤ Training Sequence ➤ Rationale Combinations of Stimulus and Response Generalizations ➤ Scheduling ➤ Contracts ➤ Highlighting Stimulus Configurations	**Professional Collaboration** Hospital/Rehabilitation Sites ➤ Areas of Competency ➤ Interaction Principles Public Schools ➤ Advantages of Collaborative Models ➤ Disadvantages of Collaborative Models ➤ Combining Pull-out and Inclusion Models

TECHNICAL (62 techniques and behaviors)	PROCESS-ORIENTED (44 techniques and behaviors)
Maintenance Things to Maintain ➤ Specific Behaviors ➤ Compensatory Strategies ➤ New Behavior Strategies	**Professional Authority** Charisma ➤ Client's Need for Charismatic Clinicians ➤ Minimizing Charismatic Experiences Competency ➤ Appropriate Use ➤ Inappropriate Use
Error Analysis General Conditions ➤ Certitude of Answers Types ➤ Unlearned Prerequisites ➤ Systematic Conceptual Errors ➤ Random ➤ Noncompliance ➤ Nonvolitional Inattention	
Correct Response Analysis ➤ Confirmation of Prior Learning ➤ Self-analysis	

SECTION 5: Summary. In the final section, the qualities and associated clinical behaviors of master clinicians are presented along with suggestions for using the material contained in this text for clinician self-management. In Chapter 10, qualities of outstanding clinicians are operationally defined in terms of skills. In other words, if we say that someone has "exquisite timing," can that be translated into specific skills each of which has behavioral components? This should be viewed as an initial effort in defining clinical qualities and therefore is subject to reasonable disagreement. In Chapter 11, a methodology of clinical analysis is presented. This can be used by clinicians or supervisors who are responsible for assessing clinician competence.

PURPOSES OF THE BOOK

The usefulness of a text may be determined by its relevance to the audiences it is designed to reach. Some texts are only for students, others for supervisors, and still others are for practicing clinicians. This book has been designed to be useful for all three audiences.

Classroom Text

One of the purposes of this book is to serve as a classroom text for gaining information on clinical skills. As a text, two different learning formats can be used. The first involves reading the chapters sequentially. The second involves structuring the reading according to the sequence of skills needed for clinical intervention.

Sequential Reading. The book is organized in terms of learning prerequisites. In other words, Section I becomes the basis for understanding Section II, Section II then becomes the basis for understanding Section III, and so on. In order to organize it in this manner, it was not possible to adhere to a more traditional approach which uses the sequence of clinical interactions as a basis of organization. For example, although *involving parents* is a skill which needs to be applied almost immediately in therapy, it is a transitional skill, and therefore may be more difficult to learn than other skills which are more basic but are used much later in therapy.

Alternative Format. The format used in this book, that of using the two continuums, may not be the preferred format for some instructors or experienced clinicians. They may wish to use a more traditional approach which is sequential, going from the skills necessary for initiating the therapeutic contact through to its termination. A format which is more sequential appears in Tables 1–4 through 1–7. The skills are classified in terms of (1) preconditions, (2) planning, (3) applying technical skills, and (4) applying interpersonal skills. Even if the alternative format is not used, it may be valuable for the student to refer back to it as each skill is discussed. The tables provide the reader with a comprehensive graphic representation of how each specific skill is related to the whole of therapy. For example, in Table 1–6 on page 20, the relationship of the modality of cues to their number are graphically represented. Additionally, because page numbers are provided for each skill, the reader can easily access the information.

Reference Text

Many readers of this text may be practicing clinicians, who while familiar with some of the skills, may be unfamiliar with others. For them, it may not make much sense to read through information they are quite familiar with from years of practice. It is suggested that they may wish to use Tables 1–4 through 1–7 as their reference guides. Additionally, the tables can provide a quick source of information when specific problems occur in therapy.

Research/Interest Text

One of the purposes of this text is to stimulate research on clinical skills, an area that, while of intense interest in other health-related professions, has been neglected in speech-language pathology. In Appendix A, articles and books of clinical and research interest have been grouped into 28 categories. Each category constitutes a unique area of research and relevance to clinical practice. This appendix will be helpful to researchers, clinicians, supervisors, and classroom instructors. Researchers can find what has already been studied in each area. Clinicians can find information about an area of particular interest. Supervisors can suggest areas to clinicians that may be instructional. Classroom instructors can construct research assignments from the categories.

Supervision Guide

Supervisors often struggle with how to explain or teach a specific skill to students. Although observation of experienced clinicians and demonstration therapy are useful, both are transient. In other words, when the event ends, so does the lesson. With videotaping the problem is lessened. However, even excellent examples of videotapes require augmentation with written materials. As a supervision guide, the text can provide student clinicians with detailed descriptions of techniques, methods, strategies, and procedures that have been clinically demonstrated to positively affect the outcome of therapy. Additionally, in Chapter 11 a self-analysis form for clinical skills is provided. With modifications to meet the needs of the site and supervisor, the form can serve as a supervision format.

TABLE 1-4

Preconditions for successful therapy

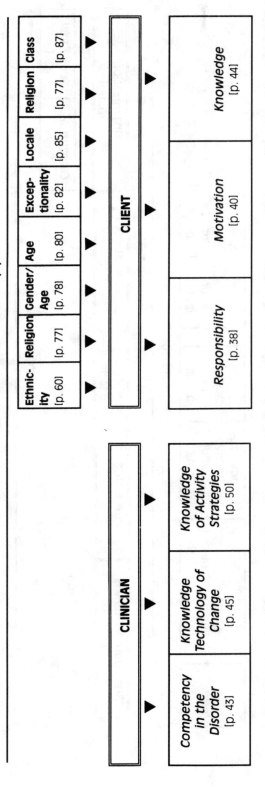

CLIENT

Ethnic-ity [p. 60]	Religion [p. 77]	Gender/ Age [p. 78]	Age [p. 80]	Excep-tionality [p. 82]	Locale [p. 85]	Religion [p. 77]	Class [p. 87]

Responsibility [p. 38]	Motivation [p. 40]	Knowledge [p. 44]

CLINICIAN

Competency in the Disorder [p. 43]	Knowledge Technology of Change [p. 45]	Knowledge of Activity Strategies [p. 50]

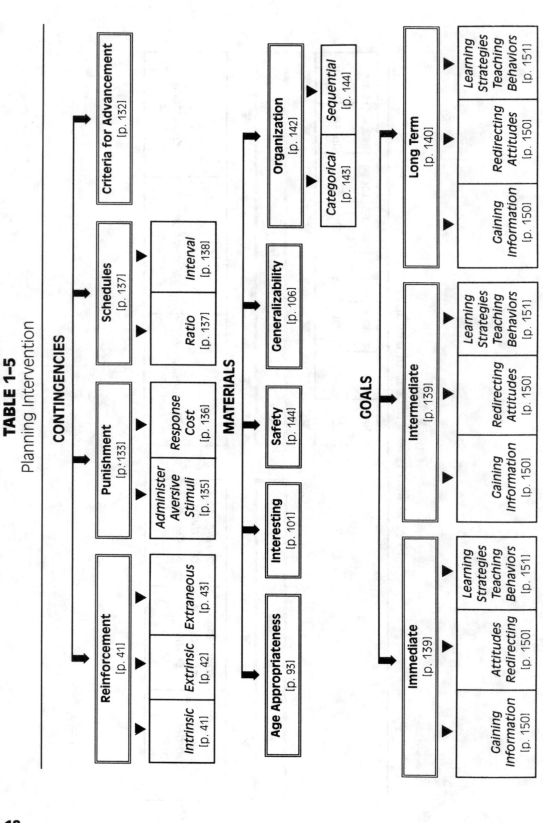

TABLE 1-5
Planning Intervention

CONTINGENCIES

- Reinforcement [p. 41]
  - Intrinsic [p. 41]
  - Extrinsic [p. 42]
  - Extraneous [p. 43]
- Punishment [p. 133]
  - Administer Aversive Stimuli [p. 135]
  - Response Cost [p. 136]
- Schedules [p. 137]
  - Ratio [p. 137]
  - Interval [p. 138]
- Criteria for Advancement [p. 132]

MATERIALS

- Age Appropriateness [p. 93]
- Interesting [p. 101]
- Safety [p. 144]
- Generalizability [p. 106]
- Organization [p. 142]
  - Categorical [p. 143]
  - Sequential [p. 144]

GOALS

- Immediate [p. 139]
  - Gaining Information [p. 150]
  - Attitudes Redirecting [p. 150]
  - Learning Strategies Teaching Behaviors [p. 151]
- Intermediate [p. 139]
  - Gaining Information [p. 150]
  - Redirecting Attitudes [p. 150]
  - Learning Strategies Teaching Behaviors [p. 151]
- Long Term [p. 140]
  - Gaining Information [p. 150]
  - Redirecting Attitudes [p. 150]
  - Learning Strategies Teaching Behaviors [p. 151]

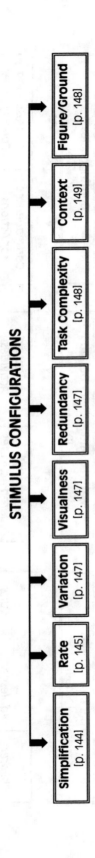

STIMULUS CONFIGURATIONS

Simplification
[p. 144]

Rate
[p. 145]

Variation
[p. 147]

Visualness
[p. 147]

Redundancy
[p. 147]

Task Complexity
[p. 148]

Context
[p. 149]

Figure/Ground
[p. 148]

TABLE 1-6

Applying technical Intervention skills

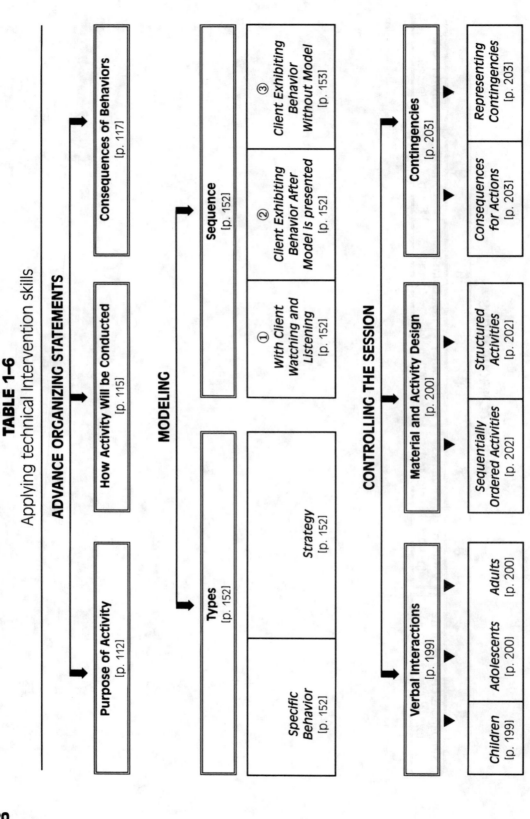

ADVANCE ORGANIZING STATEMENTS

| Purpose of Activity [p. 112] | How Activity Will be Conducted [p. 115] | Consequences of Behaviors [p. 117] |

MODELING

| Types [p. 152] | Sequence [p. 152] |

| Specific Behavior [p. 152] | Strategy [p. 152] | ① With Client Watching and Listening [p. 152] | ② Client Exhibiting Behavior After Model is presented [p. 152] | ③ Client Exhibiting Behavior Without Model [p. 153] |

CONTROLLING THE SESSION

| Verbal Interactions [p. 199] | Material and Activity Design [p. 200] | Contingencies [p. 203] |

| Children [p. 199] | Adolescents [p. 200] | Adults [p. 200] | Sequentially Ordered Activities [p. 202] | Structured Activities [p. 202] | Consequences for Actions [p. 203] | Representing Contingencies [p. 203] |

20

RESPONSE DIFFERENTIATION

Successive Approximations [p. 205]

- End Behavior [p. 205]
- Steps [p. 207]
- Components [p. 207]

Multiple Cuing [p. 212]

- Hierarchy of Abstractness [p. 212]
- Types [p. 213]
- Number [p. 214]
- Modality [p. 214]

Successive Approximations and Multiple Cuing [p. 214]

PARENTAL INVOLVEMENT

Consultation [p. 216]

① Interactions [p. 216]
② Problem Identification and Monitoring [p. 218]
③ Sharing Information [p. 218]
④ Understanding Behaviors [p. 218]
⑤ Support [p. 218]

Training [p. 223]

- Strategies [p. 219]
- Comprehensiveness [p. 219]

General Considerations [p. 219]

Procedures [p. 220]

- Observation [p. 223]
- Exact Words [p. 222]
- Joint Therapy [p. 224]
- Solo Therapy [p. 224]
- Home Therapy [p. 224]

(continued)

TABLE 1–6 *(continued)*

PROCESS OF LEARNING

Stages [p. 224]		
Apprehending [p. 224]	*Acquisition* [p. 224]	*Retention* [p. 226]

Levels [p. 227]							
① *Signal* [p. 227]	② *Stimulus/ Response* [p. 228]	③ *Chaining* [p. 228]	④ *Verbal Association* [p. 229]	⑤ *Discrimination* [p. 229]	⑥ *Concept* [p. 229]	⑦ *Rule* [p. 229]	⑧ *Problem- Solving* [p. 230]

CHANGING ATTITUDES

Discussion [p. 253]	
Client-Centered [p. 253]	*Logical Structuring* [p. 254]

Demonstration [p. 254]

MONITORING

Types [p. 256]	
Interval [p. 256]	*Signal* [p. 256]	*Event Contingent* [p. 256]

Clinician [p. 256]	
Modality [p. 256]	*Shifting From Clinician to Client* [p. 257]

Clients [p. 257]	
Nonverbal [p. 257]	*Verbal* [p. 257]

USING STRATEGIES

Considerations [p. 258]

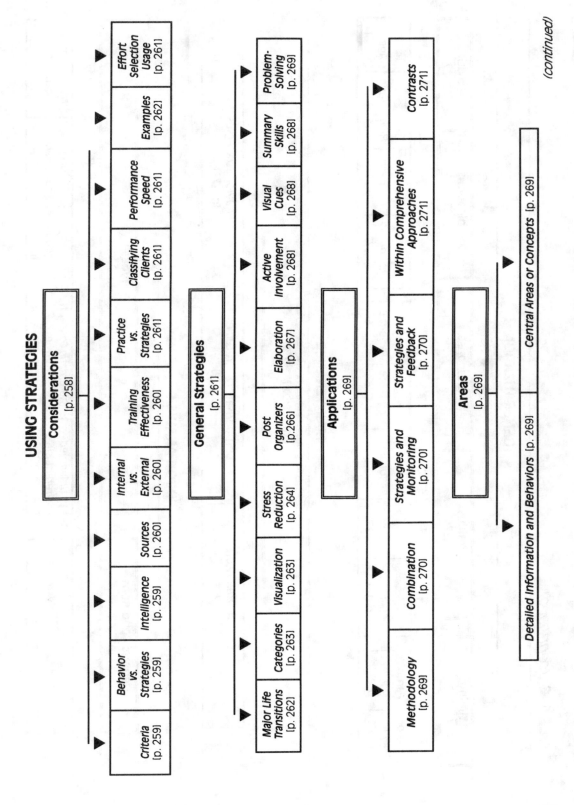

- Criteria [p. 259]
- Behavior vs. Strategies [p. 259]
- Intelligence [p. 259]
- Sources [p. 260]
- Internal vs. External [p. 260]
- Training Effectiveness [p. 260]
- Practice vs. Strategies [p. 261]
- Classifying Clients [p. 261]
- Performance Speed [p. 261]
- Examples [p. 262]
- Effort Selection Usage [p. 261]

General Strategies [p. 261]

- Major Life Transitions [p. 262]
- Categories [p. 263]
- Visualization [p. 263]
- Stress Reduction [p. 264]
- Post Organizers [p. 266]
- Elaboration [p. 267]
- Active Involvement [p. 268]
- Visual Cues [p. 268]
- Summary Skills [p. 268]
- Problem-Solving [p. 269]

Applications [p. 269]

- Methodology [p. 269]
- Combination [p. 270]
- Strategies and Monitoring [p. 270]
- Strategies and Feedback [p. 270]
- Within Comprehensive Approaches [p. 271]
- Contrasts [p. 271]

Areas [p. 269]

- Detailed Information and Behaviors [p. 269]
- Central Areas or Concepts [p. 269]

(continued)

TABLE 1-6 (continued)

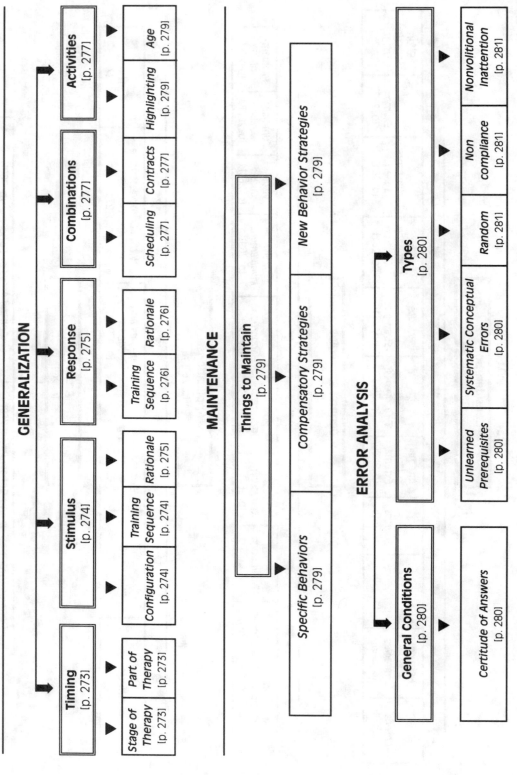

24

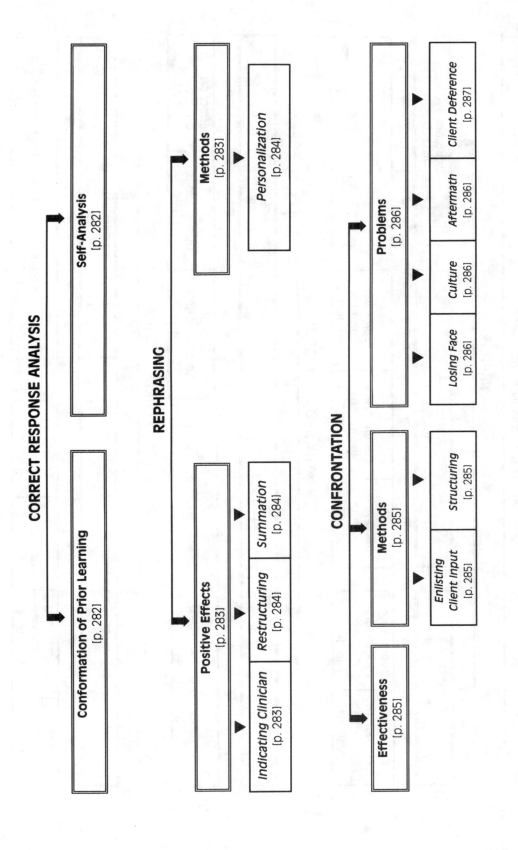

CORRECT RESPONSE ANALYSIS

Conformation of Prior Learning
[p. 282]

Self-Analysis
[p. 282]

REPHRASING

Positive Effects
[p. 283]

Indicating Clinician
[p. 283]

Restructuring
[p. 284]

Summation
[p. 284]

Methods
[p. 283]

Personalization
[p. 284]

CONFRONTATION

Effectiveness
[p. 285]

Methods
[p. 285]

Enlisting
Client Input
[p. 285]

Structuring
[p. 285]

Problems
[p. 286]

Losing Face
[p. 286]

Culture
[p. 286]

Aftermath
[p. 286]

Client Deference
[p. 287]

(continued)

TABLE 1-7

Applying process intervention skills

RAPPORT

Benefits [p. 162]
- Reduction of Defensiveness [p. 162]
- Preventing Interpersonal Conflicts [p. 163]

Methods [p. 163]
- Displaying Warmth [p. 163]
- Commonality of Interests [p. 163]
- Expressing Concern [p. 164]

Limitations [p. 164]
- Not Sufficient [p. 165]
- No Substitute for Competence [p. 165]

EMPATHY AND COMPASSION

TYPES [p. 166]
- Emotional [p. 166]
- Cognitive [p. 167]

USES [p. 168]
- Style of Communicating [p. 168]
- Qualifications [p. 168]
- Effect on Outcome [p. 168]

SPEECH CHARACTERISTICS

Intonation Patterns [p. 169]
- Age Factors [p. 170]
- Intensity and Amplitude [p. 170]
- For Effect [p. 171]
- Ending Patterns [p. 171]

Paralanguage [p. 172]
- Identifiers [p. 172]
- Characterizers [p. 172]

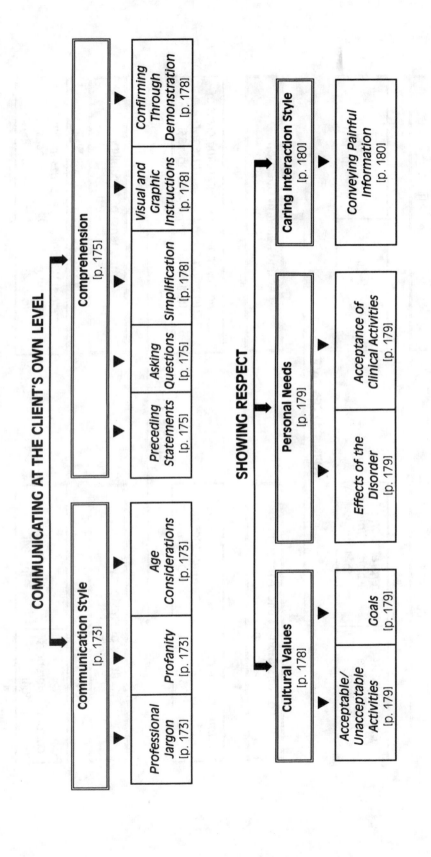

COMMUNICATING AT THE CLIENT'S OWN LEVEL

Communication Style [p. 173]
- Professional Jargon [p. 173]
- Profanity [p. 173]
- Age Considerations [p. 173]

Comprehension [p. 175]
- Preceding Statements [p. 175]
- Asking Questions [p. 175]
- Simplification [p. 178]
- Visual and Graphic Instructions [p. 178]
- Confirming Through Demonstration [p. 178]

SHOWING RESPECT

Cultural Values [p. 178]
- Acceptable/Unacceptable Activities [p. 179]
- Goals [p. 179]

Personal Needs [p. 179]
- Effects of the Disorder [p. 179]
- Acceptance of Clinical Activities [p. 179]

Caring Interaction Style [p. 180]
- Conveying Painful Information [p. 180]

(continued)

TABLE 1-7 *(continued)*

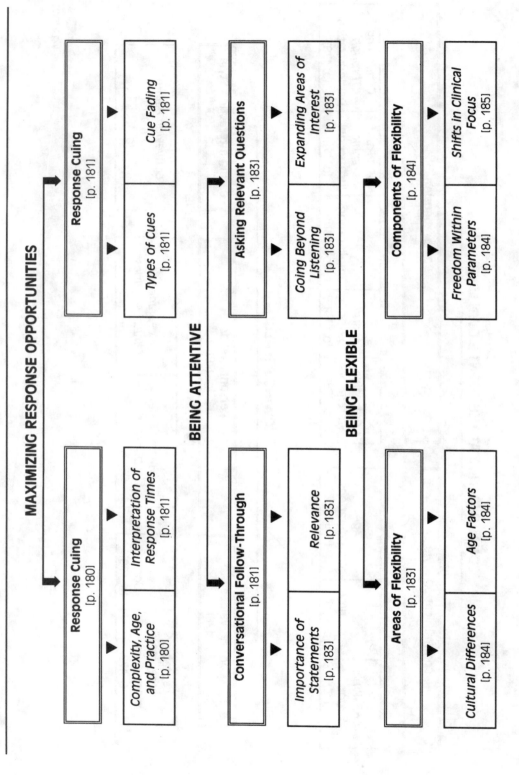

MAXIMIZING RESPONSE OPPORTUNITIES

Response Cuing
[p. 180]

Complexity, Age, and Practice
[p. 180]

Interpretation of Response Times
[p. 181]

Response Cuing
[p. 181]

Types of Cues
[p. 181]

Cue Fading
[p. 181]

BEING ATTENTIVE

Conversational Follow-Through
[p. 181]

Importance of Statements
[p. 183]

Relevance
[p. 183]

Asking Relevant Questions
[p. 183]

Going Beyond Listening
[p. 183]

Expanding Areas of Interest
[p. 183]

BEING FLEXIBLE

Areas of Flexibility
[p. 183]

Cultural Differences
[p. 184]

Age Factors
[p. 184]

Components of Flexibility
[p. 184]

Freedom Within Parameters
[p. 184]

Shifts in Clinical Focus
[p. 185]

INVOLVING CLIENTS IN DECISION MAKING

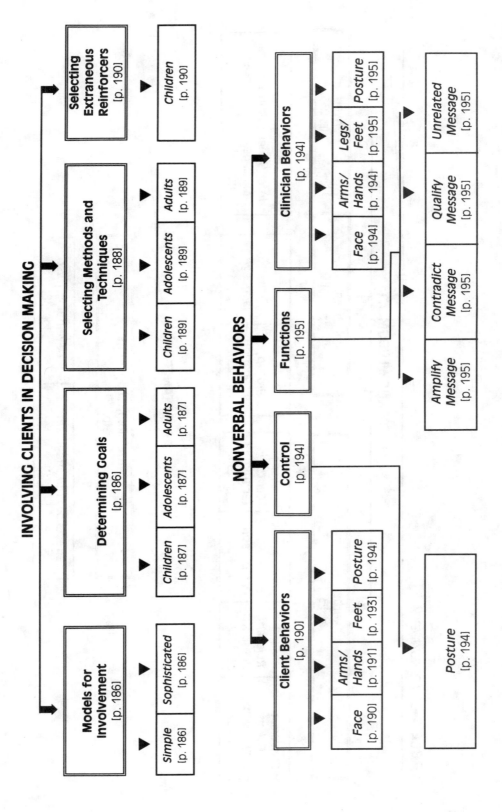

Models for Involvement [p. 186]
- Simple [p. 186]
- Sophisticated [p. 186]

Determining Goals [p. 186]
- Children [p. 187]
- Adolescents [p. 187]
- Adults [p. 187]

Selecting Methods and Techniques [p. 188]
- Children [p. 189]
- Adolescents [p. 189]
- Adults [p. 189]

Selecting Extraneous Reinforcers [p. 190]
- Children [p. 190]

NONVERBAL BEHAVIORS

Client Behaviors [p. 190]
- Face [p. 190]
- Arms/ Hands [p. 191]
- Feet [p. 193]
- Posture [p. 194]
  - Posture [p. 194]

Control [p. 194]

Functions [p. 195]
- Amplify Message [p. 195]
- Contradict Message [p. 195]
- Qualify Message [p. 195]
- Unrelated Message [p. 195]

Clinician Behaviors [p. 194]
- Face [p. 194]
- Arms/ Hands [p. 194]
- Legs/ Feet [p. 195]
- Posture [p. 195]

(continued)

TABLE 1-7 *(continued)*

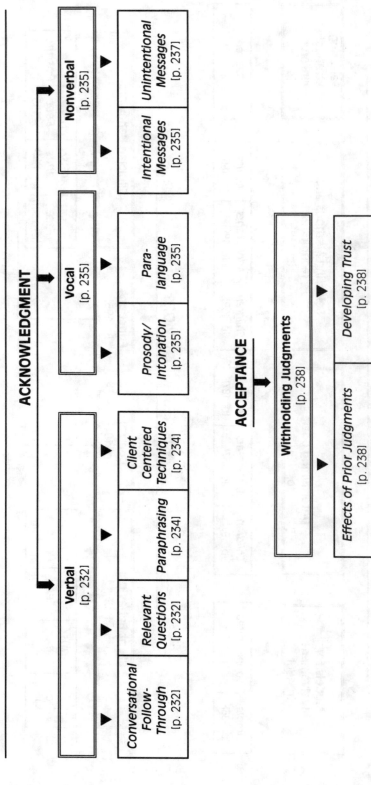

ACKNOWLEDGMENT

Verbal [p. 232]			Vocal [p. 235]		Nonverbal [p. 235]	
Conversational Follow-Through [p. 232]	Relevant Questions [p. 232]	Paraphrasing [p. 234]	Client Centered Techniques [p. 234]	Prosody/Intonation [p. 235]	Para-language [p. 235]	Intentional Messages [p. 235]	Unintentional Messages [p. 237]

ACCEPTANCE

Withholding Judgments [p. 238]	
Effects of Prior Judgments [p. 238]	Developing Trust [p. 238]

SELF-DISCLOSURE

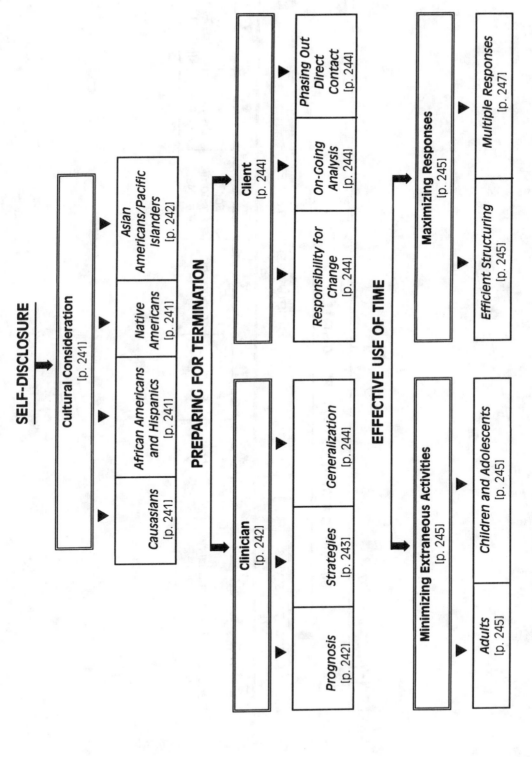

Cultural Consideration [p. 241]

- Causasians [p. 241]
- African Americans and Hispanics [p. 241]
- Native Americans [p. 241]
- Asian Americans/Pacific Islanders [p. 242]

PREPARING FOR TERMINATION

Clinician [p. 242]

- Prognosis [p. 242]
- Strategies [p. 243]
- Generalization [p. 244]

Client [p. 244]

- Responsibility for Change [p. 244]
- On-Going Analysis [p. 244]
- Phasing Out Direct Contact [p. 244]

EFFECTIVE USE OF TIME

Minimizing Extraneous Activities [p. 245]

- Adults [p. 245]
- Children and Adolescents [p. 245]

Maximizing Responses [p. 245]

- Efficient Structuring [p. 245]
- Multiple Responses [p. 247]

(continued)

TABLE 1-7 *(continued)*

MATCHING ACTIVITIES TO LEARNING STYLES

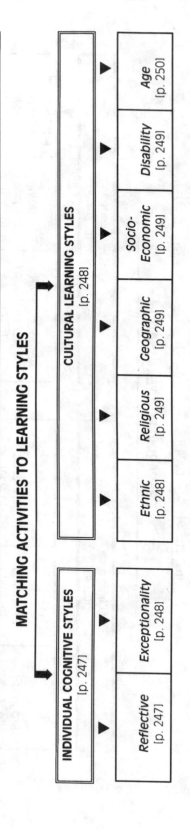

INDIVIDUAL COGNITIVE STYLES
[p. 247]

Reflective
[p. 247]

Exceptionality
[p. 248]

CULTURAL LEARNING STYLES
[p. 248]

Ethnic
[p. 248]

Religious
[p. 249]

Geographic
[p. 249]

Socio-
Economic
[p. 249]

Disability
[p. 249]

Age
[p. 250]

GROUP THERAPY

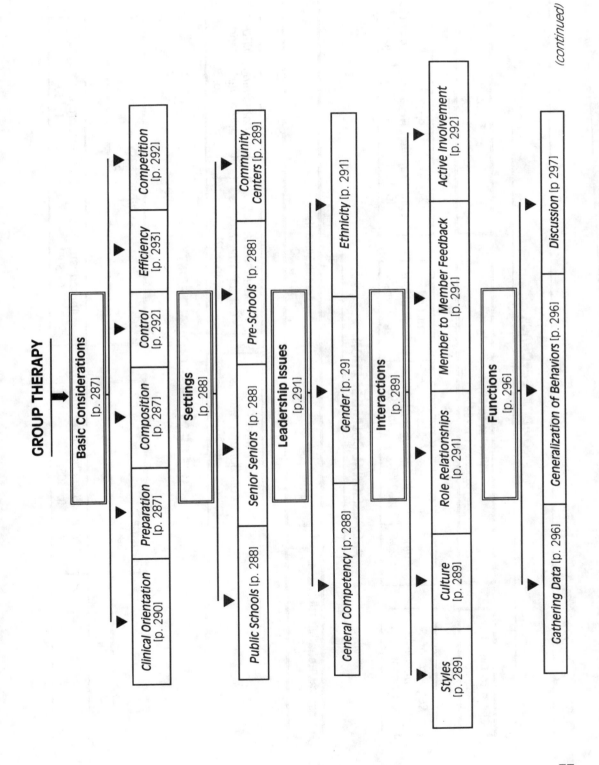

Basic Considerations [p. 287]

- Clinical Orientation [p. 290]
- Preparation [p. 287]
- Composition [p. 287]
- Control [p. 292]
- Efficiency [p. 293]
- Competition [p. 292]

Settings [p. 288]

- Public Schools [p. 288]
- Senior Seniors [p. 288]
- Pre-Schools [p. 288]
- Community Centers [p. 289]

Leadership Issues [p. 291]

- General Competency [p. 288]
- Gender [p. 291]
- Ethnicity [p. 291]

Interactions [p. 289]

- Styles [p. 289]
- Culture [p. 289]
- Role Relationships [p. 291]
- Member to Member Feedback [p. 291]
- Active Involvement [p. 292]

Functions [p. 296]

- Gathering Data [p. 296]
- Generalization of Behaviors [p. 296]
- Discussion [p. 297]

(continued)

TABLE 1-7 *(continued)*

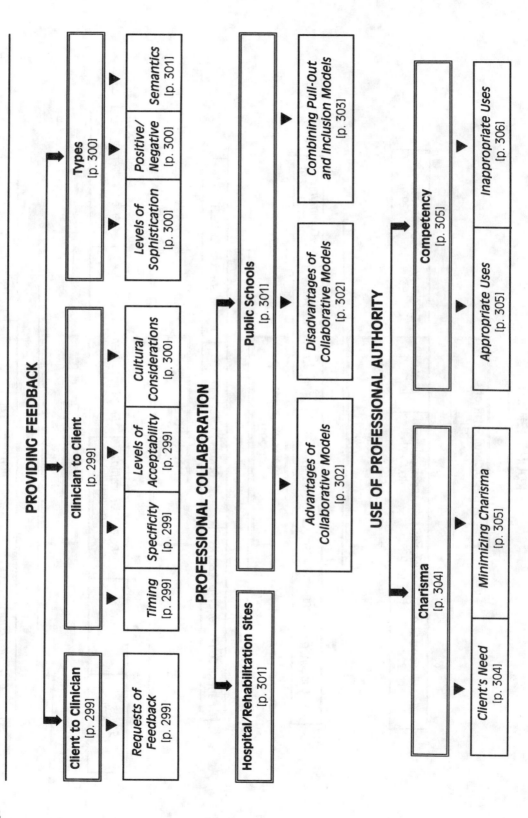

PROVIDING FEEDBACK

Client to Clinician
[p. 299]

Requests of
Feedback
[p. 299]

Clinician to Client
[p. 299]

Timing
[p. 299]

Specificity
[p. 299]

Levels of
Acceptability
[p. 299]

Cultural
Considerations
[p. 300]

Types
[p. 300]

Levels of
Sophistication
[p. 300]

Positive/
Negative
[p. 300]

Semantics
[p. 301]

PROFESSIONAL COLLABORATION

Hospital/Rehabilitation Sites
[p. 301]

Public Schools
[p. 301]

Advantages of
Collaborative Models
[p. 302]

Disadvantages of
Collaborative Models
[p. 302]

Combining Pull-Out
and Inclusion Models
[p. 303]

USE OF PROFESSIONAL AUTHORITY

Charisma
[p. 304]

Competency
[p. 305]

Client's Need
[p. 304]

Minimizing Charisma
[p. 305]

Appropriate Uses
[p. 305]

Inappropriate Uses
[p. 306]

CHAPTER
2

Principles of Change

The characteristics and requirements of change are identical, whether we are talking about personal habits, sporting activities, work behavior, family interactions, or communication disorders. Change, very simply, is the process whereby an individual, behavior, emotion, thought, or perception moves from one point to another. The simplicity of the definition hides the complexity of the event. Rarely is time taken to examine the requirements for change. Often, it is poorly understood. And usually, only a truncated version of its requirements is applied. The purpose of this chapter is to enable clinicians to develop a comprehensive understanding of the requirements of change, in general, and specifically for clients with communication disorders and their families. In order to accomplish this, four things need to be done. We need to: (1) Dispel the misconceptions about change; (2) identify the principles of change; (3) describe the technology of change; and (4) specify the components of practice activities that are necessary for change to occur. Although there will be many references to clinical studies, many of the conclusions and examples in this chapter are based on my clinical and non-clinical experiences. Therefore, the reader will hopefully indulge me in this chapter to use the first person singular in examples.

MISCONCEPTIONS ABOUT CHANGE

Life is a process of continual change. Your body, relationships, feelings, and beliefs are changing daily. Some of these changes occur slowly while others hurl forward at a frightening speed. Sometimes the changes that occur are welcomed, at other times they are met with great trepidation. Some changes occur in spite of one's self, while others occur because of involvement. As you begin reading this chapter, you start with a wealth of knowledge about the process of change that has been derived through personal experiences, some of which have been glorious and others painful. Often we tend to isolate the practice of speech-language pathology from our nonclinical experiences, assuming that what we do and experience in a clinical setting is very different from what we do and experience when the role of *clinician* is shed in favor of *wife, father, mother, friend, athlete,* or any of the other scores of roles we assume throughout the day. By doing this, years of vast knowledge are wasted, knowledge that could enhance our development as clinicians and would have been of benefit to our clients. Throughout this chapter, you should seek out instances in your own life where you attempted to change something about yourself and examine not only the outcome, but the reasons why things occurred as they did. Then utilize that knowledge for understanding how you can facilitate change within your clients. There are two misconceptions about change that are important to dispel. The first is that being motivated is a sufficient condition for change to occur. The second is that guilt increases the likelihood that change will occur.

Only Motivation Is Necessary

Therapy must begin with a desire to change, a commitment to move from point a to point b. This desire to change is often called *motivation*, and unfortunately many people believe that it is the only necessary thing for change to occur. This misconception leads to falsely crediting our clients' personalities with attributes they probably do not have when they succeed, and silently berating them unjustly when they fail. As important as motivation is for changing behaviors, it is only one of the necessary factors (Chan, 1994).

The Desire. Everybody wants to change at least one thing about themselves, and they usually attempt to change it repeatedly. How often have you started a diet or joined a health club? Each time, your determination to succeed was strong and you envisioned a "new" you in 30 days. In spite of your good intentions, you probably are still looking for the right diet or that perfect health club where trainers magically transform your body into the image of a god or goddess. The most common definitions for *desire* refer to a need to change.

This need can be expressed in many ways. One can get depressed about not having the need fulfilled or the lack of fulfillment can act as an impetus for change. Some studies have found that when individuals develop anxiety about a particular behavior, they are more likely to seek help to change it (Dugas, Letarte, Rheaume, & Freeston, 1995).

Simplifying Successes and Failures. Many people attribute success in changing to motivation and failure to a lack of personal strength or desire. Both the adulation and adoration are too simplistic. Both reduce the process and outcomes to variables that are insufficient to guarantee either success or failure.

SUCCESS
"He succeeded because he had the guts to do it."
"We all should have her level of motivation."
"It takes a person with a strong personality to stick with it."
"Highly motivated people always succeed."

FAILURE
"The only reason I didn't become fluent was that I didn't have the will."
"I could have eliminated the lisp if only I was motivated."
"If he had just put his mind to it, he could have learned the concept."
"If she was really committed to therapy, she would have improved."
"I could have remembered her name if only my personality was stronger."

You have probably heard, or even said some of these statements when looking at successful and unsuccessful attempts to change your own behaviors and those of your clients. When directed toward others, they result in feeling either adoration or derision toward that person. When directed toward one's own attempts, the person either feels proud of his or her accomplishment or terribly guilty at not succeeding;

proud because they were able to accomplish their goal out of sheer will and determination; and guilty because their weakness of character led to failure. If they based both of these self-evaluations on the belief that motivation and character were the only factors involved in the outcome, they were deceiving themselves. Their success involved more than motivation, as did their failures. If they succeeded, they probably had more knowledge about how to change than they realized. If they failed in spite of their best efforts, the failure probably had more to do with a lack of knowledge than lack of motivation.

Guilt Facilitates Change

Is there a door in your life that hasn't been fixed for 3 months that sends a bolt of guilt into you every time you have to push hard to close it? What do you think when you notice that the blouse you intended to wear today has been laying on your closet floor waiting for 2 weeks to go to the laundry? How did you feel when you realized that you forgot that lunch date yesterday that had been planned for over a month? Or realized that you didn't complete a clinic report this afternoon when you heard your supervisor asking for it? And what about your exercise schedule? What wonderful and almost believable excuse did you invent for not doing your weight training or running? When you went for your weekly music lesson how elaborate an excuse did you have to construct to convince both yourself and your music teacher that you couldn't find even a few minutes a day to practice? Unless you are a master of self-delusion, these events, and scores of others that you can probably add, have occurred repeatedly and have done little other than to impair your self-image and foster a sense of guilt because you failed. Your clients are no different than you. Not only have they suffered the same sort of embarrassments, but their list may be more devastating with attempts at increasing fluen-

cy, speaking more articulately, using a less harsh voice, retrieving the names of objects, or using appropriate linguistic forms. Regardless of the nature of the failure, both you and your clients have experienced self-deprecation caused by failure at accomplishing something that both of you felt you *should* be able to do. This failure and self-blame results in the development of feelings of guilt, which has been defined as the awareness of having done something wrong and the expectation of being punished for it.

Should Statements. "Should" statements imply that the individual already possesses all of the components required to complete a specific act or develop a new behavior. Rarely does this occur. Usually at least one critical component is missing. I remember listening to a Buddhist monk counseling a young man who was lamenting that he should have been a better father to his children, in spite of the tremendous personal problems he was undergoing. The monk, after listening quietly to the father's self-incriminating statements, said:

> You did the best you were capable of doing at that time. Given the circumstances, there was nothing else you *could* have done, regardless of what you *wanted* to do. Parents do the best they *know* how to do. You should not condemn yourself for not doing something you were not capable of doing. You did the best you could.

These wise words go to the heart of guilt. It is an emotion that has very little or no redeeming values and falsely attributes blame where none should be attributed because at least one of the components necessary for the desired change was missing.

Feelings of Inadequacy. By focusing on their failures, clients may begin developing one of the most negative of human emotions: guilt. Life is too short and filled with too many enjoyable things and experiences to spend it feeling guilty about not accomplishing them. How often have your clients berated themselves for not being able to do something they really wanted to accomplish? It could have been speaking with a more natural voice or correctly producing a phoneme or speaking fluently. Regardless of the type of activity or behavior, the feelings were identical: guilt. Why didn't I do it? Why didn't I stick with it and practice more? Why didn't I just do it and not be afraid of experiencing failure? These self-incriminating thoughts do little other than make your clients feel inadequate and hide the fact that they probably did the best they could, given their circumstances and the knowledge they possessed at the time.

Feeling guilty about failures is useless and debilitating. It can be reduced or eliminated by developing those behaviors whose absence caused it. Often we are overly zealous in blaming our clients' failures on a lack of motivation. Change requires more than motivation. It requires knowledge. The key to your clients accomplishing many of their goals is for both you and them to understand *how* to change behaviors and attitudes. The "how" is defined here as the foundations of change. It involves understanding (1) the principles of change, (2) the technology of change, and (3) the logic of activity construction. Table 2–1 shows the relationship between these three elements.

PRINCIPLES OF CHANGE

In San Francisco where I live, we are all very aware of the foundations on which our houses are built. Living on top of a series of earthquake faults does that to people. During the last major earthquake, the houses that suffered the greatest damage either did not have adequate structural integrity in their foundations or rested on ground structure that liquefied during the

severe movements of the earth. Intervention programs that involve change are no different than houses. Without an adequate foundation, they either will immediately fail, or eventually fail during periods of stress. Often, clinicians neglect to understand the foundation on which their intervention approach is based. This may occur either because they are unaware of it, or believe the time necessary for identifying it could be better spent doing other things. Regardless if the intervention program is for the enhancement of fluency, retrieval of past learned information, production of acceptable voicing, expansion of linguistic utterances, or development of phonemes, the change principles on which clinical intervention programs should be based are no different than the principles found in every other successful change program. If the program is to be successful, it should include three principles. To change, (1) clients must accept responsibility for both their current and future behaviors; (2) they must be motivated to change; and (3) they need to possess knowledge of the change process.

Accepting Responsibility for Change

If clients are to change, they must accept the responsibility for it. As a clinician, you facilitate, guide, cajole, and do any number of other things short of causing your client to change behaviors. At some level, there has to be a conscious decision to change. Without this commitment, change is unlikely to occur. A commitment to accept responsibility to change may be affected by the person's belief system, specifically their view on victimization, volition, and motivation.

Victimization. There is a growing trend in this country to champion the concept of *victimization*, where the responsibility for one's behaviors is shifted onto other people or events that may have occurred even 20 or 30 years ago.

TABLE 2–1
Foundations of Change

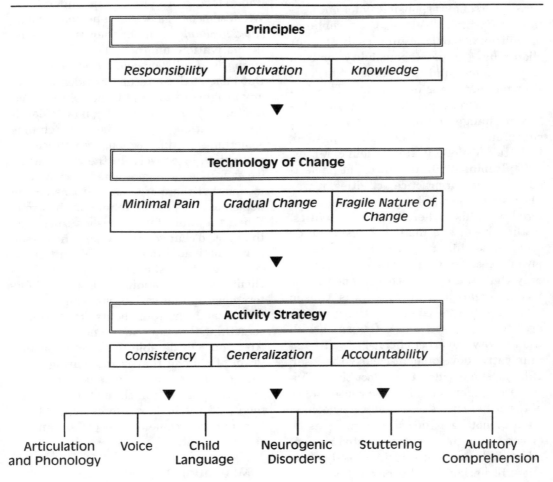

"Don't blame him for his violence, his father abused him 30 years ago."

"If he hadn't eaten all that junk food, he never would have killed him."

"You need to be understanding of my failures, remember my family's history."

"My abusiveness to my children comes from my mother's abusiveness to me."

Regardless of what one thinks about the psychological validity of the concept, if your clients adhere to it as an explanation for their current behaviors, it will negate your efforts to facilitate change. Why ac- cept the responsibility myself when I can place the blame on others? Clients who adhere to a victimization view of their communicative disorder will find it easier and less threatening to blame clinical failures on external variables, rather than critically assessing their own decision-making process. For example, a client who failed to practice a new behavior might find it easier to assert that there was too much to do at work, rather than entertain the notion that practice on his speech had a lower priority than his other activities.

Volition. The concept of *volition* refers to the act of freely choosing a course of action or behavior that one engages in. It asserts a personal responsibility for one's actions. In a clinical setting, the acceptance of volitional control implies that your clients have some responsibility for both the changes and, conversely, lack of changes that occur in their life. This is a cornerstone concept in any program of behavior change and one that is reiterated continually in our field (Chapey, 1986; Culatta & Goldberg, 1995; Klein & Moses, 1994; Rubin, 1986). If your client neglected to do certain practice activities, it was not because something or someone interfered with his or her choice of activities. Rather, he or she made a *decision* to do other things that may have been more enjoyable, less stressful, or required less energy than the prescribed therapeutic activity. Regardless of what was chosen instead of the therapeutic activity, a hierarchy of importance was established, with the activity most beneficial to their communicative development clearly the loser. If he or she decided to neglect the activities and understood that the consequence of his or her choice was that a new behavior may not be achieved as rapidly as he or she would like, he or she acted responsibly, but not necessarily wisely. The client has prioritized his or her time or interests and is willing to settle for the consequences. However, if your clients decided not to practice and blamed the program for an inability to change their behaviors, or external circumstances making it impossible for them to practice, they are deluding themselves. Life consists of events resulting from the decisions we make daily. Doing nothing about the direction in which one's life progresses is still making a choice: You are choosing to be passive and allowing people and events outside of yourself to shape you and your future.

Motivation

Motivation is a term that is probably misunderstood more often than understood. When someone says that a person is *motivated to change*, what do they really mean? Is motivation another term for *desire, strength of will,* or *conviction*? Perhaps. But none of these terms provides us with any insights as to what it means to be motivated, or more importantly, how to develop motivation in our clients to change something. In this section, we will look at motivation objectively. In the clinic, when we say someone is motivated to change, it means that there are more reasons for the person to change than to remain the same. When there are fewer reasons to change than not to change, we say that the person is not motivated to change. When this occurs, even the best clinician will fail with a client. By understanding what types of factors develop motivation, you can begin to understand why your clients are still doing something they say they do not wish to do. Also you will be able to structure a program of change that is motivating. Four categories of reasons can be used to develop a motivation for change: (1) punishment, (2) intrinsic reinforcement, (3) extrinsic reinforcement, and (4) extraneous reinforcement.

Motivation Through Punishment. I remember my mother trying to coerce me into doing various things through guilt. Whether it was a cultural predisposition, a natural maternal instinct, or a skill developed after years of practice with my father, she was a master at it! However, it rarely worked with me. And on those occasions when she was momentarily successful, I would revert back to the behaviors I preferred. Guilt, whether it comes from someone else or is self-generated, is not helpful for changing behaviors. Nor are other forms of punishment. You are attempting to change not because you like the new behavior, but rather because you fear something negative will occur if you do not change. In the case of my mother, if I did not do something, she informed me in no uncertain terms, that it would "hurt her deeply." Hurting her deeply would be punishing to me, and being a loving son, something that would be negative and to be avoided. At 9 years of age I practiced my accordion only because I didn't want to "hurt my mother deeply." I didn't enjoy practicing, and I thought the sound generated from the instrument was awful! But I continued practicing for 3 years until I realized that my mother's use of guilt was manipulative. She might be annoyed because I didn't practice, but surely there were more important things in life to be deeply hurt about than my not practicing my accordion. The minute guilt no longer was the motivating reason for practicing, I ceased doing it, because there was nothing positive about the experience. Punishment in my case was psychological. All of the clinical studies that have been conducted in the area of behavior change clearly show that, if a behavior is developed out of fear of punishment, as soon as the fear is eliminated, the new behavior quickly diminishes since there is nothing positive with which to replace it (Bandura, 1969; Skinner, 1953; Sloane & MacAulay, 1968). A good analogy is the four-way stop sign. Even though there is nobody other than you at the intersection, you still come to a complete halt. Not because you may think it makes any sense, or you feel good about it, but rather because you fear that a police officer may be hiding around the corner, just waiting for you to coast through the intersection. If in the town in which you lived, police officers could no longer give traffic citations for coasting through intersections with four-way stop signs, how often would you come to a complete stop? Probably very rarely. The same principles apply in clinical settings. If your clients are to change, they should be motivated to change because the change will result in something positive occurring for them, not because of their fear that something nega-

tive will happen if they do not. Examine your own history. Look closely at your long-term successes. Most probably came about because the change resulted in something positive occurring, not out of fear of punishment. A classic example is "cramming" for exams. The intensive period of study that immediately precedes an examination is usually done to avoid receiving a low grade. If the student were truly interested in the subject, study would occur constantly. You should use this principle in constructing intervention programs for your clients.

Intrinsic Reinforcement. Reinforcement is just another word for the receiving of a reward, but a bit longer and somewhat more technical. For clarity, you should always make a distinction between a rein*forcer* and reinforce*ment*. In the first case, a reinforcer is any *thing* that increases the likelihood that, if presented, something will occur in the future. A reinforce*ment* refers to the entire *process* where a behavior occurs and then is followed by the reinforcer. The most powerful type of reinforcement is called intrinsic reinforcement. An event or behavior is intrinsically reinforcing if the act of doing it is enjoyable. If I had enjoyed the act of making musical notes come out of the instrument, practicing the accordion would have been intrinsically reinforcing. It would have been a pleasure just to hear myself make music. The strength of intrinsic reinforcement is that it is not dependent on anything external to your client. It is an internal feeling your client gets that is so rewarding that they wish to experience it again and again. With some clients, there is intrinsic reinforcement just for the completion of a particular level of competence (Sansone and Morgan, 1992). For these few clients, it makes little difference what the act is. These are the type of individuals who thrive on competition and success. The feeling one gets through the act of lovemaking is a good example of intrinsic reinforcement. Another example for me is fly fishing. The pleasure I get from being in a beautiful place and effortlessly casting out a fly that I have tied is so strong that catching fish is almost irrelevant. When choosing a behavior that you wish to change or develop in a client, if possible find one that is intrinsically reinforcing. By doing this, you will increase the probability of your client's success. An example in aphasia therapy would be choosing the names of a client's children which he has had a great deal of difficulty in retrieving. It would be significantly more motivating for him to retrieve the names of his children rather than distant cities whose names are equally difficult to retrieve, but have little relevance to his life. The desire to acquire this ability might constitute the only motivation necessary for him to engage in a series of retrieval activities that might be difficult.

Extrinsic Reinforcement. Quite often, it is difficult to find a behavior or activity that is intrinsically reinforcing. When this occurs, seek out one that is extrinsically reinforcing. This second type of reinforcement involves receiving enjoyment from the completion of an act. If after working on a song I received pleasure when I was able to play it on the accordion without any mistakes (completion of the act), practicing would have been extrinsically reinforcing. Unfortunately, that did not happen. I have a friend whom I have been trying to teach how to fly fish. Because he doesn't have time to either learn how to cast correctly or tie his own flies, the act of placing a fly on the water is not yet intrinsically reinforcing. However, the thought of catching a wild trout is extrinsically reinforcing enough for him to be motivated to learn the skills needed to become a fine fly caster. Although less powerful than intrinsic reinforcement, extrinsic reinforcement is still a powerful form of reinforcement. An excellent clinical example of using extrinsic reinforcement is the construction of language therapy for young children. When teaching children how to appropriately use various linguistic rules, it may not be intrinsically

reinforcing for them to string various words together to create the desired utterance. However, if the production of the utterance terminates with the activation of something enjoyable, the production of the utterance becomes extrinsically reinforcing. Many years ago I was asked to substitute for a supervisor in a clinic for children with Down syndrome. The clinicians had been working on the appropriate use of the prepositions *on, under, behind* and verbs *jump, sit, stand, walk,* and *run*. Each child was shown a picture card and asked to identify either the action that was occurring or where an object was located. If they responded correctly, the clinician would praise them. Not only was there nothing intrinsically or extrinsically reinforcing about producing the correct word, but the use of praise appeared to be minimally effective because the results from each of the children were very inconsistent. Although all of the children had shown in the past they could correctly identify the pictures containing the target preposition or verb and could produce the correct response, none appeared to be motivated to engage in a desired behavior they already knew how to do. The passive activity was transformed into one that was extrinsically reinforcing when I began to engage in whatever action they described in the picture or located myself according to the preposition they used. Not only did the percentage of correct responses increase dramatically, but each of the children became fixated on what was occurring with the other children while they were waiting their turn to manipulate me through the use of language. Weeks after I had worked with them and was walking down the clinic hall, I still could hear voices yelling to me "jump," "run," "fall down." To the bewilderment of my students and the department chair, I complied with every request.

Extraneous Reinforcement. Extraneous reinforcement presents a paradox for the clinician. It is the least powerful form of reinforcement, because it is not directly related to the act or its completion, yet it is effective regardless of the client's intrinsic or extrinsic level of motivation. The most common form of extraneous reinforcement in the work place is a salary. Take, for example, the automobile plant worker who may not receive any pleasure from pressing the buttons that create an endless supply of shiny bumpers (intrinsic), nor receive pleasure from seeing the finished bumpers (extrinsic). In spite of the utter boredom he may be experiencing, he continues to work, only because he enjoys the paycheck he receives every 4 weeks (extraneous). Even though I did not enjoy making musical notes or flawlessly playing a polka, I probably would have continued practicing if my mother gave me $1 at the end of each practice session. Fortunately, that didn't happen! I remember using a guide once when I was fishing a new area in Florida. Although he was very amiable and helpful, it became very apparent that he took little pleasure in fishing. For him, the enjoyment of fishing left him years ago. Now, the only reason he guided was for the money. He confided in me that, other than on the days he guides, he never touches a fishing rod or even thinks about it. Although extraneous reinforcement is the least powerful of the three reinforcements for increasing motivation, it still can be very effective. Ten years after my guide lost interest in fishing, he still was on the water for 3 days every week. One of my most successful clients was an individual who was extraneously motivated to change. He was the controller of a major corporation and had performed very competently in that position for a number of years. The position was very technical and required a minimal amount of interaction within the corporate structure, which pleased my client, because he was a severe stutterer with blocks accompanied by facial grimaces lasting up to 15 seconds. The president of the corporation believed my client had the potential to eventually assume his position when he retired. He told my client that if he could substantially reduce his disfluencies, he would be given a vice-presidency in the company, and if upon the president's retirement he was fluent, the presidency of the corporation would be his, along with a salary that was four times what he would make as vice-president and eight times as much as he was earning as a controller. The increased status and salary were positive enough to motivate him to change. Within 2 months, the severity of his stuttering was substantially reduced. At the end of 1 year of therapy, his stuttering was under complete control. Conversely, a professional baseball player I worked with could find nothing intrinsically, extrinsically, or extraneously rewarding about developing fluent speech. With a salary in excess of $1,000,000 a year and absolutely no negative consequences because of his stuttering, he could find nothing reinforcing about developing fluent speech and quit therapy after two sessions.

Combining Various Reinforcements. We should always seek to develop activities that have all three forms of reinforcement. The stronger and more extensive the reinforcement, the more likely motivation to change will be insured. When you choose behaviors to change, be sure that at least one form of reinforcement is present. If your clients cannot find anything positive about the change you are asking them to contemplate, the likelihood that they will be successful is minimal. As important as motivation is in changing behaviors, it is not sufficient. It must be complemented by the third principle of change: knowledge.

Knowledge

How many times have you breezed through the instructions that were included in a complicated toy for your child or furniture kit for yourself and found extra parts when you completed its construction? Everything looked so simple that you felt there was no need to read the instructions. You felt sure that a cursory glance at the written instructions would be enough to complement the assembly pictures. Faced with the extra pieces you either had to go back to the beginning and attempt to reconstruct the project or throw them away, hoping that the thing would not fall apart too soon. If the kit was so simple to put together, there would not have been a need for written instructions. The instructions served as both your guide and foundation for successfully completing the task. When changing behaviors, a similar foundational basis is required for both you and your clients.

Foundation of Knowledge. Complicated behaviors, activities, and thoughts are all built on a foundation of knowledge. Great jazz musicians do not develop improvisational techniques in isolation. This incredible ability is dependent on having an intimate knowledge of individual notes, chords, and chord progressions. The basketball player who seems to effortlessly fly past the defense and miraculously send the ball through a hoop hitting only net has practiced for thousands of hours perfecting each component of his move. The artist whose painting embodies what appears to be a simple and unified design did not simply throw up spats of paint on a blank canvas. She probably spent countless hours understanding the components of the design pattern, color hues, and a multitude of design-color combinations. The furniture craftsperson who produces beautifully designed and finished tables spent many years understanding the complexities of design and the finishing characteristics of various types of wood. The opera singer who can bring an audience to tears with an aria from Puccini's Madame Butterfly

spent years practicing scale exercises and learning the intonation patterns of Italian. The complexities of these types of activities are routinely accepted. Everyone would agree that these are complicated activities that require dedication and an understanding of the basics on which the activity is grounded. But what about changing vocal volume, correctly producing the /r/ phoneme, using articles appropriately in sentences, or speaking fluently? Few people would equate a Michael Jordan "spin and dunk move" with any of these behaviors. Yet all are more similar than dissimilar to Michael Jordan's move.

Basis of Behavior Change. Changing communicative behaviors is just as complicated as developing improvisational techniques, playing professional basketball, creating a work of art, wood crafting, or operatic singing. The development of each requires knowledge of strategies, practice routines, and methods for instant retrieval. Complicated, yes. Impossible, no. Just as each of the examples in the above paragraph was achievable through a development of fundamentals, so it is possible to change your client's behaviors if a foundation of knowledge is developed. The foundations for change in smoking, weight control, physical training, attitude adjustment, language development, reduction of stuttering, memory enhancement, and a host of other areas are identical.

For example, if I am to learn how to play a musical instrument, I will need to understand how to read music and chord structures. Similarly, stuttering clients will need to know how to use specific fluency-enhancing techniques. If I am to ever become competent with the musical instrument, I will need to practice. So must the stutterer. If I am ever to play publicly without having to read the music as I play, I will need to commit the notes to memory and retrieve them appropriately. The same applies to the person who stutters when speaking in nonclinical situations. These two examples are not unique. Virtually every nonclinical and clinical example you can propose will have similar components.

TECHNOLOGY OF CHANGE

In contemporary America there is an emphasis on relying on specialists. One individual may be capable of treating only a specific type of emotional problem. Another individual may be trained only to increase physical fitness. The trend toward specialization has resulted in people believing that a specialist is necessary for addressing each type of problem they have. One person for smoking, another person for weight control, still a third person for physical training, and someone else for attitude adjustment. Each problem is viewed as something separate, something that requires special techniques and specially trained individuals. For some illogical reason, each specialist also views his or her area as something that is unique, unrelated to other areas of personal improvement. This reverence for isolation may be the result of each profession's attempt to protect its "turf." Or it may be that, when one becomes a specialist, the individual loses the ability to see the "big picture." Yet, even to the casual observer, it appears that attempts to improve in such different areas as physical fitness, interpersonal relationships, and job performance do have something in common. The thread that unites these fields and others involved in change with the area of speech-language is the *technology of change*. The phrase *technology of change* refers to how the process of change occurs. It does not involve any computer programs or cyberspace software. Rather, it focuses on the foundation on which all change occurs and the means that are used to effect it. By understanding the technology of behavior change, you can select whatever behavior you want to en-

able your client to change and be successful. By understanding *how* change occurs, you can help your client become his or her own change agent through the use of a set of techniques that have proven to be successful in a variety of scientific clinical studies. The "how" of becoming one's own change agent was beautifully described by Fritz Perls, the gestalt therapist, when he wrote about growth (Perls, 1965). For Perls, one of the most important goals of therapy was to enable his clients to grow. Growth, or maturation, for him involved the transition from environmental support to self-support. As a therapist, he would initially provide his clients with as much help, guidance, and instruction as they needed in the beginning of therapy in order for them to progress. This he called environmental support. As therapy continued, he withdrew support and required the client to exert more internal control or self-support for evaluating and developing new feelings, beliefs, and behaviors. It would be efficacious for you to assume the role of a "Fritz Perls type" therapist. Your client and his or her family initially should be dependent on you, but should shortly begin becoming their own change agents, by systematically and gradually reducing their reliance on you and assuming the responsibility themselves. By this process, clients and their families begin assuming the role of therapist. There are three components in the technology of change: (1) minimize pain and effort, (2) gradually change behaviors, and (3) protect the fragility of new behaviors.

Minimizing Pain and Effort

A number of years ago, I decided to study karate. Not for self-defense reasons, but rather because I greatly admired the beauty and effortless movement I saw when masters of the art performed either their katas (ritualized exercises) or engaged in mock combat. I enrolled in a class that was conducted by one of the leading teachers in the San Francisco Bay area. During the first class he explained that in order to do any of the kicks we would need to first stretch our muscles. As we sat on the floor cross-legged, each person's partner would grab hold of his knees and pull them toward the floor. As this very painful exercise was conducted the master yelled out "no pain, no gain," a mantra that is widely known and believed by many sports enthusiasts. Unfortunately, I believed it. I thought that the only way I could become limber enough to do the required kicks was to experience intense pain for 15 minutes at the beginning of each class for the next 8 weeks. The beauty of karate that I visualized rapidly became transformed into an activity that was associated with intense pain. Even though I was motivated to learn the art, and possessed with knowledge of why I was doing this painful exercise and that it would lead to significant results in 8 weeks, I quit after 3 weeks. The motto "no pain, no gain" may be appropriate for those who have a macho credo of life, but it is a formula for failure for the rest of us. *Too much pain, no gain!* Human beings do not continue to engage in activities that are too painful or difficult to carry out, even over a short period of time, unless the rewards far outweigh the punishment. For me, even the thought of effortless and graceful karate movements could not outweigh the intense loathing I felt for the art as I sat on the floor and tried to make my legs move in a way my anatomy never intended. Your clients are no different. Although they may be motivated to change and understand the reasons and benefits of using a specific technique or behavior, a method or behavior that is too effortful may be disregarded before it becomes effective. In the following chapters you will be shown how to gradually increase the difficulty of your client's activities, so that they never exceed the threshold of acceptable physical, emotional, or psychological pain. Change should

not be painful. Because it is easier to maintain the status quo rather than to change, resistance to change needs to be reduced. To reduce resistance, the proposed change should be only slightly more difficult, at most, from the current behavior and involve minimal physical, psychological, or emotional discomfort.

Pain and Change. Pain not only has negative effects on physical activities, but also on other aspects of behavior change. A number of years ago a stutterer sought me out for therapy. He had been seeing a very well known speech-language pathologist and abruptly stopped therapy. One of the first questions I usually ask clients is what types of therapy they have experienced in the past. After he explained what he had been doing with the therapist, I asked him to demonstrate the techniques he had been taught. Immediately, he transformed his speech from one containing severe stuttering to one that was completely fluent and normal sounding. After he had been speaking fluently for 5 minutes, I said, "Your speech is wonderful, completely fluent! Why are you coming to see me? You sound terrific. Just keep using that technique." He took a deep breath and began speaking again, this time stuttering as severely as when he wasn't using the technique.

> The technique is too hard. You have no idea what I had to do in order to use it for 5 minutes. Mentally, I'm exhausted. I can't use it for any length of time. It's just too damn hard. I'd rather speak like this (severe disfluencies) than to speak fluently using something that's so difficult.

My client's willingness to accept a way of speaking that was painful to him rather than using a technique that produced fluent speech was a revelation to me and convinced me that change should, at most, involve a minimal amount of mental discomfort.

Choosing the Easier Path. Given two paths, one easy and one difficult, we tend to choose the easier one. It's a natural human inclination. If you can get to the same place by either going over a flat road or one that has hills, gulches, and a knee-high swamp, which would you choose? If both paths are nearly identical in difficulty, your choice will depend on other factors, such as scenery or interesting things along the way. When human beings are faced with two choices, to change or not to change, a difficult *change path* may not be selected if the choice of maintaining the status quo is clearly easier. When both are of equal difficulty, a decision to change may be made for other reasons. In the clinic, it is important that the activities that are developed to change a behavior are as easy or easier than the everyday activities the person engages in that are maintaining a status quo behavior. A number of years ago, I was supervising one of my students who was attempting to develop self-help skills in an autistic child. The child would never dress herself, always staying in the last clothes that her mother had dressed her in, even when they were badly soiled. To get her to start dressing herself, we had to develop an activity that would require a minimal amount of effort, almost as little as her doing nothing. By combining two types of activities called *successive approximations* and *multiple cuing*, both of which will be discussed in a later chapter, she was gradually taught a series of small individual behaviors that required a minimal amount of effort on her part. After three sessions she was able to put on and take off her coat without help, a monumental change for this child!

Resistance to Change. We are all resistant to change, even when we say that we are not. One problem with change is that it is frightening. It involves giving up something that is known for something that is unknown. Our natural inclination is to resist it, even if what we are experiencing is less than ideal. It makes little sense to utter platitudes such as "we should welcome change," or "we have nothing to fear except fear itself," or " life is the realm of possibilities." It makes more sense to accept our client's natural fear of change and attempt to work with it or around it.

There is a certain amount of comfort in the status quo. Regardless of how dull or bad it may be, it still might be better than the unknown consequences of the proposed change. We all have a natural fear of the unknown. Clinically, there does not appear to be any significant differences in the fear level in males and females who are potential clients (Giles & Dryden, 1991). Fear is an equal opportunity attribute. There is an old joke about a dog who was laying on a nail and continued to wail in pain. A passerby who had seen the dog wailing in the same position for two days asked the owner what was the matter. The old man said that the dog was sitting on a nail. Bewildered, the passerby asked why didn't the dog move. The old man scratched his chin and said,

> Yah see, this here old dog, he's set in his ways. I guess he knows what it feels like to be sitting on that nail, and I guess he's afraid to find out what it feels like not sitting on it.

In many ways our clients are analogous to that dog. The uncertainty of the effect of change is a powerful deterrent against its occurring. Clients may not like the current communicative behaviors they are engaging in, but at least they know their ramifications. New communicative behaviors, even though they may be desirable, constitute an unknown. And the greater the uncertainty, the more difficult it will be for your clients to adopt it. This phenomenon, which we can observe in biological, sociological, and psychological settings, has resulted in the development of clinical experiments that have provided guidance to many professionals involved in personal change. Four basic findings have resulted from countless experiments:

1. The greater the amount of change, the more the resistance.
2. The less the amount of change, the less the resistance.
3. The greater the resistance, the more likely failure will result.
4. The less the resistance, the more likely success will result.

Although the logical structure and progressive nature of these findings seem simplistic, all are routinely violated in therapy, causing clients to needlessly experience failure.

Gradually Changing Behaviors

We have become the "now" generation. We want everything right now, immediately, completely, and at once! We want to build up our muscles to look like Arnold Schwartzenegger in a month, to be as supple as Jane Fonda in a week, and to be as genuine and loving as John Bradford in 3 days. Unfortunately, many of our clients believe that the process of change should also fit this paradigm.

Immediate Gratification. A number of years ago when I was trying to learn to play the banjo, I had decided that I must practice at least 1 hour a day in order to improve my playing. After accomplishing my goal on the first day I was elated. I actually achieved something that was unthinkable to me the prior week. On the second day, I was less elated at the prospect of practicing, but I did it anyway. By the third day, I began inventing excuses for not practicing. By the sixth day, my banjo was back in its case where it remained for 10 years. When I decided to attempt playing another instrument, I chose a resonator guitar or Dobro. I planned to practice for only 15 minutes a day for the first week, and then

gradually increased my practice time each subsequent week. After the first day, I still felt hungry for more practice time and couldn't wait until the next day to continue. My feelings were the same on the second, third, fourth, fifth, sixth, and seventh days. I was excited about increasing my practice time from 15 minutes to 20 minutes the following week. It has now been 6 months since I started on my new practice schedule, and I still feel excited about practicing each day. Just as I increased my tolerance to change by doing it gradually, clients need to be presented with similar situations. Change is most effective when it occurs slowly, with each new behavior grounded on past successful changes. In designing your clients' practice activities, you need to think in terms of very small, almost imperceptible steps in the progression of your clients' goals. A good rule of thumb is the smaller the step, the more likely the client will succeed.

Rapid Change. As important as success is in changing behaviors, in the clinic I have found that rapid success can be a deterrent if it is not scrupulously controlled. When people succeed rapidly, they often falsely assume that the behavior is mastered. With this delusion, they also believe that less effort can be placed on practicing the basics. Change that is rapid is very fragile and often will frighten the person who is changing and those who experience the change. As an undergraduate student, one of my professors had a deserved reputation among his colleagues and students for being mean spirited. Although brilliant in his area, his interaction with everyone was acerbic. During one weekend he came to the realization that his way of interacting with people resulted in a feeling of loneliness that had been adversely affecting his life since he became a college professor many years ago. He resolved to radically change himself overnight. On the Friday morning before his psychological awakening, he came to class dressed in his usual conservative suit and tie, critically chastised his students, and then in the afternoon sarcastically responded to his colleagues during their weekly faculty meeting. On the following Monday, after his "rebirth," he came to class wearing an unbuttoned flowing white shirt, typically worn by hippies in the 1970s, a medallion around his neck with a peace symbol, frizzed-out hair, and sandals. During his class, he tried to be sincere, listened to students, and continually responded positively to questions which the prior week would have resulted in a scathing attack. In the afternoon, he casually strolled into various colleagues' offices and attempted to be personable, asking them how they were feeling and how their families were doing. Although this attempt at transforming himself was genuine, it scared everybody, including himself. Nobody knew this "new" person or how to react to him. Being an open, kind, and hospitable being was totally foreign to the professor, although it was something he aspired to become. We are what we do. Nobody knew how to react to the new set of behaviors which mysteriously and cataclysmically appeared overnight. His attempts to change his interactions resulted in confusion on the part of some. And his colleagues were not prepared to accept his new warm interaction pattern. Within a week, the love generation clothes were shed in favor of the conservative suit, and the negative behaviors that had been a part of his life for so long returned. Do not have your clients strive for dramatic changes over a short period of time without supporting them with counseling. Without support, as quickly as changes develop, they will disappear. Behaviors should change slowly. Select little pieces of what will change, then have your client practice using them consistently until both the client and the people who interact with him or her feel comfortable. There is a Chinese adage that says, "the way to cross a large river is to feel the stones as you wade."

Protecting the Fragility of New Behaviors

Ask any recovered alcoholic how many times he or she has regressed back into the problem after achieving a short period of sobriety, or the person with a weight problem who experienced a rapid weight loss through a weight-reduction program how rapidly the weight mysteriously reappeared. New behaviors are very fragile and need constant attention and reinforcement, or they will usually diminish and eventually disappear.

Positive Rewards and Automaticity of Status Quo Behaviors. The fragility of new behaviors becomes understandable if you examine both the status quo behavior and new behavior in the contexts in which they were used. Remember, anything your client has been doing for a long period of time is intertwined within a large array of associations and may be serving a very positive function for that individual. Take, for example, a young girl who at 14 years of age believed that lisping was cute and that it enabled her to be perceived as helpless and alluring to teenage boys. The behavior, which at the time was both automatic and functional, resisted change. The young girl simply found no compelling reasons to change an automatic behavior that was rewarding. Therapy mandated by her parents proved to be utterly hopeless. Now, at 50 years of age, it detracts from her professional image, yet remains. The behavior, which is automatic, persists even in the presence of punishing consequences. Although one of the causes for the continuation of the behavior is no longer present, the other is. The *automaticity* of old undesirable behaviors significantly affects the fragility of the newly learned behavior it was meant to replace. The old behavior requires no thought and is associated with a myriad of events and people. It has a history.

Fragility of New Behaviors. The new behavior requires constant thought and arrives into the person's behavioral repertoire with as few associations as a newborn baby. Automatic is easier than volitional, associations are stronger than nativity. The more embedded the status quo behavior is in your client's subconscious, the longer it will take to change and the more effort will be needed in practicing the new behavior. In later chapters you will see how you can construct specific activities that will shift the automaticity balance from the old undesirable behavior to the new fragile one.

ACTIVITIES

Once the technology of change is understood, the information must be transformed into *action*. Being knowledgeable and motivated to change family relationships doesn't necessarily mean that the person will be able to transform them into actual activities. Just because a student is taught how to work with children in a school setting doesn't necessarily mean that she will be able to handle six children in a group all vying for attention. Knowledge and good intentions do not automatically translate into actions. Practice is required.

The Consistency of Practice. Often when clients practice, they do it sporadically or with little structure. Worksheets may be given to a client or family members with instructions generally describing the activity and possible suggestions on when to practice. Quite often, instructions are verbally conveyed through the young client, especially in school settings. Clients may be given the initial responsibility of determining when, where, and how they will practice the new behaviors. In all of these scenarios what usually results is a haphazard way of practicing and developing new behaviors. When I first started

practicing fly casting, I went to the casting ponds in Golden Gate Park in San Francisco. Not only didn't I know what I was doing, but my practice times were random. One week I practiced for 2 consecutive days for 2 hours each day, then I didn't return for another 3 weeks, practicing for only 10 minutes for 1 day. Four weeks later I cast my line for 3 minutes. My casting ability did not improve until I developed a systematic method and time structure for my practice sessions. Clients face similar situations. Without explicit guidance from the clinician, clients rarely are able to develop an effective or efficient method of automatizing new fragile behaviors. Throughout this book, the importance of structured activities will be continually emphasized.

The Structure of Practice. There was a popular television advertisement for shoes that showed various athletes doing incredible feats of strength and skill. At the end of the commercial a simple statement said "Just do it." The implication was that, to improve at something, all you have to do is begin doing it. Yes and no. Yes, if you spend your time just thinking about something, you never will do it. No, just jumping into an activity without thought probably will not result in improvement. More likely failures will occur. It is important that, when your clients engage in a change activity, its *structure* should facilitate success. In the clinic, we have found that, when activities are constructed using three basic procedures, the activities tend to help the client achieve the desired goals. These procedures are: (1) activities need to be consistently practiced, (2) activities need to be generalizable, and (3) clients engaging in change activities must be held accountable for their performance.

Consistency

There is the old joke about someone from out of town asking directions in New York

City for how to get to Carnegie Hall. The response from the wise-cracking New Yorker is "practice, practice, practice." In the area of behavior change, this is not a joke. If there is one thing that is probably more responsible than anything else for failures, it is the lack of consistent practice. Consistent practice of the behaviors your client chooses to change will result in three things. It will: (1) bring undesirable automatic behaviors to a conscious level, (2) make newly developed behaviors automatic and (3) protect the fragility of new behaviors.

Making Undesirable Behaviors Conscious.

Behaviors that your clients want to change are so ingrained in them that they often do them without realizing that they are occurring. Only after they are completed and they ask themselves, "why did I do that again?" are they aware of what they just did. Most people call these *habits*. Although the term is correct, it doesn't explain why behaviors continue to occur when we no longer want them to, or how we can stop them. Things we call habits are behaviors we have been doing for a very long period of time. They are stored in our long-term memory in a very specific way. What we remember rarely is in isolation. Rather, we remember in "chunks" of data which include the activities, objects, and feelings which are associated with the target for memory. When you remember the music you learned, you do not just remember the notes. Rather, the notes are chunked with the practice experience and possibly the emotion you felt. When a child encounters a dog for the first time and parents label it as "dog," the child stores not only the label "dog," but also its color, size, smell, disposition, and a variety of other variables. What we call habits are behaviors that were initially developed for one or more reasons. Take, for example, an individual who habitually twirls his hair. The natural reaction of the body is to relieve tension in any way that has worked in the past. With our individual, hair twirling served this function. If he continually experienced tension when meeting new people, an association would develop. A new person equals tension, and tension is reduced by hair twirling. If enough new people continually caused him to be tense, then eventually, meeting anybody new, even if they were totally nonthreatening, could cause the hair twirling to begin, even if it wasn't necessary to reduce tension. The hair twirling that became associated with meeting new people would now be an automatic behavior, out of the conscious thoughts of the individual. The behavior, which now occurs without thought, is rightly called a habit.

In the area of communicative disorders, a person may have begun pursing his lips in order to terminate a block. For example, lip pursing initially may have coincided with the termination of severe blocks. Another person may have developed negative responses to her communicatively impaired child as a way of not facing her child's limitations. Over a period of time, certain things became associated with these behaviors. For example, lip pursing for the first individual initially may have coincided with the termination of severe blocks. If the association occurred frequently, the person might begin lip pursing whenever a block began, in hope that the behavior would result in terminating the block. An unconscious association was now developed between lip pursing and blocking. This series of events are depicted in Table 2–2. In this example we can see that whenever he blocked, he found that by pursing his lips the block would be terminated. After repeating this behavior a number of times, in his mind, it now became a valuable behavior for terminating blocks. Because blocks occur during speech, it is possible that lip pursing may also become associated with speech. Eventually the lip pursing may become an automatic behavior that is triggered during speech even in the absence of blocks.

TABLE 2–2
Developing Habits

VALUABLE BEHAVIOR
Block ▸ Lip Pursing ▸ Block Termination

ASSOCIATION
New People ▸ Tension ▸ Hair Twirling ▸ Reduced Tension

HABIT
New People (without tension) ▸ Reduced Tension

When this occurs, the lip pursing has assumed that status of a habit. If this occurs, then the production of speech alone may result in lip pursing. The same type of association could be described in a mother who continually directs negative statements toward her child. Even when the child is not doing anything that would warrant criticism, the mother may be dispensing it in anticipation of something inappropriate that the child might do. If either of these two behaviors are to be stopped, the associations that have been developed over a number of years must be broken. If your clients will be attempting to replace a habit with a behavior that is more appropriate, you must enable them to identify the things that have been associated with the habit. In Chapters 6 and 8 you will be shown how to accomplish this.

Making Desirable Behaviors Automatic. Usually, when we want to have our clients stop doing one behavior, we hope that they will replace it with something

that is more appropriate. In terminating old behaviors, we must break associations that exist between the behavior and outside events. When we wish to replace it with a new behavior, we must build new associations. For hair twirling, the individual may wish to substitute a resting hand position. For negative statements, the mother may be asked to substitute a more accepting style of responding. If new behaviors are to be developed, the associations that will anchor them in your clients' subconscious must be developed through consistent practice in a wide variety of situations. With every new practice session, the amount of attention and effort necessary to perform it successfully is reduced, and the degree of automaticity is increased. *Nothing becomes automatic without consistent practice.*

Generalization

We do not develop behaviors in isolation. When we develop a behavior, many things are occurring around us. We may be doing the behavior in various settings and at times with different people. As the behavior develops, associations are made and these associations become part of our memory. The child who has a temper tantrum when unable to verbally express a desire does not engage in the behavior in a stark room with nobody present and for no particular reason. The behavior occurs in specific situations, with specific people, and for specific reasons, each of which becomes associated with the behavior in the memory of the child. These associations eventually can trigger the behavior, even when the behavior serves no useful purpose. Let me give you a clinical example. If I am working with a client who abuses her voice, I will want to teach her how to speak smoothly. Her vocal pattern is so ingrained that it is often produced without her realizing it is occurring. In the clinic, I may show her how to moderate her vocal tension to produce a smooth vocal pattern. We practice this behavior in the clinic room, in a sitting position for 45 minutes. Finally, she understands not only how to produce the desired behavior, but can demonstrate it consistently. When the session is over and she is exiting the room, she says, "Good-bye Dr. Goldberg. I'll see you next week," in as gravelly a voice as she used before we began the session! She reverted back to her original voice because we did not develop the new voice in a variety of settings. We did not generalize the behavior. The new voice was associated with the things that occurred around it: sitting quietly and describing pictures. When faced with speaking in a situation in which the new behavior was not trained, the associations in her memory with the old speaking pattern resurfaced, resulting in the gravelly voice. If she is to develop the new voice, it must be trained while standing, conversing, arguing, and so on, and with a variety of people. This is known as *stimulus generalization*, in which various types of stimulus configurations are presented and the client is expected to produce a specific response. She also must be taught how to produce various types of responses such as arguing, laughing, singing, loud talking, and soft talking with her new voice in the presence of one stimulus configuration, such as a specific person. This is known as *response generalization*, in which one stimulus configuration is present and various responses are required. It is important for you to construct activities so that the desired behaviors can be generalized. In Chapter 8 the components of stimulus and response generalization are discussed.

Accountability

Change is a very difficult process even for individuals who are both motivated and knowledgeable. You can probably identify a number of things in your life that you were motivated to change and knowledgeable regarding how it should be accomplished. Yet, provided with seemingly everything necessary for effecting change, you still failed. Quite possibly the key for understanding failures of this type resides in understanding the principle of accountability. In the clinic, I have often seen clients who want to change and know how to do it invent excuses for not practicing the behavior. It's only natural that we avoid things that are difficult, time consuming, embarrassing, or require attention that could be directed toward more enjoyable activities. There are three ways in which you can hold your clients accountable for their progress: (1) reliance on another individual, (2) unwritten internal assessment, and (3) written external assessment.

Reliance on Another Individual. In many clinical situations therapists view their role as the individual who provides feedback, encouragement, and constructive criticism to the person who desires to undergo change. This is probably important in the beginning of therapy because the client may not be in a psychological position to perform these functions. But it is the weakest form of accountability as it is being controlled and directed by someone other than the client. No therapist, no accountability. I remember one client I saw who would tell me that, when he left the session, his level of fluency was very high. After a few days, some stuttering would reappear, and by the day of our next scheduled meeting, his stuttering was back to pretherapy levels. He started our session by saying, " I'm glad I'm seeing you today, after about six days I need my fluency shot from you." What he was saying was that I was the only one holding him accountable for his fluent speech. And, as my influence abated over time, nobody, including himself, was holding him accountable. Accountability has to be internal. Although your clients may ask others to assess how they are changing, they must be the person primarily responsible for assessing progress.

Unwritten Internal Assessment.

I am sure you can identify a change in your life that you wished to accomplish and relied on unwritten internal assessments to determine how well you were doing. Diets are wonderful examples. You probably had decided that you would only ingest foods with a very low fat content and mentally determine if you were on target. Although initially you probably were successful, the amount of fat you ingested increased, eventually going beyond the level at which weight would be lost. Clients undergo a similar process of self-delusion. They try to hold themselves accountable by mentally assessing how well they are doing. Nothing is written down, and if they can remember, they rarely accurately assess their performance. It is a mistake to rely on this form of accountability, especially in the early stages of behavior change. It is too easy for a client to forget or to be kinder to himself than he may deserve. Usually, people will

choose this form of accountability over written forms because they believe that the written method unduly interferes with their activities. If that is the case, you will need to design a written form for your client that is less interfering, but not abandon it. Giving up on a written form of accountability is the first step in "backsliding."

Written External Accountability.

One excellent way of minimizing avoidance is to include something that will make your client accountable in the design of the activity. A very good nonclinical example is a budget. When someone is determined to live within a specific budget, usually the amounts that can be spent in each category are recorded. Then, with each expenditure, the amount is placed in the appropriate category. With running totals, the person always knows how well he or she is doing with the budget. A similar written external accounting is necessary in therapy. It can be something as simple as checking off each day that a client practices a new phoneme, as in Table 2–3 or as complicated as a stutterer evaluating the quality of his speech, as in Table 2–4. As you construct activities for your clients to practice their new behaviors, it is critical that their self-evaluations be in written form. By tracking their own performances, they will develop an external, objective method that will help them to develop new behaviors. You will be provided with a variety of accounting forms throughout this book that you can adapt to your clients' needs.

SUMMARY

Successful change is based on tested clinical principles, a proven technology, and an activity strategy. If your clients are to be successful in changing any behavior, they must take responsibility for that behavior,

TABLE 2-3
Simple Accountability

✓ = Practiced /r/ for a minimum of 15 minutes
x = Did not practice /r/ for minimum of 15 minutes

BEHAVIOR	Sunday	Monday	Tuesday	Wednesday	Thursday	Friday	Saturday
Produced /r/ in isolation							
Produced /r/ in words							
Produced /r/ in sentences							
Produced /r/ during spontaneous speech							

TABLE 2-4
Complicated Accountability

Evaluate each of the behaviors for every day of the week using the following 5-point rating scale.
1 = Always   2 = Sometimes   3 = Occasionally   4 = Rarely   5 = Never

	Sunday	Monday	Tuesday	Wednesday	Thursday	Friday	Saturday
Fluent Speech							
Slow Rate							
Anticipating Feared Sounds							

be motivated to change, and possess the knowledge of how to structure the change. For change to be permanent, it should involve minimal pain, occur over a reasonable amount of time, and initially be treated as a fragile entity. Permanent change requires practice that is consistent, generalizable, and accountable.

CHAPTER

3

Culture

W̲e live in a multicultural and ethnically diverse society in which individuals develop and often act in accordance
with culturally related values. With changing population demographics and the continuing influx of immigrants from Southeast Asia, Central America, the Caribbean,
and Eastern Europe, professionals in the
helping sciences have had to learn new
ways of interacting with their clients.

THE NATURE OF CULTURE

The importance of acknowledging the effects of culture on all clinical interactions
has been emphasized by various authors
(Culatta & Goldberg, 1995; Das & Littrell,
1989; Goldberg, 1993; Kayser, 1995;
Shames, 1989). Cultural sensitivity may be
one of the most critical factors in establishing a clinical relationship when clinicians
and clients are from different cultural
backgrounds. The current appeal for cultural sensitivity in the area of communicative disorders results from a longstanding
neglect of the importance of the ethnic diversity of our clients (Cole, 1992). For
many years the importance of the cultural

values of African Americans, Native
Americans, Asian Americans/Pacific Islanders, and Hispanic clients were ignored.
While many have argued that this was due
to cultural hegemony, others believe that it
may have been also due to a basic lack of
knowledge on the part of Caucasian clinicians. With the widespread acceptance of
cultural diversity, the importance of ad-
justing therapy to accommodate the ethnicity of clients began in the late 1980s.

Sensitivity to the cultural values of
Asians was forced on many clinicians with
the ending of the Vietnamese war and immigration of Southeast Asians, many of
whom, like the Mong highlanders, were
living a preindustrial existence. Their values and needs were so different from what
clinicians were accustomed to that changes
in therapy were immediately mandated,
from interactions as simple as greeting
customs to more complex issues such as
family counseling. Although the many attempts to rectify the situation have been
both well-meaning and needed, the importance of ethnicity is often simplified and
distorted. The problem is analogous to
what you may experience when moving an
overweighted cart. After loading it with

many cases of heavy objects, you must exert a tremendous amount of effort to start it moving. However, once in motion, unless you decrease your effort, the cart will likely collide with whatever is in front of it. A similar situation currently exists in many discussions regarding the importance of ethnic sensitivity. It took many years of courage and determination on the part of some individuals before the validity of ethnic values in clinical situations was even acknowledged (Screen & Anderson, 1994). Now with that acknowledgment, the importance of ethnic differences in clinical situations needs to be evaluated in the light of a broader concept of culture. Although critically important, ethnicity is only one of many cultural areas that affect the behaviors of clients.

Culture Defined

According to the anthropologist Goodenough (1987), culture is a shared way of perceiving, believing, evaluating, and behaving. When culture is viewed in this manner, it becomes apparent that it is not limited only to ethnicity but also includes different sources of shared values and methods of communication. A useful model was developed by two educators who have written extensively on cultural diversity. Gollnick and Chinn's (1990) approach to understanding cultures can serve as an important foundation for developing clinical sensitivity. They maintain that a macroculture and many microcultures exist within the United States.

Macroculture. The macroculture of the United States and all other countries consists of values on which most political and social institutions are based. For example, these are the ten values they believe are inherent in the macroculture of the United States (Gollnick & Chinn, 1990, p. 13).

1. Status based on occupation, education, and financial worth

2. Achievement valued above inheritance
3. Work ethic
4. Comforts and rights to such amenities
5. Cleanliness as an absolute value
6. Achievement and success measured by the quantity of material goods purchased
7. Egalitarianism as shown in the demand for political, economic, and social equality
8. Inalienable and God-given rights for every individual that include an equal right to self-governance or choice of representative
9. Humanitarianism that is usually highly organized and often impersonal
10. New and modern perceived as better than old and traditional

Although macrocultural values bind the population together as a whole, they are not sufficient for understanding individual value systems. Each individual is a member of a macroculture, but also shares values with members of subcultures known as microcultures.

Microcultures. Each microculture is differentiated from others by specific values, speech and linguistic patterns, learning styles, and behavioral patterns. Gollnick and Chinn list eight types of microcultures:

1. Ethnic or national origin
2. Religion
3. Gender/sexual orientation
4. Age
5. Exceptionality
6. Urban-Suburban-Rural
7. Geographic region
8. Class

From these microcultures, values emerge, and from values, styles of communication and interactions develop. Cultural identification for most Americans involves a blending of various microcultures. Take, for example, a client who was a devout

Muslim male upper class teenager who had stuttered his entire life and recently immigrated to the United States from a large urban area in Iran. No one cultural category could accurately be used to describe this client. He clearly is a mixture of various cultures. Clients come to the clinic with an amalgam of values, beliefs, and behaviors from the macroculture and their various microcultures. Although cultural identification with one microculture may dominate the values and behavioral patterns of an individual, it is rarely sufficient for understanding that person. Therefore, it is imperative that the clinician be sensitive to how various cultural components affect the communicative disorder, the client, and the clinical interaction.

Cultural Sensitivity

In many situations, a lack of sensitivity to an individual's microcultural values may result in little more than an annoyance on the part of the offended person. For example, some years ago it became popular to tell Polish jokes. Individuals with Polish ancestors may have been highly offended when someone told the joke in their presence, but if secure in their own identity, felt no life-shaping consequences. The clinical situation, however, is very different. Given the power and respect associated with the role *clinician,* everything may be of consequence.

Cultural Sensitivity Within the Clinic.
Clients enter the clinic as vulnerable individuals. They not only have a communication problem, but they have also failed to find its solution. They implicitly give permission to the clinician to probe feelings they may not have previously shared with anyone. Even more threatening, they may allow the clinician to place them in embarrassing situations or guide them in changing the way they perceive themselves and others. Because of the very intrusive and highly personal nature of the clinical inter-

action, insensitivity to any of the clients' microcultures can have serious consequences. At the very least, clients may become defensive, refusing to allow themselves to be vulnerable with an individual who does not respect or understand their values. At worst, clients may begin to evaluate their values as inappropriate, unacceptable, or worse, deviant.

One important determinant in the success of therapy are the clients' perceptions of the clinician. Clients evaluate not only the clinicians' professional competence, but also their worth as caring, protective, and supportive individuals. Many of these judgments are made on the basis of the clinicians' nonverbal and verbal behaviors, some of which are very obvious and direct, while others are extremely subtle (Butler & Geis, 1990). For example, the acceptable distance between the caucasian clinician and an Asian American client will probably be greater than if the client was an African American. The distance between the caucasian clinician and a client from the Middle East of the same sex will probably be closer than with opposite-sex clients who are Hispanic, Asian American/Pacific Islander or African American. Clients interpret the meaning of these behaviors from their own referent culture. Eye contact avoidance, for example, which is a sign of respect for authority in the Japanese culture, could be interpreted as being disrespectful in the American macroculture. The integral relationship between values and behaviors is one that is often unseen by the individual exhibiting them (Hall, 1959). Culturally sensitive clinicians must have a general awareness of their clients' cultural values and understand how their own verbal and nonverbal behaviors will be interpreted by those clients.

Cultural differences also become apparent when examining a society's philosophy and values. The cultural patterns of various regions of the world dictate specific kinds of social interaction patterns that may be confusing to some professionals and result in information being misinterpreted. For example, politeness in some Native American tribes requires that direct questions regarding a disorder not be made (LaFromboise, 1992). It is imperative that speech-language pathologists familiarize themselves with the cultural values and rules of social interchange of the populations they serve.

Speech-Language Clinician as a Cultural Anthropologist. Speech-language clinicians are not expected to be experts in anthropology. Nor can they be expected to be intimately aware of all the microcultural variables of each cultural subgroup in our country. However, sensitivity can be increased by adopting some of the concepts and methods used by cultural anthropologists (Miller, 1979). Anthropologists study the culture before beginning the field study to acquire a basic understanding of the communication and interaction patterns of the inhabitants. When the study begins, anthropologists make it clear to the individuals with whom they are interacting that there is much they do not understand and that they will probably say or do some things that may be offensive. They emphasize that their errors are made out of ignorance, not disrespect, and they would appreciate being corrected so that they will not repeat the mistakes. In addition to the general disclaimer, anthropologists also try to identify individuals who may serve as resources for their learning. Procedures similar to these have helped anthropologists such as Margaret Mead (1930) and others become accepted by societies whose cultures were very different from their own.

Speech-language clinicians can use a similar strategy for developing clinical sensitivity. The culture of the population being served should be studied. Of particular interest are greeting patterns, the communicative intent of nonverbal behaviors, how the culture views communicative disorders, usual interaction patterns between children and parents, and role expecta-

tions of professionals. This information can provide a basis for culturally sensitive clinical interactions. Many clinics and training programs identify individuals who can serve as resource persons. These can be people from the community, the clinic staff, or faculty from departments in schools of ethnic studies.

ETHNIC OR NATIONAL ORIGIN

Ethnic identity for many individuals constitutes their dominant microculture. It ties them to other individuals with a common history, values, attitudes, and behaviors (Yetman, 1985). Additionally, for individuals living in poverty, ethnic values and their sense of identification may serve as a bulwark against the obstacles parents encounter in using nurturing child rearing practices (Halpern, 1990). The commonality may involve physical characteristics, behaviors, language, values, or place of residence. In the United States, the term race is often used interchangeably for ethnicity, especially in identifying African Americans, whites, Asians, and Native Americans. Race is a term used by physical anthropologists to describe groups of people by their physical attributes. Its simplification of cultural values led UNESCO in 1950 to recommend that the term no longer be used to describe groups of people (Montagu, 1972). It therefore has no place in the description of our clients' ethnic background.

Anthropological Approach

It would be difficult for speech-language clinicians to become knowledgeable of all ethnic cultures. They should, however, become familiar with the basic behavioral patterns of the ethnic cultures from which their clients will most likely come. The east, west, and southern coastal areas, and large cities throughout the country have the most diverse ethnic cultures. For example, on the West Coast it is very likely that clients will come from various Asian, South Pacific, Central American, South American, Far Eastern, European, and African American ethnic cultures. In San Francisco for example, New Comer High School has students from over 27 ethnic cultures. The Southwest has large Native American and Hispanic populations. Chicago has been a center for eastern Europeans for many years. In the eastern part of Pennsylvania, the Pennsylvania Dutch constitute an important and large microculture. New York is home to many people from the Caribbean. Miami has the largest Cuban population outside of Havana. Population demographics are constantly changing. Speech-language clinicians practicing in a small midwestern town may find that the insular nature of their location is only a temporary phenomenon. The task of assembling culturally relevant assessment and therapy material is an ongoing process. A general source of information appears in Appendix B.

Clients do not necessarily expect the clinician to be familiar with all aspects of their culture. They do expect and should receive the clinician's acceptance of their value system and a basic understanding of the intent of their verbal and nonverbal behaviors. Many types of ethnic differences can have an impact on clinical interactions. For many Asian cultures, the public display of certain emotions with nonfamily members would be unthinkable (Cheng, 1987), whereas the same emotions might be freely displayed by African Americans (Taylor, 1992) or Hispanics (Ramirez & Castaneda, 1974). Although the feelings may be identical for each client, their culture dictates how they will be displayed. Clinicians, therefore, should not assume that because an emotion is not displayed, it does not exist. Carl Sagan, the astronomer, wrote that the absence of evidence is not the evidence of absence (Sagan, 1977). This same warning should also be applied when attempting to determine how clients feel about certain issues discussed in therapy. Macrocultural ways of displaying certain emotions may not be acceptable in various ethnic cultures.

General Considerations

When examining the experimental clinical literature regarding ethnic differences, one thing becomes very apparent. Most of the skills that have been identified as being of importance for working with clients of a given ethnic culture are not unique for that culture. The main difference for most skills is in the degree of emphasis, not in whether or not they should be used. For example, the use of flexibility has been shown to be very important when the client and clinician are of different ethnic cultures (Hector & Fray, 1987). Flexibility, however, is an important clinical skill that is appropriate for all clients whether they are from different or the same ethnic cultures. There are some exceptions to this general principle, such as the use of self-disclosure. In Chapters 4–9, 295 specific techniques and clinical behaviors are addressed. If a modification of the skill for an ethnic group has been indicated in the research literature, an explanation will be provided for how to modify the skill. What appears on the following pages is a brief summary of those special changes that may need to be made when applying some of those skills.

Flexibility. The ability to be flexible is a clinical trait that is important to have with clients of all ethnic cultures. It results in clinicians being able to change the direction of therapy based on the current needs of the client rather than adhering to a fixed position or program that does not allow for client needs. When flexibility is displayed with African American clients it conveys to them and their family an understanding of the social complexities that may have more of an influence on their lives then they would prefer (Baptiste, 1990). Many of these complexities are economic in nature, and may not be under the control of the client (Hector & Fray, 1987). The role of socioeconomic values will be discussed later in this chapter.

De-emphasize Ethnocentricity. Ethnocentricity is a term describing the trait of using one's own ethnic values as the basis for evaluating the correctness or legitimacy of the behaviors and values of another ethnic culture. An example would be using an eastern European concept of *family* to evaluate the same concept within the African American culture. Instead of viewing ethnic values as merely different, differences are often translated into degrees of correctness. The closer the different value is to that of the person doing the evaluation, the more correct it is perceived to be. In clinical situations the conveyance of this attitude results in either the establishment of barriers between the client and the clinician (Baptiste, 1990), or with fragile clients, a feeling that their ethnic values may be inappropriate or incorrect (Herbert & Cheatham, 1988). Hector & Fray (1987) found that when clinicians de-emphasized their own cultural values as being a standard of measurement, therapy had a more positive outcome.

Ethnic Matching. Some individuals believe that it is important to match clients and clinicians of the same ethnicity. Besides being a demographic problem, it may not be that important in terms of outcome measurements. Clients from various ethnic cultures were asked their preferences regarding the type of clinician from whom they would prefer to receive therapy (Goldberg & Romeria, 1990). Ethnic matching was important when no other variables were present. However, when given the choice of having a clinician of the same ethnicity with a given level of competency and a clinician of a different ethnicity but of greater competency, the overwhelming choice was the clinician of different ethnicity and greater competency.

The only significant importance of ethnic matching seems to be in the retention of resistant or uncommitted clients. Retention rates were found to be higher with Asian Americans and Pacific Islanders (Takeuchi, Mokuau, & Chun, 1992) and with African Americans and Hispanics (Sue et al., 1991) when there was ethnic matching between clients and clinicians.

African Americans

African Americans along with Hispanics occupy a disproportionate position in the lower socioeconomic structure. Being poor, regardless of one's ethnicity, results in economically associated behaviors such as being consumed by providing the basic necessities of life, protecting one's family from violence, and trying to provide children with whatever is necessary to avoid the cycle of poverty. Although economic advances have been made in the last 20 years by African Americans, a significant number of clients are economically disadvantaged. Living conditions affect one's values, whether the person resides in affluent suburbs such as Shaker Heights in Ohio or economically depressed areas such as the south side of Chicago. These values are brought into the clinic and need to be considered in the design of any intervention program. For example, we know that African American children worry more about school, health, and safety than children from other ethnic groups (Silverman, LaGreca, & Wasserstein, 1995). Acknowledging the importance of these concerns may be important in understanding the reactions of some African American children to some clinician statements and behaviors.

The literature indicates that there are nine specific skills that should be emphasized when working with African American clients. There may be others of importance, but these were the only ones that have been studied extensively and objectively verified. A summary of these appears in Table 3–1.

Expectations. It is important for clinicians to clearly state their expectations of the client and determine what the client expects of them. Although this should be done with all clients, it has an added importance when the client is an African

TABLE 3–1
Experimental Justification of Culturally Specific Clinical Skills—African Americans

Skill	Justification	Citation
Establish Expectations	Clearly Indicate clinician expectations and determine client expectations. Tendency to terminate when expectations are not met or behaviors are evaluated using undiscussed clinician expectations.	Willis, 1988
Develop Rapport	Development of rapport is critical. Distrustful of caucasian clinicians based on past experiences.	Watkins & Terrel, 1988; Watkins et al., 1989; Griffith, 1986; Watkins et al., 1989
Use Reciprocal Approach	Use reciprocal and supportive approach rather than authoritative approach. Most effective clinical style.	Kalyanpur & Shrideve,1991; Kalyanpur & Rao, 1991
Accept Values	Need to communicate an understanding and acceptance of family issues and values. Family is important in intervention.	Baptiste, 1990, Hector & Fray, 1987; Boyd-Franklin & Shenouda, 1990
De-emphasize Ethnocentricity	De-emphasize ethnocentric therapeutic bias. Convey acceptance of cultural differences.	Baptiste, 1990; Herbert & Cheatham, 1988; Hector & Fray, 1987
Disclose Personal Information	Increases client disclosure.	Berg & Wright-Buckley, 1988
Be Flexible	Convey acceptance of social complexities.	Baptiste, 1990; Hector & Fray, 1987
Acknowledge Role of Religion	Church/religion is an important social institution affecting many values.	Boyd-Franklin, 1989; Jones, 1990; Willis, 1988; Boyd-Franklin, 1989
Acknowledge Role of Family	Demonstrate understanding that individual family roles are adaptable. Circumstances may require family members to switch roles.	Boyd-Franklin, 1989

American and the clinician is not. Willis (1988) found that there was a tendency to terminate when expectations were not met or behaviors were evaluated using undiscussed clinician expectations. By having a frank discussion of what clinicians and clients expect of each other at the beginning of therapy, the likelihood of premature termination due to misunderstandings can be reduced. Clinicians should focus their discussion of expectations in two categories: routine issues and the client role in therapy. Since both should be dealt with in the initial interview session, care should be taken in how the issues are presented. Preferably both should be addressed near the end of the first session after the clinician has begun to establish a trusting relationship with the client. If it is presented before the relationship has begun, there is the danger that the client may misinterpret the clinician's reason for discussing the issue. Namely, that the clinician may hold inappropriate stereotypes of African Americans.

When presenting any of these issues, it is important for the clinician to verify the client's acceptance of each statement before proceeding. To assume that it is agreeable to the client may enhance the impression that this will be just another "white-black professional relationship," where the caucasian professional dictates and the African American client accepts. Clinical relationships that are based on this perception are surely doomed either to failure or minimal progress. Routine issues should cover areas such as the days and times when therapy begins and ends, the procedures for canceling therapy, and procedures for sending and receiving information to and from other professionals.

There are many things that the clinician may expect clients and their families to do in order to increase the likelihood that therapeutic progress will occur. These are termed *role expectations*. They generally involve specifying behaviors clients and their families are expected to do both in the clinic and at home. Just as clinicians have expectations of their clients and their families, clients also expect clinicians to perform certain services and act in certain ways. It is important to discuss these not only near the end of the first session but at various times throughout therapy. The fact that clients or their family members may not express any expectations of the clinician does not necessarily mean they do not exist. During the initial session, they still may be reluctant to express them, or they may be new to the therapeutic process and really do not know what to expect from the clinician. Therefore, clients should be asked about their expectations of the clinicians. This could be the opening to some meaningful dialogue between them.

Development of Rapport. Many caucasian clinicians believe that they should not be held accountable for the racist attitudes and behaviors of their ancestors and current individuals who hold ideologies that they abhor. They believe that it is unfair and totally unjustified for them to be lumped together with racist individuals by African Americans only because they share the same skin color. After all, isn't this what bigoted whites do to African Americans? Although the feelings are justified and make sense on a personal level, they are irrelevant in the clinic. Perceptions are more important than reality. It makes little difference to African American clients whether clinicians support or disagree with their values and aspirations if that individual's primary contact with caucasians historically has been negative. As a survival technique, it makes sense to initially assume the worst about a person. This results in the use of defense mechanisms that have been developed over years of strife and may have aided the person in maintaining self-respect. Unfortunately, it has negative consequences in the clinic. One of the clinician's primary tasks is to begin developing rapport with a client. Various researchers have found that based on past experiences, the majority of African American clients are initially distrustful of caucasian clinicians (Griffith, 1986; Watkins and Terrell, 1988; Watkins, Terrell, Miller, & Terrell, 1989). These experiences were both on a personal and professional level. If any significant changes are to occur within the clinical setting, rapport must be established between clinicians and their clients and family members in order to reverse or minimize the effects of past negative experiences. The development of rapport is not something that just magically occurs in the clinic. It results after very specific events transpire between the client and the clinician. In Chapter 5 the components of rapport are discussed.

Reciprocal and Supportive Approach. Various approaches can be taken in therapy, ranging from being very authoritative to nondirective. Some approaches are more acceptable in some ethnic cultures than in others. Kalyanpur and Rao (1991) found that the most effective approach to use with African American clients was one that was both reciprocal and supportive. An approach that is reciprocal is one that provides for a maximum amount of client input. Decisions are not unilaterally made by the clinician, but rather result from an interchange between clinicians and their clients and family members. It is a consultative role that the clinician serves. The supportive aspect of the approach is one that is more complex and requires a greater sophistication on the part of the clinician in order to correctly identify attitudes and feelings that should be supported and those that should be challenged. In Chapter 7 this topic will be addressed extensively.

Importance of Family. For many clinicians, the concept of *family* is a self-contained unit consisting of mother, father, and children. In the African American community, this is too restrictive a concept (Baptiste, 1990), and some would argue

that it no longer adequately describes *family* in any ethnic culture. The "African American family" is an extended concept that may include individuals living in the client's home and individuals living at other residences. Family within the African American culture refers not only to related members within a physical structure, but also responsibilities that members have to each other. In the clinic you may have a grandfather, aunt, cousin, brother, and mother taking turns bringing a young client to the therapy. Each views their responsibility for the welfare of the child as being equal, and therefore their roles need to be acknowledged and accepted.

Disclosing Personal Information. The relationship that exists between client and clinician is that of professional provider and consumer. Regardless of how equal one may wish to have it, by its very nature there are built-in inequalities. Often these inequalities may interfere with the therapeutic relationship. These differences often involve socioeconomic issues. Clients, who clearly have something about themselves requiring change, are seeking the assistance from an individual who will be in a position of evaluating them. This relationship for clients of all cultures is one that is threatening. Evaluation is a frightening process whether it is done by a clinician, teacher, or even a well-meaning relative. It is even more so if the evaluator comes from an ethnic culture that has historically been perceived by the person being evaluated as using evaluations in a way that is regarded as assaulting the person's cultural values. This may be especially true when the evaluator is a caucasian clinician and the individual being evaluated is an African American client. For example, a school district in California was under a court order to reduce the number of African American children who were identified as requiring special education services, because the proportion of African American males in special education was significantly greater than the school population demographics. Many believed that referrals were being made through the use of inappropriate testing procedures and for reasons of disruptive behavior rather than demonstrable special education considerations. Within this suspicious milieu, it became extremely difficult to identify any African American males as needing special education services, regardless how legitimate the reasons.

If there is a fear of being unfairly evaluated in therapy, clients and their families may be reluctant to disclose information that places them in a vulnerable position. Unfortunately, this may be precisely the information the clinician needs to develop an effective intervention plan. Berg and Wright-Buckley (1988) found that when clinicians disclosed personal information about themselves the likelihood that African American clients will disclose personal information about themselves increased.

Acknowledging the Role of Church/ Religion. For the African American community, the role of the church and religion historically has been of prime importance. In the past, it was one of the few institutions that escaped white domination. Throughout slavery and the early 1900s, the church not only was responsible for sustaining the spirituality of the community, but often was at the pivotal point of social support and change (Boyd-Franklin, 1989). Throughout the 1960s the majority of African American leaders in the civil rights movement were ministers or active members of church organizations. Although this role currently is shared by individuals with no direct church affiliations, it still has a position of dominance for many African Americans (Jones, 1990). Although many individuals may not associate themselves directly with any church, their values are directly related to it (Willis, 1988). Therefore, when treating African American clients and their fami-

lies, the role of the church as one of the central bases of all behaviors needs to be acknowledged (Boyd-Franklin, 1989).

Religion seems to have an impact on the degree of separatism African Americans may feel toward white society. While members of traditional African American dominations (i.e., Baptists and Methodists) express a stronger African American identity than non-church-affiliated African Americans, they encourage a more inclusive relationship with whites than do African Americans who either have no church affiliation or are Muslim (Jones, 1990; Spaights, 1990; Wade & Bernstein, 1991).

Family Roles. When dealing with families, clinicians may expect that the role of each family member is well-defined and static. A mother may be perceived as being responsible for taking care of the house, a father responsible for economically sustaining the family, a grandmother for doing occasional chores in the house, siblings for playing with each other and doing menial chores, and aunts and uncles for occasional visiting and being pleasant. Staid and unchanging role relationships are more appropriate for societies in which adversity is minimal. However, within the African American community, social and economic adversity is still more prevalent than in many other ethnic cultural groups. Thirty percent of African American families are poor compared to 9% of white families. As a group, there are 14 million African Americans in the labor force with 2 million unemployed (Chideya, 1995). This constitutes a 14% unemployment rate as compared with a 6% unemployment rate for whites. Some sociologists believe this to be one of the seed causes for problems that plague the African American community (Halpern, 1990).

Because of what may be required to meet economic necessities, the roles of family members in the African American community are more variable than in other ethnic communities (Boyd-Franklin,

1989). Therefore, the clinician should not assume that the person responsible for bringing in a child one day, or working with him at home, will necessarily be the same individual responsible for this assignment the following week. The clinical implication is that the clinician must be prepared to substitute various family members both within therapy and for home generalization activities.

Native Americans

Many individuals have an idealized vision of Native Americans as mystical individuals whose ties with nature transcend all societal concerns. This concept, besides being false, does little to establish a positive therapeutic relationship. Possibly not having a realistic understanding of Native American cultural values may have much to do with minimal contact, false film depictions, and cursory knowledge of the writings of their great warrior-philosophers. Native Americans need to be understood both within a historical perceptive and an environmental context.

Historical Perspective. Most people have some familiarity with the subjugation of the Native American tribes throughout the 1800s. The loss of land, the great battles won and lost, and the countless treaties that were broken. However, there is less of an understanding about how the policies of the United States Indian Bureau in the early 1900s directly affected the values found in many Native American clients who are currently seen in therapy (Herring, 1992). During the early 1900s Native American children were forcibly removed from the reservation and sent to schools where native languages were forbidden and cultural values were scorned. When they returned to the reservation, they did so as individuals who were stripped of their identities. When traditional values are devalued, social disorganization follows (Sullivan, 1983). These in-

dividuals, who no longer had a Native American cultural identity and were rejected by the white society, were the individuals who resorted to alcohol addiction, became unemployable, and had difficulty maintaining families. With few traditional values to pass on to their children and nonacceptance by the caucasian society, problems were passed on from one generation to the next. Individuals with traditional values usually have minimal dysfunctional behaviors.

Rural and Impoverished. A significant number of Native Americans live in rural impoverished areas. The cultural values associated with being *rural* and having a *lower socioeconomic status* need to be considered when understanding Native American values. Native Americans have a disproportionate number of deaths related to alcoholism, accidents, homicides, pneumonia, influenza, diabetes mellitus, and tuberculosis (Marshall, Martin, Thomason, & Johnson, 1991). All of these health problems are correlated with rural impoverished living. When Native Americans move from rural to urban settings, many social problems occur since their cultural values involve rural values. Many of the behaviors which are considered appropriate in a rural setting are not only inappropriate in urban settings, but can result in very negative consequences. For example, a trusting friendly Native American transplanted from the Flathead reservation in Montana to the poorest area of Portland might have as much difficulty functioning as the highly sophisticated caucasian urbanite who wakes up to find himself in the Highlands of Laos. The problems are particularly heightened with older disabled individuals. Being disabled and old engenders a sense of isolation in the individual. It is even more of a problem for Native American elders who are traditional and have been relocated away from their community (Weeks & Cuellar, 1983).

Acculturation. Not all Native Americans adhere to cultural values to the same degree. For example, in four generations of one family, not only did each generation have different affinities for cultural values, but vast differences existed within the same generation. The eldest member of one family was a revered woman in her 80s who still adhered to traditional Native American values and was one of the few people in the tribe who was able to speak and understand the native language. Her daughter, who was in her 60s, had been forcibly removed from the reservation when she was a child and sent to an Indian Bureau boarding school. She eventually returned to the reservation, stripped of her native culture, and eventually developed an alcohol problem. Now, in her 60s, she had regained her native values but still bore the scars of her forced acculturation by caucasian society. Her two daughters, who were in their 30s, were very different. While both lived within the caucasian and Native American worlds, one was significantly more interested in living by traditional values than the other. She was committed to passing traditional values on to her teenage daughter who, as all teenagers do, was struggling with identity problems. The more Native Americans are acculturated into the Anglo culture, the less they identify with traditional values and more with the Anglo macroculture. There are 14 clinical skills that should be emphasized when working with Native Americans. These appear in Table 3–2.

Emphasize Wellness. Clients do not come to therapy because they are communicatively intact. Obviously, they come to be treated for a problem or disorder. Therefore the terms that we use tend to have a negative orientation: stuttering, voice disordered, aphasia, language delayed, and so on. Although these terms are appropriate and meaningful for us as pro-

fessionals, they present cultural difficulties for Native American clients (Levy, 1988). This is related to the Native American view of wellness and disease. For Native Americans, the orientation to health issues is that of wellness (LaFromboise, 1992). One is basically healthy unless the natural harmony with nature is disrupted. When a disruption occurs, the focus is on what can be done to restore the harmony, not on how to eliminate the disorder. Although one could minimize the differences between striving for wellness and eliminating a disorder to semantics, the difference for Native Americans is real and reflects a cultural lifestyle. Therefore, it is incumbent on the clinician to speak in terms of either restoring or teaching normal behaviors.

Understand Rural Issues. The vast majority of Native Americans live in rural areas, most of which are located in the West and Southwest (McShane, 1987). The quality and style of rural living is substantially different than that of suburban and urban areas. The usual defensive postures and suspicion appropriate in urban societies not only serve few useful purposes in rural areas, but can be misinterpreted as being hostile. The pace of rural living is also slower than that found in urban settings. Whereas in urban areas there tends to be an isolation among residents, in rural areas with fewer services available, people tend to rely on each other. Along with rural living also comes reduced economic opportunities. For that reason, you will usually find lower incomes and higher degrees of poverty for individuals who live in rural areas.

Directive Therapy. Few people are completely directive or nondirective in their therapy (Culatta & Goldberg, 1995). Generally there is a mix of the two, the portions of which change with the circumstances encountered. During one part of

TABLE 3-2

Experimental Justification of Culturally Specific Clinical Skills—Native Americans

Skill	Justification	Citation
Emphasize Wellness	Emphasize wellness rather than disability. Cultural orientation is toward positive rather than negative.	LaFromboise et al., 1990
Avoid Labels	Many type of labels have either negative or no meaning within culture.	Levy, 1988
Understand Rural Issues	Most Native Americans live in rural areas.	McShane, 1987
Use Direct Therapy	Nondirective therapy is disliked. Use directive forms of therapy.	Darou, 1987
Be Flexible	Flexibility implies respect for culture.	Darou, 1987; Lockhart, 1981
Use Group Therapy	Very effective form of therapy since it is compatible with cultural values.	Edwards & Edwards, 1984; DuBray, 1985
Observe Nonverbal Behaviors	Attention should be paid to nonverbal behaviors. Reliance on sending and receiving messages.	Katz, 1981
Do Not Use Self-disclosure	Do not rely on self-disclosure for obtaining information; not characteristic of Native American culture.	Lockhart, 1981
Avoid Authoritarianism	Do not use an authoritarian style or give excessive advice; it engenders distrust.	Lockhart, 1981
Use Culturally Appropriate Reinforcement	Reinforcement needs to be adapted to culture. Reinforcing contingencies may be different for Native Americans.	Goldstein, 1974
Focus on the Present	Present time orientation is more important than either past or future.	DuBray, 1985
Use a Holistic Approach to Therapy	Therapy should be constructed in large themes.	Yates, 1988; Denis, 1974
Acknowledge the Importance of Nature	Nature is an integral part of cultural life.	
Acknowledge the Importance of Family	Family is considered to be everyone in clan.	DuBray, 1985; Little Soldier, 1985

the session, the clinician may believe that it is necessary to be very directive when either trying to convince a client about a specific point or guiding a client through a communicative exercise. Later in the same session, as the client begins enfolding a series of life-shaping events, the clinician may become very nondirective, allowing the client to determine what should be discussed. Although some nondirective therapy is appropriate for Native Americans, it should be minimized. One study found that when nondirective therapy was the overriding approach, the client's assessment of the session was negative (Darou, 1987). Conversely, when the sessions were directive, clients found them to be more acceptable.

Group Therapy. Other than in school settings, the majority of speech-language therapy is conducted in dyads consisting of the clinician and the client. When group therapy is used, it is usually done for practical reasons or to practice and generalize new behaviors. Rarely is group therapy considered to be a primary therapy setting for cultural reasons. However, because Native Americans view the group as the main focus of identification, group therapy should be the first choice of therapy (DuBray, 1985; Edwards & Edwards, 1984). The group serves as a support structure for clients. However, when using group therapy, clinicians need to be aware how the behaviors of Native Americans may differ from those of caucasians. For example, when the clinician is talking, the gazing activity of clients between members of the group is not a sign of inattention. Rather, the group members are looking at each other to convey an acceptance of what the clinician is saying (Edwards & Edwards, 1984). It is a form of group consensus.

Nonverbal Behaviors. Speech-language clinicians tend not to observe what their clients are doing nonverbally (Goldberg, 1993). This is probably due to a lack of training in the area and the use of

tables in therapy, which significantly reduces the number of nonverbal behaviors that can be observed. When a client is providing unambiguous information to the clinician verbally, the importance of observing nonverbal behaviors may be minimized. However, when clients reduce the amount of verbal output or are reluctant to share certain feelings with the clinician, important information can be conveyed through nonverbal behaviors. With Native Americans, there is a great reliance on receiving and sending messages through nonverbal channels (Katz, 1981). Because a Native American is verbally quiet does not necessarily mean that important messages are not being sent to the listener-observer. Information is constantly being conveyed through nonverbal behaviors. Therefore, it is necessary for the clinician not only to observe what information clients are conveying nonverbally, but also to be aware of their exhibition of nonverbal behaviors. This is also true with African Americans and Asian/Pacific Islanders. The eyes in particular are used to covey many messages.

Self-Disclosure. With some clients, the disclosure by clinicians of problems or feelings they have may reduce the reluctance on the part of the client to divulge painful or embarrassing information. This technique, although appropriate for clients from certain cultures, is inappropriate for clients who are Native Americans. With Native Americans, the disclosure of embarrassing or painful information is antithetical to their cultural values (Lockhart, 1981). Therefore, the clinician should not only refrain from engaging in this behavior, but also should not expect the client to do so. Other means for obtaining information need to be found. For Native Americans the use of analogies is very effective. For all clients the use of general examples would be appropriate. An example for an aphasic client who is reluctant to learn a new way of communicating would be to talk about how difficult everyone finds it to learn new behaviors.

Authoritarian Style. Although an acceptable role for the clinician is that of someone who directs the course of therapy, care needs to be taken so that it is not misinterpreted as authoritarian when working with Native Americans. By being perceived as authoritarian, attempts at developing trust will be threatened (Lockhart, 1981). This can occur when the clinician begins giving advice to the client. The perception of authoritarianism is minimized if the client is involved in important decisions. By allowing clients to have input into the agenda of the session, therapy can become client-centered, yet not perceived as nondirective. This was found to be an acceptable style of therapy by Native Americans (Alson & Simphiwe, 1992).

Selection of Reinforcing Contingencies. Therapy should be intrinsically, extrinsically, and extraneously reinforcing. We know that the use of reinforcing contingencies is important for clinical progress. There seems to be an assumption on the part of some clinicians that the selection of these reinforcing contingencies is transcultural. That is, reinforcing contingencies for African Americans, Hispanics, Asian Americans/Pacific Islanders, Caucasians, and Native Americans are identical. For Native Americans with a strong sense of *traditional values,* this may not be true (Goldstein, 1974). The key term here is traditional values. The more traditional the values of the client, the more likely that reinforcing contingencies will differ.

Focusing on the Present. The philosopher Krishnamurti (1970) wrote that most individuals are so concerned about the past or the future that they spend little time focusing on the present. Instead of enjoying an activity when it is occurring, they are already thinking about what will happen when it ends or an event that occurred pri-

or to its beginning. For Native Americans it is a cultural imperative to focus on the present (DuBray, 1985). In a clinical setting this would be translated into structuring activities and discussions that are directed toward the present and the process, rather than on eventual goals.

Holistic Approach to Therapy. One important feature of Native American culture is the reliance on holistic approaches to understanding, rather than approaches which are reductionist. This can take many forms. Native Americans place a great deal of importance on intuition for understanding (Yates, 1988). Therefore, clinicians should not rely on abstract conceptualizations for explanations. A more effective approach is to use concrete descriptions to make reference to a person's past experiences, and incorporate global concepts into explanations. Often the use of parables, symbols, analogies, and stories is very effective (Denis, 1974). This narrative style is also thought to be very effective with all ethnic groups in developing client-clinician bonds (Vitz, 1992). The holistic approach is also apparent in an orientation for visual over auditory explanations (Yates, 1988). When explaining something to a client, instead of just verbalizing it, use visual and graphic representations.

Importance of Nature. The role of nature in structuring time and relationships in Native American society cannot be overstressed. As a society, we tend to be very time-oriented. Appointments are made by the clock and the calendar. Few would argue that any other form of commitment is possible in an advanced technological society. Yet, within the Native American culture, time is a more nebulous concept, with activities often related to nature. When asked when a retreat for parents of children with communicative disorders would occur, a Native American speech-language clinician responded that it would be scheduled "sometime in May. We would like to have it during the planting time, so that the rebirth of family relations coincides with the rebirth of the plants." Although this form of scheduling would make little sense to caucasian parents, it presented a powerful symbol to the Native American parents who were being asked to change their interaction with their children from one that was negative to one that would facilitate communication growth.

Importance of Family. Previously it was noted that for the African American community, a caucasian concept of family was too restrictive. The Native American concept of family goes even beyond that of African Americans. At a powwow on the Flathead Indian Reservation, the family of a Native American speech-language clinician was introduced to the author. It consisted of all the members of the clinician's clan, a unit which included any individual who was even remotely connected by lineage. Individuals who, in caucasian society, would not be even thought to be related, were considered to be on equal family status as aunts and uncles. For Native Americans, the family, which is at the level of a clan within the tribe, is of utmost importance (DuBray, 1985). The welfare of the family is placed above that of the individual (Little Soldier, 1985).

Religion. In many Christian religions, evangelical and missionary behaviors are designated as positive religious values. These have no place in Native American religions. Religion for most traditional Native Americans is an intensely personal experience. Although many of the traditional dances, symbols, and ceremonies have been well documented, others are known only to tribal members. More importantly, the feelings associated with religious experiences are topics that often are not discussed within the tribe, and never with outsiders (Friedlander, 1995). Therefore it is important that issues of religion are not initiated by the clinician.

Hispanics

The term "Hispanic" is a federal designation used to identify individuals of Spanish or Latin descent. The term is inclusive of Central Americans, South Americans, some Caribbean Island countries, and Spain. The term obviously is too inclusive to be descriptive of all of these populations. In a discussion concerning the term, a speech-language clinician in Costa Rica adamantly maintained that the culture of Costa Ricans was as different from that of Mexico as Mexico was different from the United States. Whether or not the comparisons are accurate, of importance is that whenever a term is too inclusive, important distinctions are often ignored. What appears in Table 3–3 are general considerations that clinicians should be aware of when treating Hispanic clients. Although fewer culturally specific skills are listed on this table than the other ethnic skill ity there are fewer. Rather, fewer skills have been documented in the research literature.

Importance of Family. Just as was discussed earlier with African Americans and Native Americans, the role of the family is very important in all Hispanic cultures (Baptiste, 1990). The importance of the family as a supportive unit is often attributable to fact that in many situations it constitutes the only institution that an individual can turn to for comfort, support, and safety. This tends to be an oversimplification of its importance. If the role of families in the Hispanic societies found around the world is examined, it becomes apparent that the extended family unit has importance regardless of the adversities found in the society. These findings could lead one to believe that the western concept of a limited family structure is more the exception, in a world-wide context, than the rule.

TABLE 3-3
Experimental Justification of Culturally Specific Clinical Skills—Hispanic

Skill	Justification	Citation
Importance of Family	Important for rapport.	Baptiste, 1990
Flexibility	Important for conveying respect for culture.	Hector & Fray, 1987; Baptiste, 1990
De-emphasize Ethnocentric Therapeutic Biases	Important for conveying respect for culture.	Baptiste, 1990
Indicate Clinician Expectations and Determine Client Expectations	Tendency to terminate when expectations are not met or behaviors are evaluated using undiscussed clinician expectations.	Willis, 1988
Acknowledge Role of Religion	Church/religion is an important social institution affecting many values	Baptiste, 1990

Flexibility. Although being flexible is a clinical trait that is important to have for all clients, there is an added dimension when clients have limited communicative ability in English. In many areas, children who are seen in the public schools and their families may have limited English abilities. Unless clinicians are fluent in Spanish, alternative methods may need to be devised to accommodate the communication difficulties of clients and their families. When flexibility is displayed with Hispanic clients who may or may not have difficulty with English, a message of cultural sensitivity is conveyed which greatly facilitates the development of rapport (Baptiste, 1990).

De-emphasize Ethnocentricity. Hispanic individuals undergo constant pressures to acculturate to American society. Although the greatest pressures involve issues relating to language, social values are also of concern. Often the source of these pressures are individuals who are identified as people who have authority, power, or are professionals. Not only are speech-language clinicians professionals, but by

the nature of the clinical relationship, are thought to possess both authority and power. If clients and their families associate the speech-language clinician with individuals who they believe are attacking their culture, barriers can be established which may prevent positive changes occurring in therapy (Baptiste, 1990). Clinical studies have shown that when clinicians de-emphasize their own cultural values and incorporate the values of the client in therapy, more positive outcomes are likely to occur (Hector & Fray, 1987).

Expectations. In the section on African Americans, it was stated that clinicians should clearly state their expectations of the client and determine what the client expects of them. The same is true for Hispanic clients and their families. With both African Americans and Hispanics, there was a tendency to terminate when expectations were not met or behaviors were evaluated using undiscussed clinician expectations (Willis, 1988). By having a frank discussion of what the clinician and client expect of each other at the beginning of therapy, the likelihood of premature termination due to misunderstandings can be reduced.

Views on Disability. An individual's cultural perspective can affect how he or she views a disability. An important element of all Hispanic cultures is religion. Therefore, when trying to understand how the ethnicity of Hispanic clients affects their values and beliefs, the importance of religion needs to be included, especially in terms of their views of disability. One study found that Hispanics who had a family member with mental retardation reported that it increased their religiosity (Heller, Markwardt, Rowitz, & Farber, 1994). They also believed that it was a religious obligation to take care of that family member, and the additional care that was required was not viewed as burdensome as it was with non-Hispanic families. Not only these, but additional factors were found in a study of Mexican American attitudes toward disability (Smart & Smart, 1991). For those individuals, a stoic attitude toward life and the importance of the family were significant factors in preparing them to meet the needs of their disabled family member. The usual assumption of clinicians is that individuals with disabilities impose burdens on their families, regardless of the level of caring. It appears that what is burdensome may be related to cultural influences. Therefore, the assumption that all disabled individuals impose some form of hardship on families needs to be validated before clinicians formulate intervention protocols based on the belief.

Asian Americans/Pacific Islanders

Although there is a tendency to group all Asian Americans and Pacific Islanders together, distinct differences exist between Filipinos, Chinese, Japanese, Vietnamese, Laotians, Samoans, Malaysians, Indians, and the other individuals whose ancestors come from the Pacific Rim, Asia, and Southeast Asia. Yet, they

have much in common. In this next section, both similarities and individual differences will be presented. A summary of appropriate skills to use with Asian Americans/Pacific Islanders appears in Table 3–4.

Family. In virtually all Asian American/Pacific Islander cultures, the family is a central unit that overrides most social and personal decisions (Berg & Jaya, 1993). Family needs, therefore, take precedence over individual needs. In therapy, clinicians should structure discussions about the client's communicative disorder and intervention procedures in terms of the effect on the family. When advocating for the child, the clinician must remain aware of the cultural importance of the family unit.

Avoiding Public Shame. The public display of anything that is considered "not normal," can result in a feeling of shame or humiliation for clients (Tedeschi & Willis, 1993). For example, in Japan, the presence of stuttering is considered to be the result of abnormal psychological functioning. The stigma placed on clients who stutter and their families has resulted in many stutterers actually leaving the country to receive treatment and eliminate family shame. This feeling of shame may also be experienced by families who have immigrated to the United States a number of years ago. These feelings seem to affect the willingness of Asian Americans/ Pacific Islanders to seek therapy. One study found that, although there was a general reluctance to seek professional help for personal problems, women were more amenable to seeking help than men, and those who were highly acculturated (strongly identify with the culture) were less likely to seek help than those who were less acculturated (Gim, Atkinson, & Whiteley, 1990). In therapy, care should be taken to minimize the amount of disordered behaviors clients are asked to display in a clinical group or publicly. A better approach would be to focus on

TABLE 3-4
Experimental Justification of Culturally Specific Clinical Skills—Asian Pacific Islanders

Skill	Justification	Citation
Emphasize Family Needs	Family needs take precedence over individual needs.	Berg & Jaya, 1993; Steiner & Bansil, 1989
Avoid Doing Anything that Results in Feeling of Shame	Very debilitating and antitherapeutic.	Tedeschi & Willis, 1993
Be Direct	Difficulty in dealing with ambiguity in therapy.	Chan et al., 1988
Do Not Rely on Emotional Self-Disclosure	Difficulty in expressing and verbalizing emotions in therapy.	Chan et al., 1988
Assert Authority	Results in more effective therapy.	Tamura & Lau, 1992
Direct Therapy Toward Interconnectedness of Relationships	Interconnectedness is more important in culture than differentiation.	Tamura & Lau, 1992
Utilize Appropriate Nonverbal Behaviors with Clearly Understood Meanings	Important in defining social relationships.	Tamura & Lau, 1992
Deemphasize Ethnocentric Therapeutic Biases-	Important for conveying respect for culture.	Baptiste, 1990
Focus on Pragmatic Solutions	More acceptable than exploration of feelings.	Berg & Jaya, 1993; Berg & Miller, 1992
In Group Therapy Focus on Traditional Activities and Practical Information	Most effective form of group therapy.	Kinzie et al., 1988
Use Flexibility in Therapeutic Approach	Important for conveying respect for culture.	Hector & Fray, 1987; Baptiste, 1990; McQuaide, 1989
Use Directive Therapy	More effective than nondirective therapy.	Exum, 1988

the development of either compensatory behaviors or new behaviors that replace the disordered one.

Directness. Directness is an important value in the Chinese culture (Chan et al., 1988). Vague allusions to problems or their impact should not be made. Rather, the clinician should deal with them in a straightforward manner. However, directness is not appropriate for other cultures. For example, Filipinos regard confrontation and directness as rude and impolite; thus, clinicians should initially refrain from asking direct and confrontational questions (Agbayani-Siewert, 1994). This same concern for directness and confrontation has been attributed to Japanese clients. It is an Asian tradition to solve problems through negotiation and mediation, not through head-on confrontation. However, nondirective forms of therapy are not as effective as more directive ones (Exume & Lau, 1988).

Pragmatic Solutions Rather Than Emotional Self-Disclosure. When Asian families contact service providers, the contact tends to be crisis-oriented, brief, and solution-oriented; thus insight and growth-oriented approaches are not recommended (Berg & Jaya, 1993). In none of the Asian American/Pacific Islander cultures is emotional self-disclosure an acceptable behavior. Pragmatic solutions, not exploration of feelings, tend to be valued by Asian clients (Berg & Jaya, 1993). Clinicians should focus discussions and clinical activities on strategies for correcting the problem (Berg & Miller, 1992).

Authority. The family and social institutions of most Asian American/Pacific Islander cultures are highly structured and hierarchical both in terms of role relationships and behaviors. Within a clinical context these formalities should be respected. One notable exception to the family hierarchical structure exists in the Filipino culture. When working with Filipino American couples, clinicians should interact with both sexes on an equal basis and not defer to the male (Agbayani-Stewart, 1994). As with other cultural variables, the importance of formal structures for Asian Americans/Pacific Islanders will depend on the acculturation of the clients and their families. With most clients, there is a blend of traditional and western values (Tamura & Lau, 1992).

Although authority is a clinical trait that can be used negatively in therapy, it can be useful when dealing with Asian American/Pacific Islander clients. Clinicians are expected to act with authority, and deviations from this role expectation can impact upon therapy. If clients assume that a competent clinician will act with authority, the more democra-

tic clinician may be perceived as incompetent. Therefore, it is important that clinicians act in accordance with their clients' cultural expectations for the exercising of authority. This does not mean that a dictatorial role should be assumed. Rather, clinical decisions should still be made by first asking for input from the client, then formulating a course of action, and finally asking the client if it is acceptable.

Individual and the Group. In most Asian American/Pacific Islander cultures the group is more important than the individual (Tamura & Lau, 1992). This results in the development of an interconnectedness of relationships. When changes occur in an individual, it affects all group members. When explaining concepts, constructing intervention protocols, and implementing therapy, the importance of the group should be emphasized. This can take the form of enlisting the help of the group or family in delivering therapy. It could also be the justification of therapy in that the amelioration of the disorder will have a positive impact upon the family or larger group.

Nonverbal Behaviors. Nonverbal behaviors and postures are very important in many Asian American/Pacific Islander cultures for establishing the formality of role relationships (Tamura & Lau, 1992). This becomes most evident during greeting activities. For example, when greeting Asian clients there should not be any physical contact, with the possible exception of a handshake, which many Asian immigrants have adopted as a courtesy to western cultures (Dresser, 1996). Although bowing in many Asian societies serves the same function as handshaking, it goes beyond it. The manner in which a bow is performed reveals the social relationship between the interactants. For Japanese clients, since the relationship between client and clinician is not one of equals, Japanese clients will bow lower and longer to clinicians who greet them with a bow. While bowing, they will lower their eye gaze. When unfamiliar with the greeting customs of clients, allow them to initiate the process.

Group Therapy. Group therapy is a very helpful form of therapy for Asian Americans/Pacific Islanders (Kinzie, Leung, Bui, Ben et al., 1988). During group activities the focus should be on traditional activities and practical information. During the activities, care should be taken so that clients are not embarrassed by their disorders. In Chapter 9, the various functions of group therapy are discussed. A very common one is the expression of emotions. Although this is very acceptable in some cultures, it is not in others. For Asian American/Pacific Islanders with strong traditional values, the public display of emotions, even within a very supportive group structure, is not appropriate. The group, however, can serve other important functions such as a situation in which new, non-dysfunctional behaviors can be practiced and generalized.

Blending of Macro and Ethnic Microcultures. Rarely are Asian American/Pacific Islander clients seen in the United States who have only Asian American/Pacific Islander ethnic cultural values to the complete exclusion of western cultural values (Durvasula & Mylvaganam, 1994). Clients bring both sets of values into the clinic. It is incumbent on the clinician to develop an understanding of how traditional ethnic values can coexist with those that are more western in orientation.

RELIGION

During an average week in the United States, approximately 42% of all adults attend a church or synagogue, and nearly 143 million individuals claim an affiliation with a religious group (Gollnick & Chinn, 1990). For many people, religion is a formal institution that has little influence on the development of their values and behaviors. For other people, it can serve as the culture having the greatest impact on their lives, affecting everything from child raising to business practices. With changing demographics, clinicians need to acquire a practical understanding of religious beliefs that may be new and different to them. They should also avoid the pitfalls of bias and stereotyping which often accompany superficial knowledge of a culture (Georgia, 1994).

Relationship to Therapy

Awareness of a client's religious values can be important in avoiding embarrassing situations. Knowing that a client has strong Mormon values would prevent the clinician from offering a cup of coffee, as this beverage is forbidden by Mormon doctrine. Even having a Halloween party during the time designated for therapy might offend some fundamentalists who view the holiday as a form of Satanic worship. Similarly, scheduling an important clinical event on Yom Kippur would be viewed as insensitive by even mildly religious Jews. Although some people are quite open and even evangelical about their religious beliefs, others are very private. Therefore inquiries regarding religious values should be limited to those that have a direct effect on therapy, such as scheduling, activities, and child-rearing practices.

Selecting Clinical Activities

Every year at a university on the West Coast, a departmental activity was scheduled on Yom Kipper, the holiest day of the year for devout and even moderately religious Jews. Although no disrespect was intended, one faculty member yearly expressed her annoyance at the insensitivity or ignorance of those who persisted to do the scheduling. It would be similar to asking Christians to attend a function on Easter morning. Clinic and school schedules tend to be accommodating and sensitive to Protestant and Catholic holidays but often ignore Jewish, Greek Orthodox, and Muslim holidays. It takes only a little research on the part of clinicians to identify the major holidays of their client's religions. It may be as simple as looking on a calender that highlights various religious holidays.

Food and Drink

There are some basic lifestyle considerations that clinicians should be aware of when dealing with clients who have strong religious feelings (Markowitz, 1994). For example, Orthodox religious Jews and Muslims will only eat food that is kosher. During certain times of the year, Jews will not eat food that contains yeast, and Muslims fast from sunrise to sundown during the month of Ramadan. Mormons will not drink caffeinated beverages or ingest alcohol. Muslims will not drink alcohol. Dispensing Halloween candy to children whose parents are fundamentalists would be considered insensitive to their culture. With a little bit of research, clinicians should be able to avoid simple errors that could significantly impact therapy.

Discussions About Religion

There appear to be acceptable and unacceptable ways of discussing religion with clients. One study found that there were no negative consequences when counselors either supported a client's view about the relationship of Christian values to their behavior or ignored it and chose to focus instead on family influences (Morrow, Worthington, & McCullough, 1993). In the same study, negative consequences did result when religious values were directly questioned. For clinicians, the application is direct. If the religious values of clients are thought to be irrelevant for therapy, or even antithetical, it is best not to question them, but rather to redirect discussion to-

ward other areas. For a very few clients, religious issues may have a direct impact on therapeutic progress. In one interesting case, an orthodox Jewish woman did not want to take a necessary medication because she believed that it was not kosher for Passover (Markowitz, 1994). A simple consultation with a rabbi took care of the problem. In cases where there is a conflict between religious values and clinical progress, it has been suggested that the individual's minister or rabbi be consulted if the client agrees (Presley, 1992). The involvement of the client's spiritual leader often can lead to the resolution of the conflict.

GENDER

The gender history of the United States has been one of clearly defined behavioral expectations (Fazier & Sadker, 1973). Little boys were expected to be dominating, strong, good in the sciences, and love baseball. Little girls were expected to be sweet, nice, lovable, great spellers, and collectors of cute dolls. The behaviors taught to children were considered to be the method of indoctrinating values that would carry over to adulthood (Stockard & Johnson, 1980). As the social values of America changed, the expectations of children's behavior also changed. Values that once were considered to be "male" and "female" now have less rigidly defined boundaries for both children and adults.

Use of Language

Listeners often judge the attitudes of a speaker based on the words chosen to express ideas. For at least the last 20 years the trend in both professional and social contexts is to use more inclusive words, in order to reflect a less sexist society. For example, "humankind" instead of "mankind," "congressperson" instead of "congressman," "server" instead of "waitress," and hundreds of other examples too numerous to mention.

The effects of sexist and less inclusive terminology in clinical contexts differs with both the age and sex of clients. Generally, the use of this type of terminology was found to be most offensive with younger clients and clients who were female (Rubin & Green, 1991). It is best to avoid it with all clients.

Selection of Clinical Materials and Activities

Although some psychologists believe that many gender-specific traits are "hard wired" into our genetics (Barfield, 1976), others see the blending of masculine and feminine traits as the logical extension of progressive societies (Sadker, Sadker, & Steindam, 1989). There is some evidence to suggest that, when children are seen individually, there are minimal differences in their behaviors that can be identified as gender specific (Maccoby, 1990). Differences become more apparent in social settings. These differences seem to be related to the socializing influences of the family and culture at large (Meyer, Murphy, Cascardi, & Birns, 1991). In one study of children ranging in age from 3;5 to 6;8 years, significant differences were found (Cramer & Skidd, 1992). Boys were more likely to use male-stereotyped styles of domination and intrusion, while girls were more likely to use female-stereotyped styles of affiliation and inclusion. The male gender-specific behaviors were related to perceived physical competence and peer acceptance, while female gender-specific behaviors were related to perceived cognitive ability.

Other characteristics become more apparent with older children. Male adolescents (12–14 years) were found to be more attentive to issues of control, while female adolescents tended to focus more on the social aspects of a problem (Martinez, 1992).

In treating children, one needs to be aware of inherent behavior characteristics, societal influences, and parental orienta-

tions. What may have been considered to be "tom-boyish" or "sissy" behavior 20 years ago is now viewed as acceptable and appropriate. Activities should be designed for the gender values of the children and their families, not the clinician. Activities and materials selected by clinicians should not be a reflection of their personal values and social preferences. Rather, they should be related to the clients' and families' needs and preferences.

Perceptual Orientation

It would be reasonable to conclude that if two people, both with normal visual acuity, observe the same thing, what will be seen will be identical. Yes and no. Although at a sensory level, there will be no differences in what is registered in the cornea or transmitted to the occipital lobe, the perceptual and conceptual functioning of the brain may transform a simple image into something that is radically different in the two individuals. It appears that at least at the perceptual level there may be gender-related differences. An interesting study examined the differences between female and male undergraduates to remember routes on a novel map (Galea & Kimura, 1993). Males made fewer errors and took fewer trials to reach criterion. Females remembered more landmarks both on and off the route than did males and had superior memory for landmarks. Males outperformed females in knowledge of the Euclidean properties of the map. For both male and female subjects, spatial ability was related to landmark recall. It is difficult to generalize the specific findings of this study to clinical interactions. However, of importance is the understanding that, at least on a perceptual level, male and female clients may be different.

Conceptual Orientation

Just as there are findings that men and women may perceive things differently, so are there findings that they think differently about many things. One important area for clinicians to be aware of is how male and female caregivers view the disabling conditions of their children. One study found that, not only did mothers think more about the disabling condition of their children, but they also had a more realistic conception of its nature than did the children's fathers (Schultz, Kemm, Bruce, & Smyrnios, 1992). If the findings of this Australian study are applicable to families of disabled children in the United States, clinicians should be more vigilant in including fathers in their family counseling. Not only do fathers need to be encouraged to be involved in therapy, but frank discussions with them may be necessary concerning the nature of their child's disability and future prospects.

Disability

It appears that a family's view of disability may be partially related to the importance its ethnic culture places on gender (Westbrook & Legge, 1993). Although each ethnic culture has its own general views about disability, the magnitude or superficiality of the problem may depend upon the gender of the disabled individual. In Asian countries where male children are valued more than female children, a disabled son is viewed with more tragedy than a daughter with a similar problem. The more traditional the family, the more likely this attitude will have an effect in therapy. Clinicians need to be aware of these cultural influences before making judgments on the family's level of caring. Although both male and female disabled children are loved equally, the life expectations for male children are greater. Those expectations are destroyed with the disability. A family's commitment to clinical involvement may initially be greater for male children. The clinical commitment to involvement for female children can be enhanced, not by confronting cultural differences, but rather by enabling the family to see the advantages to the whole family of their involvement in therapy.

Homosexuality and Lesbianism

The gradual acceptance of homosexuality has allowed many men and women to openly express their sexual preferences. Many years ago the American Psychological Association removed homosexuality and lesbianism from its list of personality disorders; yet for many people the sexual preference of gays and lesbians becomes the one behavior that overrides an individual's values and beliefs. Just as stutterers are not their behavior, homosexuals are not their sexual preference. The values found in heterosexual parents and clients are the same as those found in homosexual parents and clients. In rare occurrences, the sexual preference of a client may be a factor in clinical intervention, for example, an individual who wishes to change his or her vocal range because of a transsexual operation. It is much more likely that it may be a factor affecting the clinician's responsiveness and understanding of the client or parents of a client. The concern that gay fathers or lesbian mothers feel for their communicatively impaired children is no different than the concern felt by heterosexual parents. In almost all cases, the sexual orientation of clients or their parents will have little or no effect on therapy, regardless of the sex or sexual orientation of the clinician (Moran, 1992).

AGE

Certain cultural values are associated with age groups. Whereas older clients find a comfort in activities that are stable, teenagers may look for the opposite. For them, change is desirable, and stability is to be avoided. As a society, we tend to identify individuals as belonging to one of eight age categories (Kalunger & Kalunger, 1986):

1. infancy   (birth–2 years)
2. early childhood   (3–5) years)
3. middle childhood (6–8 years)
4. late childhood   (9–12 years)
5. adolescence   (13–19 years)
6. early adulthood   (20–39)
7. middle age   (40–65 years)
8. elderly   (beyond 65 years)

For the sake of simplicity, these categories will be reduced in this section to four: Childhood (up to 12 years), adolescence (13 to 19 years), adulthood (20 to 65 years), and elderly (over 65 years).

Values

Age-related values are determined primarily by experiences. For example, the 4-year-old child's view of the importance of money is very different from that of the 70-year-old retiree who must sustain herself on $450 a month. The age-related values of clients will affect their belief systems and clinician's choice of clinical materials.

Age and Guilt. The amount of guilt and its sources appears to vary with age (Williams & Bybee, 1994). Younger children appear to feel more guilty about things they have no control over, and sources tend to be related to extended family members and siblings. With age, parents still remain the main source of guilt. At higher grade levels, the percentage of students reporting guilt from aggressive, externalizing incidents decreases, whereas those mentioning guilt over internal thoughts and inconsiderateness increases. Guilt over flouting rules peaks at the 8th grade. Male students reported more guilt over externalizing behaviors than female students, whereas female students reported more guilt over violating norms of compassion and trust. Regardless of the source of guilt or the events it is related to, guilt is something that should be minimized or eliminated. It adds nothing to the therapeutic process because it focuses the clients' attention on events which occurred in the past. It is best to redirect thoughts to behaviors that can now be changed. The preceding data suggest that what clients may feel guilty about is related to age. Although only some clients enter into therapy with guilt that is related to their communicative disorder, an awareness of its relationship to age will enable clinicians to become more sensitive to its presence. An approach that has been shown to be successful, especially with middle school children, is the use of stories, metaphors, role playing, and simulations (Kottman, 1990) since they may find it difficult to express their feelings about the effects their communicative disorders have on their lives.

Selection of Materials. The clinician must be aware of age-related values not only in interactions, but also in the selection of appropriate clinical material. Choosing stimulus material for an adult aphasic from a child-oriented language kit may be effective in terms of the linguistic concepts to be taught, but it may inadvertently convey to the client a disrespect and condescension that can interfere with therapy. Some test instruments are designed only for one specific age range, such as children (Shine, 1980), adolescents (Deshler, Shumaker, & Lenz, 1984), or adults (Woolf, 1967). A few authors modify instruments to be appropriate for more than one age range. One example of sensitivity to age factors is found in the Goldberg-Culatta 5 Steps to Fluency Program (1997). Goldberg and Culatta designed three different sets of interview questions for children, adolescents, and adults. Although the information sought by the interviewer is identical for all ages, each set of questions uses age-appropriate terminology, phrasing, and concepts.

Behaviors

Age not only affects clients' values, but it also affects the types of behaviors clients display in clinical contexts. Three important ones are related to reaction time, optimism, and resistance.

Reaction Time. Although it is generally accepted that the reaction time of younger subjects is quicker than that of older subjects, practice changes the equation. One study found that with practice, reaction times of older subjects were significantly reduced (Rogers & Fisk, 1990). For clinicians this means two things: First, with new activities, additional time should be allotted for the elderly to respond before answers are provided. Second, just because the initial additional time to respond is necessary, the stereotype of a slow elder should not be developed. With a little practice, reaction times of the elderly become similar to those of younger individuals.

Presence and Absence of Optimism. Optimism in therapy is a belief on the part of clients that positive change is a possibility. The absence of optimism in the elderly is a serious problem that is thought to be analogous to the concept of *failure to thrive* usually associated with the physical development of infants. However, recently the term is being applied to the elderly who are hospitalized after a major physical problem (Newbern, 1992). These patients' physical problems result in severely diminished environmental, social, and functional capacities. Some clients who have suffered a stroke fall into this category. For these clients, traditional aphasia therapy may be inappropriate until other more basic areas of functioning, such as nutrition and socialization, are addressed. For these clients, intervention needs to be multidimensional and coordinated with many professionals.

Resistance. The type of resistance to therapy displayed by clients may be related to age values. Not all clients wish to be in therapy. Adults who view their life as essentially over may not believe that the benefits gained by speech-language therapy are worth the effort. Some adults who have suffered a stroke and are very depressed have little interest in therapy, even though they have consented to it. Their consent may be an accommodation made to their family or an activity that can diminish endless boredom. Adolescents who are going through an identity crisis and sexual transformation are concerned with their image. The adolescent who is pulled out of her class or has the clinician work with her in the class may be very resistant to therapy. In both situations, the attention drawn to her may be embarrassing. Unless the communicative disorder is substantial, children often cannot see any value in the experience. Children may not see any value in correcting the way they speak since it is not apparent to them or their friends that a problem exists.

Regardless of the type of age-based resistance, it was found that, when clinicians are perceived by resistant clients as understanding, interested, and concerned, resistance diminishes and in many cases is transformed into active involvement (Patterson, 1990). The same approach is suggested with children and adolescents who present themselves as aggressive and angry individuals (Davis & Boster, 1992).

EXCEPTIONALITY

Clients with communicative disorders confront their problems as soon as they attempt to understand another individual, respond, or ask for something. In the presence of people, it cannot remain a hidden disorder. When faced with a problem, an individual can accept it, compensate for it, or attempt to eradicate it. Regardless of the solution chosen, the choice results in the development of values that may be infused throughout the individual's behaviors. For many disabled individuals, humiliation is faced on a daily basis which may lead to hurt, anger, and depression (Kirshbaum, 1991).

Values

Exceptionality is not often thought to constitute a culture with specific values. However the experience of being different can be so substantial that it becomes a primary cultural identification for some individuals. Being identified as a *disabled individual* involves the development of values and beliefs which at times seem to be contradictory.

Dilemma of the Disabled. Some disabled individuals continually are involved in the dilemma of wanting to have accommodations made for the disability, yet wishing that society would minimize emphasis on the disability (Esten & Willmott, 1993). This dilemma can result in the development of values that are conflicting. An aphasic client, for example, would like to have his wife communicate for him, but also wants people to provide him with the time necessary to formulate and produce his thoughts. Unfortunately, for some disabled individuals, their exceptionality can become their predominate microculture, overshadowing all other cultural values (Szivos & Griffiths, 1990). The adult stutterer who has been unable to control his speech may see life as a series of events on which he has little effect. The aphasic client who was an articulate professor before his stroke may now view all interactions as painful vignettes, all designed to humiliate him. The young child whose language disability prevents her from telling her parents she is in physical pain may come to believe that physical pain is a normal part of life, to be accepted and endured.

A model for counseling disabled individuals, which was proposed by Keany and Glueckauf (1993), may be valuable for speech-language clinicians to use with clients whose primary cultural identification is their disability. They have suggested that, if the disabled are emotionally and intellectually to go beyond the effects of their condition, four areas need to be addressed. The first is that their value system must be enlarged beyond the scope of values associated with the disability. In other words, exceptionality should be viewed as only one microculture. The second is that the disability should not be used to define themselves. Individuals are not their disability. Third, the disabling effects of the problem need to be contained. There should be a focus on what can be done in spite of the disability. And fourth, instead of comparing themselves with nondisabled individuals, emphasis should be placed on their own intrinsic worth.

History of Failures. Continual communicative failures can lead to emotional scarring. Often the pain these clients carry is masked by inappropriate behaviors. It may involve acting out a behavior by a child who does not know how to respond verbally. Or adults, who after experiencing numerous failures in communication, retreat into their disability, developing an insular shield that is impervious to even the most caring clinician. It is important for clinicians to address this problem immediately. This can be easily accomplished by structuring therapy in a way that quickly results in success. In Chapter 6, two methods are provided which have clinically been demonstrated to be effective. These are called *successive approximation* and *multiple-cuing*.

Self Evaluation Based on Societal Reactions. The cultural values of exceptionality also develop from the reactions of society to the individual with the disorder. All too often individuals are viewed as their disabling condition, as someone to be pitied or avoided, to bear the brunt of jokes. One study of junior high and high school students has shown that reactions differ with age and gender (Darrow & Johnson, 1994). Females showed more positive attitudes than males toward a wide variety of disabilities. And the older the students, the more likely that they would be accepting of a disability. As a society, we have progressed significantly over the past 25 years—from viewing disabled individuals as helpless wards of the state to the current view which is that most disabled individuals can be mainstreamed into society and live productive semi-independent or independent lives. Although this view is considered the most appropriate one, the common reaction of many people to the disabled is one that still denies them full equality. It is a belief that is transformed into behaviors toward the disabled that make it difficult for them to perceive of themselves in a way other than a "disabled person," rather than a unique individual who, among other things, has a disabling condition. As a result of either being isolated from a larger community through nonacceptance or a lack of understanding, individuals with similar disabilities may form associations or communities that have as strong and well-defined value systems as other types of cultures. The deaf culture is one example.

Relation to Other Cultural Influences. Often you hear someone saying that a disabled individual has "gone beyond his disability." The implication is that, in spite of a disabling condition, he or she has been able to achieve something. Although this may occur because of an individual's personal strengths, it may be the result of other cultural influences. For example, in a study of profoundly deaf Native Americans, it was found that issues of importance were related to traditional tribal values rather than attachment to deaf culture (Eldredge & Carrigan, 1992). For these individuals, deaf culture was not as important as traditional Native American values.

Ethnic cultural influences may affect the acceptance of a goal of independent living. Disabled advocates in the United States have emphasized the importance of developing independent living skills for the disabled. Although this goal is desirable and

compatible with the macroculture of the United States, it may be a concept that is unimaginable in some Asian societies (Miles, 1992). In many Asian societies, the responsibility for individuals with disabilities belongs to the family, not to larger societal units. If clinicians wish to prepare disabled Asian American/Pacific Islander clients for independent living, their families will also need to be prepared for the transition.

Preference for Disabled Clinicians. Disabled individuals not only prefer clinicians with disabilities, but the preference is even stronger for those that share the same disability (Nosek, Fuhrer, & Hughes, 1991). Disability, like ethnicity, can serve as a strong identification for its members. When a group, rightly or wrongly, believes that it has been historically mistreated by other groups, it is more likely that they believe only members of their own group can be sensitive enough to both understand their problems and treat them competently. Clinicians who are not disabled can minimize the effects of this initial distrust by displaying the appropriate sensitivity to the client's condition and providing competent services that have been mutually formulated with the client.

Behaviors

Many of the behaviors exhibited by disabled individuals result from societal reactions to the disabling condition (Lee & Rodda, 1994). The reactions are rarely simple and may involve both prejudiced attitudes and realistic assessments (Beckwith, 1994).

Interpersonal Relationships. Disabling conditions adversely affect an individual's ability to interact with the general population. There are two sources for the problem. The first is the disabling condition itself. An individual confined to a wheelchair or required to use crutches may be physically isolated from interacting with other individuals. A person with aphasia who has difficulty understanding sentences will not be able to engage in conversation. The esophageal speaker will have difficulty feeling fully included in the rapid banter of friends who are engaging in a comical exchange. A child with a language disorder may not know the pragmatic language rules that are necessary for inclusion in a play group of peers. However, in addition to the limitations imposed by the condition, others are needlessly added by society (Lindstrom & Kohler, 1991). Disabled individuals experience as much isolation as a result of societal attitudes as they do from their conditions and environment. Through ignorance and prejudice, the able-bodied population reacts to disabled individuals in ways that are differential. Either individuals with disabilities are treated as if they were unable to interact normally with the able-bodied population, or they are greeted with outright prejudice.

Social Acceptance. Currently, there is a greater emphasis on involving disabled individuals as much as possible in all societal institutions and experiences, ranging from modifications of bus entry ways to inclusion of severely disabled children in normal classrooms. All of these efforts involve the restructuring of either physical entities or service delivery systems. As important as they are, they are not sufficient for increasing the social acceptability of the disabled individual. Critical to acceptance are the attitudes of individuals who are in contact with the disabled (Forlin & Cole, 1994; Law & Dunn, 1993). When attitudes are negative or condescending, the likelihood that the disabled will develop normalizing attitudes and behaviors is minimal.

Gender. Earlier, it was noted that some ethnic cultures view the disabilities of male and female children differently. This is also true of the macroculture. Eleventh graders responded to a survey regarding attitudes toward males and females with disabilities (Weisel & Florian, 1990).

Attitudes toward females with disabilities were less positive than attitudes toward males with disabilities. These less positive attitudes were expressed more by boys than by girls. It appears that disabled males are perceived in a more positive light than disabled females. This disturbing finding may be a corollary of a macroculture's sexist view of the potential societal contributions of men and women. In other words, because men may be viewed as having more potential to contribute to society, their disabling conditions are viewed as a greater tragedy than those of women.

GEOGRAPHIC

With increasing mobility, it has become increasingly difficult to identify unique geographical value systems. The "sophistication" of the East Coast, the "laid-backness" of the West Coast, the "hospitality" of the Southwest, the "congeniality" of the South, and the "straight-arrowness" of the Midwest are stereotypical labels whose edges have been blurred by the relocation of individuals and acceptance of macrocultural values. Although blurred, some distinctions still exist. Often the importance of these regional differences is ignored in clinical contexts. In the past, when we were a fairly immobile population, people generally trained and practiced in the region they would live. At one university in California, the student enrollment in the graduate program in speech-language pathology over a 10-year period went from 95% enrollment from within the state of California to 50% enrollment of California residents. Most of the students graduating from the program continue to begin their practices in California. For many, coming from the Midwest and the South, some of the values they were accustomed to in interactions were either absent or modified by people living on the West Coast. Understanding the nature of these regional differences helped these new clinicians avoid misinterpreting their clients' behavior.

URBAN-SUBURBAN-RURAL

Although regional geographic lines have been blurred, distinctions among urban, suburban, and rural life styles remain more intact. The physical necessities and restrictions of these environments result in the development of cultural values.

Urban

For many people, cities can be a source of wonder, excitement, and stimulation. For clients who live in socioeconomically disadvantaged neighborhoods, the city may also be a source of daily concern and terror. Because crime is disproportionately located in the areas of cities where the poor live, it is reasonable to assume that clients who reside in these areas will have developed survival values that may affect the development of a trusting relationship in therapy. Fortunately, many of these behaviors can be modified by knowledgeable clinicians (Brondolo, Baruch, Conway, & Marsh, 1994).

Aggressiveness. Often, children who live in the poorer sections of cities that are experiencing high levels of crime develop aggressive attitudes as a survival technique (Brondolo, Baruch, Conway, & Marsh, 1994). These are often defensive attitudes created in relation to a hostile environment that threatens them daily. Even with the best of intervention techniques, used by the most competent clinicians, many of these children will not benefit from therapy (Hains & Fouad, 1994). Improvement of communicative ability is just not something very high up on their list of priorities.

Stress. Life for children and adolescents in urban settings may be fraught with experiences that can cause enormous stress (Cowen, Wyman, Work, & Iker, 1995). The severity of the problem is magnified when its sources involve unsolvable problems. Given the enormity of the problems, it is understandable why many of the children who are seen for therapy in school settings place a very low priority on speech and language therapy.

Suburban

Although there are values associated with the suburban living style, their relationship to therapy has not been extensively studied. An underlying assumption appears to be that the better economic quality of life experienced by those who live in the suburbs results in no special considerations therapists need to make when treating these individuals. This probably is a fallacy. Any variable that affects one's culture needs to be considered, even those that are not aversive. This same void of factual information is also evident for middle- and upper-income socioeconomic status. In the absence of factual clinical data, the reader is directed to more general sociological treatments of suburban life styles.

Rural

Two features that have been cited as significantly affecting the values of rural clients are being isolated and impoverished (Fiene and Taylor, 1991). Although many rural clients are neither, these features are prevalent at least for the majority of rural dwellers. Of importance to the clinician is the effect each will have on therapy.

Isolation. The tranquility associated with rural living has its price. With an isolated living style also comes a lack of services. In any major city a quick glance in the Yellow Pages under "Speech Therapy" will result in scores of individuals, hospitals, and rehabilitation sites. The choices can be substantial both in terms of the number of clinicians and their specialties. In rural settings, the communicatively disordered individual often must travel great distances to acquire services. *Rural America* is not found only in the hills of West Virginia or the mountains of North Carolina. Rural America is a living condition that can be found outside almost every major city in the United States, and therefore all clinicians should be familiar with rural values. For example, a client who lived outside of Eureka, California drove 150 miles each way once a week to receive therapy in San Francisco, because there were no therapists who specialized in stuttering in the Eureka area. The isolation found in rural communities affects not only the provision of services from speech-language clinicians, but also other related services. Coordinating services for clients who require multiple services can be difficult, when services are located a significant distance from each other. To facilitate coordination, it is suggested that the speech-language clinician work very closely with the individual or professional who made the referral, so that the client can be viewed within a family and social context (Gesuelle, Kaplan, & Kikoski, 1990). Follow-up contacts after the termination of therapy are even more problematic. For some clients, traveling great distances for a short maintenance check is burdensome. Clinicians may need to use more imaginative ways of assessing the clients' ability to maintain behaviors, such as telephone conversations, audiotapes, and videotapes.

Poverty. A disproportionate percentage of rural dwellers are impoverished (Fiene & Taylor, 1991). Given limited personal financial resources and minimal or nonexistent insurance reimbursements, therapy needs to be cost-effective. The luxury of slowly and systematically implementing an intervention protocol may not be possible with poor rural clients. Therapy should focus on teaching coping strategies that clients can use either on their own or with the help of family members after short-term therapy is terminated. An intervention program with a specific number of sessions should be developed for clients who must either travel long distances for therapy or are restricted to a limited number of visits due to limited federal, state, or personal funding.

SOCIOECONOMIC CLASS

The socioeconomic class that one identifies with can have a significant influence on the development of values, forms of interaction, and language usage. The sociologist Max Weber (Parsons, 1947) believed that the values of individuals were shaped primarily by the socioeconomic class to which they belonged.

Place of Socioeconomic Values

For Weber, to understand why people act as they do, one must first understand their socioeconomic position in society. The effect of socioeconomic class values on the individual's behaviors has been documented in many studies, ranging from the occurrence of neurosis and psychoses (Hollingshead, 1958) to the prevalence of stuttering in children (Morgenstern, 1956). It is a common assumption that problems in therapy are related only to lower socioeconomic values: that the values of those with less money, power, and position may be less conducive to positive outcomes than values of those who are economically and socially better off. This is not the case. Stereotyping the positiveness and negativeness of class structures makes as little sense as stereotyping ethnic cultures. There is variability in both. While the parents of one child who is economically well off may hold the importance of developing communication normalcy as a high value, other parents in the same socioeconomic class may find it irrelevant, given all of the advantages available for their child. Likewise, while one parent living in abject poverty may be so consumed by her personal dilemma that she does not see the importance of speech therapy, another mother in a similar situation may give up basic necessities to provide help for her child.

Although the individuality of clients cannot be overemphasized, certain types of problems statistically are more likely to occur in one socioeconomic class than in another. Insensitivity to socioeconomic values leads to problems not only in therapy but also in diagnosis. A misdiagnosis can occur when an evaluation instrument is normed on one socioeconomic culture and then applied to another that is very different. In these cases, the instrument may create the communicative disorder.

Style of Interactions

Clients who are from lower socioeconomic classes may occupy positions within the macroculture that limit their power and control over their lives. The longer one occupies a position of socioeconomic powerlessness, the more likely it is that the feelings of limited control will generalize into other areas of the person's life. Clients with communicative disorders may come to view their problem as one that is beyond their control and either develop a sense of hopelessness or inappropriately rely on the clinician for change. It has been suggested that these nonproductive attitudes can be changed by clinicians using a conversational strategy that emphasizes the client's ability to exert control over all aspects of therapy (Ventres & Gordon, 1990). In discussing the effect a disorder has on the life of the client, terms that emphasize the ownership of the behavior should be used rather than terms that objectify it. For ex-

ample, instead of allowing a client to say "the aphasia stops me from remembering," the client should be reinforced for using a construction such as "with my problem its hard to remember."

Conversely, clients who have always wanted to exert control over their own lives, but have not been given the opportunity to do so, may embrace the chance to be intimately involved in restructuring their own behaviors or those of their children.

Occupation

The effect of occupation on the development of values and behaviors is a phenomenon that has been recognized by sociologists for many years. It can shape values as well as preferred styles of interaction. Take, for example, an elementary school teacher who spends 6 hours a day, 5 days a week, for 9 months every year, instructing 6-year-olds on what they can and cannot do. As a client, she may present the impression of someone who is more interested in talking and controlling the session than listening. Similarly, the individual who is never afforded the opportunity to act independently in a job may appear confused when asked to choose between tasks. For these people, clinicians are asking them to function in a way that is not only unfamiliar to them, but would have resulted in negative consequences if they did so in their job. Although it is important to understand how clients' occupations shape their interactions, it is equally important not to stereotype clients based on what they do for a living. In his book, *Working,* Studs Turkel (1992) has over 100 people describe their jobs and how they feel about them. Two very revealing stories are told by a waitress and a telephone operator.

Everyone says all waitresses have broken homes. What they don't realize is when people have broken homes they need to make money fast, and do this work. They don't have broken homes because they're waitresses.. People imagine a waitress couldn't possibly think or have any kind of aspiration other than to serve food. (pp. 390–391)

It's a strange atmosphere. You're in a room about the size of a gymnasium talking to people thousands of miles away. A lot of the girls are painfully shy in real life. You get some girls who are outgoing in their work, but when they have to talk to someone and look them in the face, they can't think what to say. They feel self-conscious when they know someone can see them. At the switchboard, it's a feeling of anonymousness. (pp. 65–66)

Relationship to Premature Termination

Lower socioeconomic status is highly correlated with lower levels of education. Because better paying jobs require higher levels of education, the poorly educated individual is more likely to find lower paying jobs. The correlation between lower socioeconomic status and less education is clinically important when identifying mothers who are at risk for prematurely terminating therapy for their children. It appears that there is a reverse correlation between premature termination and levels of education (Sirles, 1990). In other words, the less education a mother has, the more she is at risk for prematurely taking her child out of therapy.

Nutrition

With poverty comes the reduced ability of parents to feed their children. Although starvation is not a widely known phenomenon in the United States and most western countries, the effects of poor nutrition on children may be less recognized. A study was conducted in rural Kenya to determine the effect of nutrition on the cognitive abilities of children. It was found that better nutrition was correlated with increased at-tention during classroom activities, better verbal comprehension, and increased cognitive abilities (Sigman, Neuman, Jansen, & Bwibo, 1989). Although few of the children seen by speech-language clinicians would be classified as *starving*, an alarming number are malnourished. For these children, traditional speech-language therapy may need to be complimented with an interdisciplinary approach involving health care providers. Hungry children do not learn well for both neurological and psychological reasons.

Homelessness

Homelessness is a phenomenon that appears to be increasing in our society and is not limited to the hopelessly addicted or mentally ill. All too often, homeless families are appearing at shelters and in food lines. Most families attempt to send their children to schools and provide for them as best as is possible. Children who are homeless and require services of the speech-language clinician in public schools are a special challenge. In addition to their communicative disorders, these children may be suffering from malnourishment, may not live in an environment in which generalization is feasible, most have an overriding fear that their homelessness will be discovered resulting in social stigma (Walsh & Buckley, 1994). As the number of these children increases, possibly there will be more of an interest in meeting their special needs, both in public school settings and at social welfare settings that provide them with medical services.

SUMMARY

Cultural sensitivity is not the panacea many adherents of multiculturalism maintain it to be. Cultural sensitivity is nothing more than the acceptance of differences as valid components of an individual's identity. These differences should be viewed by the observer as differences without hierarchies. The child-rearing practices of Native Americans, African Americans, Hispanics, Asian Americans/Pacific Islanders, and the ancestors of eastern and western Europeans are different, with no inherent ranking as to their appropriateness or quality. The customs associated with Muslim traditions of Ramadan are no stranger than the kosher laws of Jews, the baptism rites of Protestants, or the sacraments of Catholics. That is not to say that specific practices of all cultures have the same effect on communication disorders. On the contrary, the cultural values of various societies vary dramatically in how they affect the communicative behavior of their members. For example, in Japan, stuttering is viewed as a disorder related to psychological problems and is an embarrassment to the family of the stutterer. In Egypt, stuttering is believed to be something Allah has given to a person to test them and their family. Stuttering therefore to an Egyptian is nothing to be ashamed of, but it also is not something that should be treated by speech-language clinicians.

Fairbanks (1954) developed a concept of communication that looked at noise as anything that disrupted the successful sending and receiving of information. In the Fairbank's model, these were things such as faulty transmission lines, difficulties in coding messages, and anything that interfered with the decoding of messages. Possibly, viewing cultural sensitivity in a similar framework in clinical situations can provide a model that goes beyond the controversies regarding the legitimacy of cultural differences and focuses on the successful remediation of communicative disorders. Without being culturally sensi-

tive, clinicians themselves introduce "noise" into the clinical processes which can effectively interfere with the transmission of information to and from clients and their families and can adversely affect the comprehension of these messages. Interference is reduced or eliminated when variables that disrupt the process are eliminated. Elimination of the variables is directly related to the cultural sensitivity of clinicians.

Cultural sensitivity often can be reduced to asking the right questions. It is impossible to be knowledgeable regarding all cultures. Although one may know the preferences for children between the ages of 4 and 10, the needs of the elderly may be a mystery to even the most caring clinician. One of the easiest ways to become sensitive to the cultural needs of clients is simply to use the following statement/question format: "Today I would like to do _____. Will that be okay with you, or would you like to try to do it differently?" If you have established a solid clinical relationship with your client, the use of questions usually will result in honest answers.

There is something disarming about the individual who admits ignorance and asks for help in gaining knowledge. When initially working with a client whose culture is different from yours, you should feel free to admit your ignorance, and ask the client to help you understand him and his culture. Few people are sufficiently knowledgeable in all of the many cultures clients bring to a therapeutic relationship. And no one can predict how the cultures of a client will interact and ultimately develop the set of values that must be accounted for in developing intervention protocols.

SECTION II

FOUNDATIONAL SKILLS

C H A P T E R
4

Technical Foundational Skills

skill is *foundational* if it serves as the basis for learning, understanding, and applying more complex skills. It is technical if it is defined by a precise condition and specific interaction steps. In this chapter, four categories containing 508 techniques and behaviors will be presented. All of these skills should be learned by new clinicians, preferably before they begin therapy. Practicing clinicians may find that some of these skills are unfamiliar to them, since their importance does not appear in the speech-language pathology literature. If familiar, justifications for their use have been based either on intuition or clinical experience. In this chapter, as all others, if there is a research justification for using a skill, it is cited. Therefore, this chapter may be equally as appropriate for practicing clinicians as it is for student clinicians.

MATERIALS AND ACTIVITIES

By understanding why certain objects or activities work, clinicians can develop a

strategy that can be used for many clients within a given age range. By only being familiar with certain objects and activities, clinicians are limited to only knowing the interest value of a specific material. When designing or selecting materials and activities, clinicians should consider the following variables: (1) age, (2) interest factors, and (3) generalizability.

Age Appropriateness

Clients range in age from infancy through old age, so no one set of materials and activities will be appropriate for all. Yet there is always the desire to be efficient and make an activity or a set of materials appropriate for a wide age range of clients. It would be much easier if one set of generic materials could be developed that would be appropriate for all clients. Unfortunately, very few, if any, materials are so wonderfully adaptable. There is nothing more humiliating to an adult than to be presented with material appropriate for a child or adolescent. There is nothing more boring to a child than to be provided with material appropriate for adults. When selecting materials and activities that are age appropriate for clients, clinicians should focus on identifying the *type* of materials and activities that are suitable for different age ranges, rather than concentrating on identifying a specific game, object, or activity. For the sake of simplicity age appropriate materials and activities will be divided into three categories: (1) children, (2) adolescents, and (3) adults. Obviously there will be differences within each group, and it is assumed that the suggestions that follow should be modified to meet individual needs.

Children. Although most of the content and sources of information will be derived from their parents, alternative sources are available. These are provided in Table 4–1. Often the choice of what to use in therapy with children is dictated by what is available. Most of these materials are commercially made and familiar to many children. An informal survey of five public school sites and one university clinic found that over 70% of the therapy material available and consistently used involved some sort of board game. Although board games initially are of interest to many children, most are limited in terms of the embedded critical features that can hold children's attention for a long period of time. Additionally, they have few generalizable features. There are eight critical features that children tend to respond to in materials and activities. These will be presented below. The more of these features an activity has, the more likely the child will respond positively to it. At a minimum, every activity or material used in therapy should have at least one critical feature. In Table 4–2 the critical features are listed. Some common examples are provided for each critical feature. Prior to using an activity in therapy it is a good idea to first try it with another child. If that is not possible, engage in the activity with another person who can simulate the type of behaviors associated with

the age of the child you will be seeing in therapy. If that is not possible, assume the role of both clinician and client and run through the activity by yourself. When simulating a child, try to engage in behaviors that would indicate boredom, noncomprehension, or disruptive behaviors. By doing this, you will be in a position to anticipate most types of problems that may occur during its actual application.

Children enjoy *mobility,* whether it is only one part of their body or actually physically moving around the room (Duchan, Hewitt, & Sonnenmeier, 1994). Many of the classic children's games have this as their predominant focus and have not changed for generations. "Hide and go seek" is one example. By interspersing activities with a mobility feature within activities requiring mental concentration, cognitive fatigue can be reduced. For example, if a child is attempting to expand the length of her utterance from two to three units through the use of a linguistic strategy, the target responses could involve descriptions of activities that the child will be able to perform following the successful use of the strategy. By alternating between a purely cognitive task and one that is physical, children seem to stay on task longer.

Children love to build and *construct.* Observe infants who are just beginning to develop the ability to grasp objects and manipulate them. It is a natural activity for children to engage in constructive activities. Putting things together to create a new entity is both exciting and intriguing for the child. From one type of object, another unique one is formed. That is probably the appeal of toys such as Lego blocks whose popularity and acceptance have endured for the last 25 years. Various types of construction activities can be used with children, from placing the facial features on a Mr. Potato Head to the elaborate construction of a Lego airplane. Of importance in the use of constructive activities is that the child's need

TABLE 4–1
Areas of Discussion for Children

Games
- [ ] Board Games
- [ ] Creative Activities
- [ ] Games of Movement
- [ ] Group Games

Stories
- [ ] Cartoons
- [ ] Sesame Street
- [ ] Carmen San Diego
- [ ] Barney
- [ ] Child-Oriented Situation Comedies
- [ ] Disney Channel Movies and Series

Sports
- [ ] Soccer
- [ ] In-Line Skating
- [ ] Swimming
- [ ] Baseball
- [ ] Basketball
- [ ] Gymnastics
- [ ] Football
- [ ] Hockey

Miscellaneous
- [ ] Ballet
- [ ] Tap
- [ ] Bicycling

Communicative Disorder
- [ ] How it affects the person
- [ ] How children react to it
- [ ] How adults react to it
- [ ] How family reacts to it
- [ ] Television
- [ ] Children's Books
- [ ] Records/CDs
- [ ] On-Line Computer Services

to complete an activity does not interfere with the goal of the activity.

The opposite of the construction process is *destruction*. For children, the process of destroying something is not necessary negative or a sign of frustration. Rather, it can be viewed as an attempt at control (Piaget, 1972). Few children have much control over their lives. They are usually told when to eat, sleep, play, work, stand, walk, and talk. As they get older, more control is given to them by their parents and other adults, sometimes reluctantly. Given the limitations placed on them, it is understandable then that they not only would be fascinated by opportunities to express their limited power, but also seek it out. In therapy, this can be harnessed by allowing children to destroy something they have constructed. Block towers are prime examples.

The materials you choose should have an element of *movement*. This is the counterpart of physical mobility. It can be as minimal as moving a game piece along a path or having a marble move through a maze of holes. Movement gives the activity a dynamism which tends not to be present when the activity is static, such as using pictures as stimulus materials for constructing linguistic units or pronouncing target phonemes. Additionally, the movement aspect of an activity can serve as an indicator of behaviors performed or correct responses.

TABLE 4–2
Critical Activity Features for Children

Mobility (reduces mental fatigue; engages child)
☐ Walking around the room to specified points

Construction (a favorite activity; adds dimension of forward movement to therapy)
☐ Block tower
☐ Legos
☐ Mr. Potato Head
☐ Paste facial parts onto a facial outline

Destruction (gives control)
☐ Block tower
☐ Legos

Material and Activity Movement (engages child; adds dimension of forward movement in therapy)
☐ Moveable pieces to a board game
☐ Moveable pieces to any game

Completion (sense of fulfillment; achievement)
☐ Activities should have discrete end points
☐ Activities should require a minimal amount of time

Flexibility (sustains interest in the material/activity)
☐ Bottle caps
☐ Sticks
☐ Pieces of multicolored paper
☐ Balls
☐ Blocks
☐ Paper plates and cups

Surprise (maintains attention)
☐ Items kept in a bag
☐ Shoe boxes full of items
☐ Give list of available items at beginning of therapy, but not the sequence order

When choosing an activity, you should be sure that if there are any constructive aspects to it, the child will have sufficient time to *complete* it. There are few things as frustrating to a child than to be allowed to begin a project and then be forced to stop it before it can be completed (Piaget, 1963). Not being allowed to complete a project often will result in the child developing resentment toward the clinician. For example, an autistic child was given a sheet of paper and allowed to color it with a crayon after she said "Linda color." Although the activity was well thought out by the clinician and involved extrinsic reinforcement (the completion of the verbal activity was reinforcing), it became problematic when the client wanted to complete coloring the entire sheet of paper before proceeding to the next production of "Linda color." In this case, the reinforcing activity became the focal point of therapy, rather than the production of a linguistic goal. Therefore, it is important that activities involving construction are designed so that their completion does not interfere with the therapeutic goals of the activity. For example, the use of clay in an activity can be a disaster, since the intended object never seems to be completed. The malleability of the medium lends itself to ever changing forms. Painting also fits into this category. Although some clinicians attempt to place a time limit on constructive activities, problems still persist. Children are less attuned to time parameters than they are by the parameters imposed by the activity itself. A game is not really over when a bell rings; it is over when someone wins. A picture is not completed until it is completed, regardless of how long it takes. A play scenario is not done until the intended themes are fully expressed.

Flexibility should be an important feature of material and activity design. On any Christmas morning, watch the excitement of children as they open their presents and are amazed at the wonder of complex toys that seem to do incredible things all by themselves. Two weeks after Christmas observe how often the toy is used, if it even can be found. Activities and materials that can only do one thing tend to lose their interest for children in a relatively short period of time. This should be considered in the selection of materials. If you will be using something whose functions and use are fixed, do not spend much time on its construction or expect the child to remain interested in it for an extended period of time. The effects of disregarding this principle are exemplified by a new clinician who was assigned to work with a young autistic child. Over the weekend, she spent over 20 hours constructing what she called "a coat of many pockets." It was a magnificent jacket on which had been sewn over 50 pockets. The pockets were at various angles, sizes, shapes, and colors.

Some even had pockets within themselves! The clinician was sure that she had developed the ultimate clinical tool for this child. When therapy began and the clinician began her pocket activity, the child turned away and started to play with a box of tissues. Objects which are flexible hold the child's interest for a much longer period of time since they can become something new when a current activity becomes boring. For example, a common bottle cap involves no construction, yet can serve many functions, some of which are listed below:

tiddlywinks	flying saucer
facial imprint marker	game marker
noisemaker	spinner top
face to be painted	sun
receptacle for throwing (in peas)	

Creativity in constructing and selecting materials and activities should be focused more on designing in flexibility and less on "wowing" the child.

Most children are excited by the unknown, whether it involves the outcome of a story or the next object that will be used in therapy. This critical feature of *surprise* can be easily incorporated into most therapy activities. One clinician routinely kept everything that is to be used in therapy for the session in a large brown paper bag. Although the child knew the goal of therapy, he never was sure what would be used to accomplish it. The clinician would never select the item. She would have the child put his hand into the bag and pull out an object that would then be the vehicle through which therapy would be delivered. By changing some of the objects each week, the element of surprise was always present and the child always was eager to engage in the therapeutic activity.

Although many would argue that the *competitive* urge is universally found in children, cultural data suggest the opposite. Traditional Native American values as well as those of various Asian cultures stress cooperation and group effort rather than competitiveness and individualism. The acculturation of children from these ethnic cultures to American macrocultural values will determine how important competition is in therapy. For example, the Native American child whose traditional cultural values have secondary importance may find cooperative group activities boring when compared with the possibility of winning at a game. Sometimes the use of competition can be negative if a child consistently is placed in a losing position and, as a result, devalued by the rest of the group members. An altered form of competition combines group cooperation and individual competitiveness. This is a form of competition where a child competes only with him- or herself. By keeping data on past performances, the child can attempt to achieve higher scores or percentages than in a previous session. A very simple and effective technique is to use a graph, where the correct responses are plotted along the x axis (horizontal) while the y axis (vertical) is used for session dates.

Adolescents. Without question, adolescents pose the greatest challenge for clinicians. Their worldview, values, and beliefs are undergoing a transformation from those of a child to those of an adult. The process for many is painful and usually confusing. With this altered state of being, many adolescents are not only reluctant to be involved in therapy, but also may view clinicians as adults who neither can understand them nor have the vaguest idea what interests them (Lenz, Ellis, and Scanlon, 1996). The problem tends to be further exacerbated when the client and clinician are of different sexes. Just as with children, activities and materials should involve specific content that can be derived from common sources. Although materials for younger adolescents may involve games

and activities with some similarities to those used for children, older adolescents and teenagers are reluctant to engage in anything that is associated with younger children. Word games or activities that involve cognitive processing, such as solving verbal puzzles, are appropriate. However, with many adolescents, therapy can be worked directly into conversations. The items listed in the left column of Table 4–3 constitute possible areas of discussion. The items in the right column are sources of information that you can use to familiarize yourself with the content areas.

Ideas for adolescent activities may be generated from an understanding of the types of friendship expectations they have of their peers. In a study conducted by Zarbatany, Ghesquiere, and Mohr (1992), the expectations adolescents had of friends did not differ across sexes, but varied with the type of activity. For competitive activities, friends were expected to perform behavior supportive of self-evaluation, such as ego reinforcement and preferential treatment. Therefore, clinicians should structure competitive activities in a way that will glorify or reinforce excellence. For noncompetitive activities, relationship enhancing expectations such as inclusion, common interests, and acceptance were cited. For activities that would be considered academic, peer support and help should be utilized.

Adolescents may find areas that have even the slightest overtone of sex to be off-limits for discussion with adults, especially if the clinician is of the other sex. Sexual identity for many adolescents is one area that undergoes the greatest amount of change. They are beginning to develop an awareness of the opposite sex that may be confusing and involve social taboos. Certain topics of conversation tend to result in nonresponsive answers and interactions, such as dating, sexual identity, and discussions of what they would like to do when "they grow up." It is best that topics of discussion and activities focus on what is

TABLE 4–3
Areas of Discussion for Adolescents

Music
- [ ] Rock
- [ ] Rap
- [ ] Jazz
- [ ] Folk
- [ ] Classical

- [ ] Television
- [ ] Magazines
- [ ] Records/CDs
- [ ] Books
- [ ] On-Line Computer Services

Television Shows
- [ ] Oriented Towards Teens
- [ ] Soap Operas

Sports
- [ ] Local School
- [ ] Extra-Curricular

Dance Clubs
- [ ] Location
- [ ] Type of Music
- [ ] Age Requirements

Communicative Disorder
- [ ] How it affects the person
- [ ] How it affects family members
- [ ] How it affects school activities
- [ ] How it affects social relationships

Adults
- [ ] Opinion of
- [ ] Relationship to

Family
- [ ] Relationship to
- [ ] Family Members

current and of immediate interest. Some suggestions for content appear in Table 4–3. You can use this table as a check sheet in reviewing the client's file or analyzing the first session.

The sources for content are similar to those for children and adults. A relatively easy method of learning more about things that interest adolescents is to watch any of the many television shows that have been programmed for adolescents. However, you should be aware that the values and behaviors of most television adolescent shows tend to depict middle-of-the-road, mainstream values that may not be applicable to clients with dissimilar cultures. Movies may be a better source of relevant information, because their producers seem to be less reluctant to examine controversial issues and more willing to tackle ethnically related issues. As with adults, on-line computer services may be a valuable source. There are increasingly more adolescent "chat boards" on the Internet in which adolescents seem to be more willing to share their beliefs and feelings with each other.

Adults. Probably the easiest materials and activities to make age appropriate are those for adults, because clinicians can use themselves as reference points. If you consider the activity too immature or boring for you, it probably will be so for your clients. Activities will generally involve conversations and simulations for practicing specific communicative behaviors. When designing these activities, you should think in terms of their content and source. Table 4–4 provides a quick reference list of materials and activities. In this table, you will find suggested areas of discussions for adults. In your advance planning, use this form to identify areas of discussion that would be appropriate for your client. Check off the boxes that may be appropriate. Activities for adults should be centered around discussions, direct work on the communicative disorder, and simulations. The items listed in the left column of Table 4–4 constitute possible areas of discussion. The items in the right column are sources of information that you can use to familiarize yourself with the content areas. When identifying activities for adults, focus on those areas that have been most affected by the communication disorder.

Content merely means that which will be discussed or simulated. It is evident in Table 4–4 all of these areas are rather common and should not require any specialized training or extensive research. All can be easily used as the basis of conversations or simulations. The seven areas represent only possibilities for topics. It is best to rely on clients to choose those that are of the most interest to them and areas in which simulations will be most beneficial. After determining areas that are of interest to clients, you should begin a minimal research of sources that will provide you with at least enough rudimentary knowledge to hold a simple conversation, construct a simulation, or ask the most appropriate questions. A new and interesting source of appropriate information can be found on any of the on-line computer services. Some have encyclopedia features, while all provide Internet access featuring bulletin boards on thousands of topics. Often, being able to phrase reasonable questions about topics of interest to clients is sufficient to begin practicing the new communicative behaviors in a more natural context.

When designing activities that the client will engage in outside of the clinic, care should be taken that they are compatible with the social support systems clients have at their disposal. Generally, there are four categories of social support for adult clients. The first is ethnic community centers. For many clients, especially recent immigrants or clients with strong ethnic cultural identification, the community center serves many very important needs. The second category is religious institutions. Clients who have strong religious affiliations tend to structure a significant amount of their free time in church, mosque, or synagogue activities. These do not only occur on a designated day of worship, but throughout the week. The third is organized social organizations such as social service clubs, sports clubs, and private clubs. Although these may be important for clients, they tend to occupy a more minor role in their lives. The last category is agencies which provide a service to clients such as a communicative disorders clinic. Although these agencies may provide critical activities for the client, they involve a relatively minor amount of the time. While young and mature adults may be involved in an abundance of social support systems, elders generally have significantly fewer support systems (Florsheim & Herr, 1990). In some cases, one of the most important aspects of therapy is to link the elder client with a social support system.

Interesting Information

Many clinicians collect and construct various games and activities that they hope will be interesting to clients. Intuitively, it

TABLE 4–4
Areas of Discussion for Adults

Family
☐ Relationships
☐ Activities of Family Members

Work
☐ Place of Employment
☐ Functions of Job

Current Events
☐ National Issues
☐ Foreign Affairs

Sports
☐ Local
☐ State
☐ Professional

Politics
☐ Local
☐ State
☐ National

Communicative Problem
☐ How it affects the person
☐ How it affects family members
☐ How it affects job activities
☐ How it affects social relationships

Leisure Activities
☐ Hobbies
☐ Sports
☐ Relaxation
☐ Discussion
☐ Magazines
☐ Books
☐ Television Programs
☐ Pictures
☐ On-Line Computer Services

just makes sense to use interesting materials. This belief has been substantiated through research. When designing interest into materials and activities, age characteristics should be considered, such as the effects of clinician efforts on perceptions, how they affect long-term memory, how they expand neural nets, and how they affect generalization.

Age. Sources of interesting material for adults, adolescents, and children appear in Tables 4–5 through 4–7. There will obviously be an overlap between materials that are interesting and materials that are age related. By making materials and activities age appropriate you have already completed the first step in choosing interesting information. For *children,* your first source in finding specific interesting information is the children's parents. The second source are clinic reports. And the third source is the children themselves. In Table 4–7, each source of information is listed in the vertical columns.

When probing the interests of *adolescents,* care should be taken that you are not perceived as being intrusive. If you are practicing at a public school, it is relatively easy to find activities on the campus that have an immediate interest for clients. You may also wish to ask the clients' teacher to share with you the activities that are currently holding an interest for students. Additionally, each of the items listed in the age section of this

TABLE 4-5
Sources of Interesting Information for Children

PARENTS "I will be working with ____ next week. It will help me if you could tell me if he likes to do anything in the following areas."	**CLINIC REPORTS.** First look for direct statements of the child's interest in terms of specific activities and critical features. Then look for activities that were associated with efficient and effective therapy.	**CHILDREN.** One of the best ways of determining what the child is interested in is to give them an opportunity to choose. Assemble a large assortment of toys and games that cover the range of critical features. Note what activities are chosen and the length of time of activity engagement.
Toys _____ _____ _____ _____	Toys _____ _____ _____ _____	Toys _____ _____ _____ _____
Activities _____ _____ _____ _____	Activities _____ _____ _____ _____	Activities _____ _____ _____ _____
Television/Video/Movies _____ _____ _____ _____	Television/Video/Movies _____ _____ _____ _____	Television/Video/Movies _____ _____ _____ _____
Story Telling/Make Believe _____ _____ _____ _____	Story Telling/Make Believe _____ _____ _____ _____	Story Telling/Make Believe _____ _____ _____ _____

TABLE 4–6

Sources of Interesting Information for Adolescents

List topics of interest in the appropriate boxed areas.

Material Gathered from Teachers	Material Gathered from Conversation
School Sports	School Sports
School Activities/Clubs	School Activities/Clubs
Classroom Activities	Classroom Activities
School Social Events	School Social Events
Rival School Activitles	Rival School Activitles
	Family
	Music
	TV/Video/Music
	Dance Clubs
	Sports
	Cars
	Communicative Disorder
	Adults

TABLE 4–7
Sources of Interesting Information for Adults

Material Gathered from Written Reports	Material Gathered from Conversation
Family	Family
Job (present or past)	Job (present or past)
Hobbies	Hobbies
Books	Books
TV/Movies/Videos	TV/Movies/Videos
Leisure Activities	Leisure Activities
Current Events/Politics	Current Events/Politics
Cultural Values/Activities Ethnicity _____ Religion _____ Geographic _____ Socioeconomic _____	Cultural Values/Activities Ethnicity _____ Religion _____ Geographic _____ Socioeconomic _____

chapter under "Adolescents" are appropriate. In Table 4–6, you can list the activities in the corresponding boxes. It may not be appropriate to delve into cultural behaviors with adolescents. During this time in their lives, they are struggling with many issues, including cultural identification. It is quite possible that questions relating to issues that are still not resolved will result in either little information being provided or the development of a negative view of the clinician as just another probing, questioning adult.

A significant amount of information about an *adult's* interest can be obtained just by carefully examining past therapy and diagnostic reports. These should contain personal information that can serve as the initial conversational starting point. Suggested areas to note are provided on the left side column in Table 4–7. Once conversations begin, additional areas of interest can be determined. As clients converse with you, note areas of interest that can be used in the column on the right side of Table 4–7. You should note that the very last rows refer to cultural values. Not all areas of a client's culture are appropriate for discussion. For example, Native Americans do not like to talk about their religion to non-Native Americans. Therefore, with Native Americans, questions about religion should not be asked. Care needs to be taken when choosing socioeconomic values to discuss. A better approach is to first determine the client's socioeconomic status, then focus on activities that are associated with that class. For a retired individual who is wealthy, a discussion of cruise activities or country club events is appropriate. For the single mother on welfare, a discussion of the difficulty in finding affordable child care may be a topic for an in-depth discussion. Of importance here is the way in which discussions of cultural topics are initiated. By focusing on specific activities associated with the socioeconomic class, clients will be more ready to converse about them, than if asked directly to talk about their values.

Effects of Interesting Material. Five positive effects result from the use of interesting material. The first is that it creates *positive perceptions of clinicians* since clients believe that clinicians have enough concern about them to select materials and activities that are interesting. The clinician obviously took the time necessary to individualize the materials. Perceptions are important in therapy. Some would argue that perceptions may even be more important that reality (Goldberg, 1993). In an interesting study done with college students, an attempt was made to determine what characteristics students attributed to outstanding teachers. Since clinicians also function as teachers, some of the findings of the study are applicable. One key component of outstanding teaching was that the teacher used materials that were interesting to the students (Meredith, 1985). The subjects in the study believed that the interest taken by the teacher to use materials that were interesting to them was an

indication of a sincere desire to effectively convey ideas. The similar phenomenon occurs in therapy when clinicians select materials that are interesting to their clients.

The second positive effect of using interesting material is that it *engages reluctant clients*. Often clinicians are faced with clients who have no interest in being in therapy. A child may be there because a parent insists on it, the adolescent because a teacher suggested it, an adult because it was recommended by the psychologist providing therapy to her child. In all cases involving reluctant clients, it becomes critical that the material and activities chosen be of interest. Although the reader has been provided with suggestions for activities and materials in the section on age considerations, these suggestions are not sufficient for guaranteeing interest. Not all adolescents and teenagers are interested in cars. Not all children are interested in surprises. It is necessary after limiting the selection of activities and materials to appropriate age categories, to identify specific interests for the client. It has been shown that by using materials and activities that are of interest to clients, even the most reluctant individual may become cooperative and benefit from an instructional activity (Thames & Reeves, 1994). The therapeutic goals become secondary to the activity. Although not the most desirable of circumstances, it often can result in the goals being met, almost by osmosis.

The third effect of interesting material is that it *facilitates long-term memory*. If new behaviors are to be learned and later retrieved, they must be retained in the individual's long-term memory. When retrieval problems occur, the difficulties are often attributed to cognitive problems. Although this might be true for some clients, the importance of the materials and activities used to initially teach the concept cannot be overlooked when assigning contributive factors for long-term memory problems. The use of interesting material facilitates long-term memory, both in cognitively impaired and cognitively normal clients. Studies have shown that the use of interesting materials may result in as much as a 60% increase in retention of ideas when compared to the use of uninteresting material (Smith, 1993). Therefore, if clinicians wish to enhance the retention of information or the use of specific behaviors, it is incumbent on them to use materials and activities that are interesting to their clients.

The fourth effect of interesting material is that is *expands conceptual nets*. Learning rarely is an isolated event. When we learn something, that concept is usually related to other things. For example, when learning the concept of *red*, we would not expect the client just to think of red in isolation of other things. Colors are associated with various objects, objects are associated with functions, and functions associated with the satisfaction of needs. The *red* a client visualizes may be the color of a car (object) that is used for transportation (function) that takes her to the clinic (need). The more associating clients can do, the more expansive is the learning. It was found that activities and materials that were of interest to a learner resulted in the individual not only mastering the material, but doing so at a depth and breath that far exceeded materials and activities of less interest (McCarthey, Hoffman, Christian, Corman et al., 1994).

Finally, the fifth effect is that it *facilitates generalization*. The purpose of teaching anything in the clinic is not to have clients merely produce the desired response or behavior in a controlled setting. Rather, it is to enable them to use that concept or behavior in nonclinical, unstructured settings. In comparisons between irrelevant and relevant material and activities, it was found that through the use of relevant material, learners began generalizing what was learned in a teaching environment to other areas of their lives (Barksdale-Ladd & Thomas, 1993; Dent & Seligman, 1993). When selecting

materials and activities for clinic use, the first question clinicians should ask themselves is whether the materials and activities are relevant to the clients' lives outside of the clinic. If they are not, different materials and activities need to be used.

Generalizable Materials

The technical definition of *generalization* was developed by Stokes and Baer (1978). Generalization according to them is "the occurrence of a relevant behavior under different, non-training conditions (i.e., across subjects, settings, people, behaviors, and/or time) without the scheduling of the same events in those conditions as had been scheduled in the training condition." Simply put, generalization of new communicative behaviors occurs when clients can use their new speaking pattern outside the clinic, in a variety of situations and with a variety of people. Often in the literature, the terms *transfer, carryover,* and *generalization* are used interchangeably. Usually they refer to the display of a behavior in a new setting. In this text *generalization* will be used instead of either *transfer* or *carryover,* because it has a standard definition.

In Tables 4–8 through 4–10, four areas of functioning are cited under which a variety of generalization activities are listed. Some of the activities are listed under more than one category. Each of these activities should be modified in order to consider the special needs of the situation. For example, "speaking on the phone" appears in at least three categories for all age groups. For stutterers who have difficulty on the phone, telephone activities in each area should be constructed. At the bottom of the form is the list of cultural variables that should be considered when identifying generalizable material.

Research Literature. Various studies examining the long-term effectiveness of activities and materials have shown that the more generalizable the activities or

TABLE 4-8
Areas to be Identified for Child Generalization Activities

FAMILY	SCHOOL	SPORTS/LEISURE	SOCIAL, ETC
❑ Asking questions	❑ Asking questions	❑ Asking questions	❑ Asking questions
❑ Speaking on phone	❑ Asking for help	❑ Asking for help	❑ Speaking on phone
❑ Asking for help	❑ Conveying thoughts	❑ Conveying thoughts	❑ Asking for help
❑ Conveying thoughts	❑ Expressing thoughts	❑ Expressing thoughts	❑ Conveying thoughts
❑ Expressing thoughts	❑ Expressing feelings	❑ Expressing feelings	❑ Expressing thoughts
❑ Expressing feelings	❑ Understanding directions	❑ Understanding directions	❑ Expressing feelings
❑ Understanding directions	❑ Remembering to use strategies	❑ Remembering to use strategies	❑ Understanding directions
❑ Remembering to use strategies	❑ Understanding conversation	❑ Understanding conversation	❑ Remembering to use strategies
❑ Understanding conversation	❑ Retrieving names	❑ Retrieving names	❑ Understanding conversation
❑ Retrieving names	❑ Writing	❑ Writing	❑ Retrieving names
❑ Writing	❑ Speaking with teachers	❑ Counting money	❑ Writing
	❑ Speaking with peers		❑ Counting money

In each area, list those cultural characteristics of the client that will require modifications in the selection of generalizable activities.

Ethnicity/National Origin
Religion
Gender/Sexual Orientation
Exceptionality
Urban/Suburban/Rural
Geographic Region
Socioeconomic Class

TABLE 4-9
Areas to be Identified for Adolescent Generalization Activities

FAMILY	SCHOOL	SPORTS/LEISURE	SOCIAL, ETC
❏ Asking questions	❏ Asking questions	❏ Asking questions	❏ Asking questions
❏ Speaking on phone	❏ Asking for help	❏ Asking for help	❏ Speaking on phone
❏ Asking for help	❏ Conveying thoughts	❏ Conveying thoughts	❏ Asking for help
❏ Conveying thoughts	❏ Expressing thoughts	❏ Expressing thoughts	❏ Conveying thoughts
❏ Expressing thoughts	❏ Expressing feelings	❏ Expressing feelings	❏ Expressing thoughts
❏ Expressing feelings	❏ Understanding directions	❏ Understanding directions	❏ Expressing feelings
❏ Understanding directions	❏ Remembering to use strategies	❏ Remembering to use strategies	❏ Understanding directions
❏ Remembering to use strategies	❏ Understanding conversation	❏ Understanding conversation	❏ Remembering to use strategies
❏ Understanding conversation	❏ Retrieving names	❏ Retrieving names	❏ Understanding conversation
❏ Retrieving names	❏ Writing	❏ Writing	❏ Retrieving names
❏ Writing	❏ Speaking with teachers	❏ Counting money	❏ Writing
	❏ Speaking with peers		❏ Counting money

In each area, list those cultural characteristics of the client that will require modifications in the selection of generalizable activities.

Ethnicity/National Origin	
Religion	
Gender/Sexual Orientation	
Exceptionality	
Urban/Suburban/Rural	
Geographic Region	
Socioeconomic Class	

TABLE 4–10
Areas to be Identified for Adult Generalization Activities

FAMILY	WORK	SPORTS/LEISURE	SOCIAL, ETC
❏ Asking questions	❏ Asking questions	❏ Asking questions	❏ Asking questions
❏ Speaking on phone	❏ Asking for help	❏ Asking for help	❏ Speaking on phone
❏ Asking for help	❏ Conveying thoughts	❏ Conveying thoughts	❏ Asking for help
❏ Conveying thoughts	❏ Expressing thoughts	❏ Expressing thoughts	❏ Conveying thoughts
❏ Expressing thoughts	❏ Expressing feelings	❏ Expressing feelings	❏ Expressing thoughts
❏ Expressing feelings	❏ Understanding directions	❏ Understanding directions	❏ Expressing feelings
❏ Understanding directions	❏ Remembering to use strategies	❏ Remembering to use strategies	❏ Understanding directions
❏ Remembering to use strategies	❏ Understanding conversation	❏ Understanding conversation	❏ Remembering to use strategies
❏ Understanding conversation	❏ Retrieving names	❏ Retrieving names	❏ Understanding conversation
❏ Retrieving names	❏ Writing	❏ Writing	❏ Retrieving names
❏ Writing	❏ Speaking with supervisors	❏ Counting money	❏ Writing
	❏ Speaking with supervisees		❏ Counting money
	❏ Speaking with co-workers		

In each area, list those cultural characteristics of the client that will require modifications in the selection of generalizable activities.
Ethnicity/National Origin
Religion
Gender/Sexual Orientation
Exceptionality
Urban/Suburban/Rural
Geographic Region
Socioeconomic Class

materials used in the clinic, the more effective they will be in developing behaviors outside of the clinic (Cuvo & Klatt, 1992; Sriram et al., 1990; Swanson & Stillman, 1990; Vu, Barrows, Marcy, Verhulst et al., 1992). This requires the use of materials and activities in the clinic that have similarities to those that occur outside of the clinic. For example, when working with an adult aphasic who is having difficulty retrieving number concepts, it would make more sense to work on the counting of money, giving change, and simulating the purchase of objects requiring a specific amount, rather than just using a numbers drill book. Approaches that use functional methods are more effective with these clients than those that have no context (Hartley, 1995). With a child who has a language disorder, the selection of words to initially teach should involve concepts that will be encountered daily. For example, the words "milk," "more," and "potty" would have more generalizability than the word "giraffe" or others with which the child would have little contact.

Age Variables. Generalization activities should be derived from those activities which were identified as being interesting to clients. All should be age appropriate. The generalization activities for *children* appear in Table 4–8. Contact both the child's teacher and parents to determine how the communicative disorder affects each of the listed areas. Although children may be able to identify a few of the areas in which they have the greatest problems, they tend not to be able or willing to identify all of the appropriate areas.

The generalization activities for *adolescents* appear in Table 4–9. Although materials for communicatively disordered adolescents should also be directly related to areas in their lives where their impairment causes the biggest problems, some areas are more appropriate than others. You might find that adolescents will identify situations that do not necessarily cause them the greatest problems, but rather situations in which they feel most comfortable. For example, some adolescents may not wish to engage in generalization activities with their families, even if the problems are severe there. Initially, allow the client to select areas in which they wish to work. After they have achieved success in these areas, you should begin suggesting activities in situations they are reluctant to engage in, but which you know is affected by the disorder.

Generalization activities for *adults* appear in Table 4–10. Most adults with communicative disorders can easily identify areas in their lives that are most affected by their problem. Therefore, allow them to choose the types of generalization activities they would like you to construct for them.

Types of Materials and Activities

The development of new speech and language behaviors in a controlled clinic environment can be accomplished through various activities and materials. Those that are most effective have a direct relationship to clients' everyday lives.

Pictures and Games. Although pictures of objects can be effectively used for developing vocabulary and improving articulation, it has limited generalizing ability when compared with other types of materials (Bleile, 1995; Duchan, 1984). For example, if clients are having difficulty correctly producing a phoneme, the use of picture cards may be used to teach the correct production of the sound. Clients however, do not use pictures when speaking outside of the clinic. Similar problems are encountered with the use of most commercially available board games. Although children do play games, and therefore a game situation becomes an appropriate setting for generalization, clinicians tend to place too much reliance on them. Children do not spend the majority of their time outside of the clinic playing board games. If the purpose of the game is to simulate unstructured conversation, then it is appropriate. However, it should not be used as the primary method of either teaching or generalizing behaviors. Children speak when engaging in conversations and during functional activities. If for any reason clinicians choose to use either pictures or board games, they need to realize that an additional step is required for generalization to occur: a transition must be made from the artificial material and activities to those that occur in children's everyday lives (Goldberg, 1993).

Real or Simulated Objects. It is more efficient to begin with material that is immediately generalizable rather than introducing an additional step. In later therapy, for example, instead of using pictures of balls, blocks, cars, and chairs to teach these concepts, it is better to use the real objects. When it is not possible to use real objects, such as with the concepts of *stove* and *refrigerator,* the use of simulated or miniature stoves and refrigerators is significantly better than the use of pictures of these objects.

Simulated Activities. A simulation is an approximation of an event that contains the most relevant aspects of that event. Although the events are contrived, they can be an important component of therapy. Suggested areas of simulations for adults, adolescents, and children can be found in Tables 4–11 through 4–13. Simulations serve as a bridge between highly structured activities and normal nonclinical activities. They allow clinicians to control certain features that may be important for learning to take place. The following example of a simulation for an adult involves teaching the skills necessary for speaking fluently over the telephone.

The client has always had difficulty speaking fluently to strangers on the phone. The clinician elected to use a form of prolongation to begin shaping fluency. During the initial teaching of the behavior, the client was taught to prolong while holding the telephone to his ear. Then, with the clinician also holding a phone, the client and clinician simulated a telephone conversation. Finally, using two phones that were connected, the client called the clinician and simulated asking for information from a directory assistance operator. The key elements of the simulation were the use of a telephone and a dialogue similar to the type that would be used outside of the clinic.

ORGANIZATION STATEMENTS

Therapy should begin with telling the client: (1) what the purpose of the activity will be, (2) how the activity will be carried out, (3) why the activity is being done, and (4) the consequences of both correct and incorrect responses. By doing these four things, clients develop a sense of focus and purpose that greatly facilitates learning (Balluerka, 1995). Advance organizing statements should be used prior to the beginning of every activity, *regardless of the number of times clients have engaged in it.* These statements should include *what* will be done, *how* it should be performed, *why* clients are doing it, and for young clients, the *consequences* of both correct and incorrect responses. Model statements for adults, adolescents, and children appear in Table 4–14.

Purpose of the Activity

By explaining to clients the purpose of the activity, they are able to focus their attention on the task at hand. Two important consequences result. The first is that success rates increase and the second is that what is learned is better retained.

TABLE 4–11
Child Simulations

AREAS OF SIMULATION	POSSIBLE ACTORS	POSSIBLE ACTIVITIES
School	Teachers Volunteers Students Administrators Clerical help Maintenance help	Asking questions in class Peer interactions in class Activities on the playground Conversations in office Conversations in hallway
Play Activity	Peers Younger children Older children	Independent activity Shared activity Cooperative activity Taking turns Asking for directions Taking directions Asking for help Directing others
Family	Parents Siblings Relatives Others living in the home	Independent activity Shared activity Cooperative activity Taking turns Asking for directions Asking for help Directing others Dinner time Bed time Watching television Describing the day's activities
Store	Parents Siblings Relatives Peers Sales people	Asking for something Describing something Responding to a question
Miscellaneous	Parents Siblings Relatives Peers Known adults Unknown adults	Riding in the car Walking on the street During a sports activity

Increase Success Rate. It has been shown that providing even simple focusing statements before an activity begins not only diminishes the response time between the presentation of the stimulus and the response (Willingham, Koroshetz, Treadwell, & Bennett, 1995), but also increases the success rate for both easier and more diffi-

TABLE 4–12
Adolescent Simulations

AREAS OF SIMULATION	POSSIBLE ACTORS	POSSIBLE ACTIVITIES
School	Teachers Volunteers Students Administrators Clerical help Maintenance help	Asking questions in class Peer interactions in class Activities on the playground Conversations in office Conversations in hallway
Sports Activities	Peers Younger children Older children	Independent activity Shared activity Cooperative activity Taking turns Asking for directions Taking directions Asking for help Directing others
Family	Parents Siblings Relatives Others living in the home	Independent activity Shared activity Cooperative activity Taking turns Asking for directions Asking for help Directing others Dinner time Bed time Watching television Describing the day's activities Arguing
Store	Parents Siblings Relatives Peers Sales people	Asking for something Describing something Responding to a question
Miscellaneous	Parents Siblings Relatives Peers Known adults Unknown adults	Riding in the car Walking on the street

cult cognitive tasks (Snapp & Glover, 1990). For example, before beginning an activity designed to increase the proficiency of pro- ducing a specific sound, the child should be told the purpose of the activity: "Mary, we are going to be saying the /r/ sound now."

TABLE 4-13
Adult Simulations

AREAS OF SIMULATION	POSSIBLE ACTORS	POSSIBLE ACTIVITIES
Work	Supervisors Peers Supervisees Customers Other workers	Asking questions Peer interactions Supervisor interactions Supervisee interactions Customer interactions Face-to-face interactions Telephone interactions
Sports/Leisure Activities	Peers Authorative individuals Individuals to be coached, etc.	Independent activity Shared activity Cooperative activity Taking turns Asking for directions Taking directions Asking for help Directing others
Family	Parents Spouse Siblings Relatives Children	Independent activity Shared activity Cooperative activity Taking turns Asking for directions Asking for help Directing others Dinner time Bed time Watching television Describing the day's activities
Store	Spouse Sales person	Asking for something Describing something Responding to a question
Miscellaneous	Parents Siblings Relatives Peers Known adults Unnown adults	Riding in the car Walking on the street

Increase Retention. Focusing also increases the retention of material in general (Gillstrom & Ronnberg, 1994) and the specific items to which an individual is directed to concentrate (Miller & Davis, 1993). There are various ways to direct a client's focus. The manner in which it is performed will also affect outcomes. In one study, it was found that visual cues used as focusing devices acted equally as

TABLE 4–14
Advance Organization Statements

You should use three types of statements that will allow your clients to focus their attention on the learning activity. These statements should be used prior to beginning each activity, regardless of the number of times the activity has been used. What appears below are only suggested statements. Modify them in any way that is appropriate. What is important is that clients are told what will occur, how it will be performed, and why they are being asked to do it.

AGE	WHAT	HOW	WHY	CONSEQUENCES
Adults	Now we are going to do _____.	This activity will have _____ parts. Initially you will _____ , then, and finally _____	The reason we are doing this is that it will enable you to _____	NONE
Adolescents	Now we are going to do _____.	There are _____ things you will be doing. First you _____ , then _____ , and finally_____	The reason we are doing this is that it will help you to_____	ONLY YOUNGER If you do it right then _____. But if you say it wrong then _____.
Children	Now we are going to do _____.	You will _____	We will do this because it will help you _____	If you do it right then _____. But if you say it wrong then _____.

well on responses that required an auditory behavior or one that was motoric (Ward, 1994). However, visual cues were more effective when motoric responses were expected.

Conduct of the Activity

Often clients may have concerns about the type of activities in which they will be asked to engage. Instead of providing the explanation while they are engaging in the activity, it is better to describe it prior to beginning the activity. Descriptions should involve both the sequence of events and their components.

Components of Activities. All activities have at least a beginning, middle, and end. For many activities, this is all that will need to be explained or demonstrated to clients. For others, however, each individual step may need to be discussed. The more unusual, threatening, or different the activity, the more explanation and details should be provided. Knowing what will occur often significantly relieves clients' anxiety of what to expect. The use of a graphic representation can be very effective, especially for clients with cognitive problems. The representation can have various levels of abstraction. Blank cards can be used merely to indicate where in a sequence an activity is. Or it can be more literal, using graphic representations or words. For example, if three sequential behaviors are required to correctly produce a target word, the clinician or client could move his or her finger from one card to the next as the behavior is being produced.

Timing Sequence of Activities. For more severely involved and behaviorally disordered children, sequencing can be more global and related to time. For example, for a child who has difficulty either doing an activity for a specified amount of time or wishes to do it beyond the allowed time span, "beginning," "middle," and "end" cards could be used. This can also be done for the entire session, blocking out segments of the session into specific units.

Justification for the Activity

Mysteries are appropriate for novels, but not for therapy. Clients need to be informed about why they will be engaging in an activity that may be either embarrassing or difficult. The principle to use is that if the clients' cognitive abilities allow for it, always explain the reason the activity is being done. When clients know why they are doing an activity, they tend to be less resistant and become more actively involved with changing their own behaviors. Three reasons can be given to a client for why an activity is being done: (1) to change a behavior, (2) to improve communication, and (3) to reduce the negative consequences of the disorder.

Specific Changes in the Behavior. Often clients cannot see the relationship between a specific activity and the remediation of their communication problem. This is particularly evident when many steps are involved in shaping the behavior. The best form of explanation in these cases is to demonstrate each step in the program which takes clients from where they are in their behavior pattern to where you would like them to be. For example, when working with a client who has an articulation problem, clinicians may wish to use a number of steps starting with auditory discrim-

ination and ending with using the target sound in unstructured spontaneous speech. If the clinician begins with auditory discrimination and does not explain its relationship to the production of the target in spontaneous speech, the client may not realize its importance. In fact, the client may view it as a waste of time. However, if the clinician explains, and possibly demonstrates its value and place in therapy, it is more likely that the client will be able to understand its importance.

Effects on Communication. Often activities that are done in therapy, although not directly related to a change in a specific behavior, have far-reaching consequences for the use of that behavior. Unless clients can understand the relationship, they may not see its value. For example, clients who stutter not only need to learn how to speak fluently, but also be able to use their new speaking pattern in a variety of situations. One of these situations involves interruptions. The clinician may wish to interrupt clients during therapy to prepare them for speech in nonstructured situations. If clients understand that this is the intent of the activity, they are less likely to be annoyed at the clinician.

Reduction of Negative Consequences. Negative consequences often are associated with speech and language disorders. Although these are usually understood by adults and most adolescents, children may have difficulty understanding the relationship. If clinicians can explain it to them in a simple way that reduces the onus of having a disorder, and redirects the source of the problem, even very young children can be enlisted into the therapy process. The following dialogue with a child who has a phonological problem can serve as an example.

Clinician: You know how sometimes people keep asking you to

	say the same thing over and over again?
Child:	Yah.
Clinician:	Does that make you angry when they do that?
Child:	Yes.
Clinician:	Well, I'm going to show you how to say words a little differently, so no one will ask you to say things over and over again. How does that sound to you?
Child:	Good!

Consequences of Behaviors

It is especially important for children to understand the consequences of all behaviors before the activity begins. If consequences are instituted after an activity begins, clinicians create the impression that they are arbitrary, since the consequence was not specified before the activity began. A consequence checklist appears in Table 4–15.

Desired Behaviors. If extraneous reinforcers will be used in therapy, clinicians need to specify what they will be and the responses required for receiving them. This should be done before the activity begins. It is important for consistency that clinicians adhere to the rules they establish. Clinicians should explain to parents what will be used as extraneous reinforcers. If they object to the choices, it is better that the objection occurs prior to beginning therapy than after it begins.

Undesirable Behaviors. Two types of undesirable behaviors can occur in therapy. The first is that the target behavior is not produced in spite of a client's best efforts. The client should be informed what, if anything, will happen when the target behavior is not correctly produced. The second type of undesirable behavior is one that is maladaptive. This simply means that it is a behavior that interferes with the learning process. It can be something as minor as inattention or as substantial as leaving the room. For clients who are not disruptive, there may not be any need to specify what the consequences are for maladaptive behaviors. As with the use of extraneous reinforcers, all decisions regarding the use of punishment should be discussed with the parents prior to their use.

USING APPROPRIATE OPERANT TECHNIQUES

Operant conditioning is a term applied to the systematic process of either teaching a new behavior or eliminating an established one through the application of consequences. It is not a stand-alone approach to treating speech and language disorders, but rather a technique that can be used with a variety of approaches. In the past, practitioners in many fields applied the technique as if it constituted a fully integrated clinical approach. Failures with adolescents and children were usually attributed to not being able to find the appropriate reinforcing and punishing contingencies. However, recent studies with children have indicated that, even when significant behavioral changes are made, the absence of a more comprehensive approach can result in less effective therapy (Sayger, Szykula, & Laylander, 1991) and premature termination (Nangle, Carr-Nagle, & Hansen, 1994). It appears that many parents do not only want to have their children's specific behaviors changed, but also seek help in addressing family problems that are related to the behavior (Rettig, 1993).

TABLE 4–15
Consequence Checklist

	Desired Consequence	Undesirable Consequence
Activity	Additional time in activity New activity Modification of activity	Reduce time in activity No new activity Modification of activity
Extraneous Reinforcer	Reinforcer provided	Reinforcer withheld Reinforcer/token taken back
Information Given	Parent Teacher	Parent Teacher

Basis for Using Operant Techniques

A famous historian said that those who fail to understand history are doomed to repeat it. The history of operant conditioning provides insights to the current problems the technique encounters because of past attempts to use it by individuals with little knowledge.

History. Operant conditioning in the field of psychology was pioneered by the animal research of B.F. Skinner. Although Skinner had been publishing his research since the 1930s, the most vehement opposition to his work started in the mid-1950s after the publication of his book *Science and Human Behavior* (1953). There were various reasons for the initial adverse reactions. Because Skinner had developed his theories of behavior from experimentation on animals and birds, many people believed that his laws of behavior did not apply to human beings. After all, we not only have vastly greater cognitive abilities than rats and pigeons, but also possess free will. If people possess free will, how is it that any deterministic laws can apply? And, the argument continued, since Skinner's experiments were conducted within a laboratory under controlled conditions with all extraneous variables eliminated, they did not adequately address the vagaries associated with everyday behaviors. His critics maintained that since human beings interact within continually changing conditions, extraneous variables could not be controlled, and it would therefore not be possible to state scientific laws regarding human behaviors. Succinctly put, the argument was presented that "pigeons are not people." Throughout the 1950s and 1960s researchers in all areas of human behavior began testing the scientific laws developed by Skinner. What they found was startling, even to those who opposed Skinner's viewpoint. In many ways, the behaviors of human beings could be controlled and predicted with almost the same degree of certainty as could the behavior of pigeons. With their findings, the attack became twofold, one practical and the other ethical.

Relevance of Animal Research. The argument from practicality was that the sterility of an experimental condition does not lend itself to the everyday settings in which practitioners in psychology and speech-language pathology must function. It may be possible to reinforce a child's attention in a therapy room with a piece of candy, but this would not work in a classroom of 35 students. Proponents of operant conditioning countered that the introduction of independent variables does not negate a law of human behavior, but rather the variables require the practitioner to account for them in the development of intervention strategies. The opponents of operant conditioning were left with few persuasive arguments when the application of operant clinical strategies began resulting in successes. Shames and Sherrick (1963) demonstrated that stuttering could be minimized by the use of operant techniques. Holland and Matthew's (1963) article on the use of teaching machine concepts in speech pathology and audiology introduced the field to the scientific application of operant principles. Sufficient research had been done by the mid-1960s when Sloane and MacAulay (1968) were able to provide specific operant techniques that could be used in the areas of speech and language therapy.

Over-applications. With conclusive evidence that operant conditioning could be applied effectively to human beings, it became a panacea for attempting to solve all behavioral problems in the 1960s and 1970s. Some proponents believed that the techniques were in and of themselves sufficient for remediating everything from self-destructive behaviors to complicated linguistic constructions (Lovaas, 1965, 1966). People with little or no training in linguistics applied operant procedures to teach long and complex sentences by rote memorization to children. Although able to produce the sentences on demand, they rarely, if ever, produced unique utterances. In institutions for the retarded and emotionally disturbed, poorly trained caregivers viewed operant conditioning as a way of changing behavior through the application of aversive stimuli. If nothing else, this indicated that they lacked even a basic understanding of the

tenets of operant conditioning. Many people became outraged by the use of confining time-out boxes and sensory-deprivation rooms. The adverse notoriety these institutions gained through the inappropriate use of punishment created a public outcry against operant conditioning. Even the use of reinforcement in humane, noninstitutionalized settings was criticized. Many parents, clinicians, and educators believed that children should not produce behaviors simply to receive a tangible reward. They were afraid that children would begin expecting rewards for behaviors that "children ought to do just because it's right."

Ethical and Moral Concerns

The irrational fear of operant conditioning was best exemplified in Skinner's novel *Walden Two* (1948) when a member of the operant society was explaining its principles to a visitor:

> It's a little late to be proving that a behavioral technology is well advanced. How can you deny it? Many of its methods and techniques are really as old as the hills. Look at their frightful misuse in the hand of the Nazis! And what about the techniques of the psychological clinic? What about education? Or religion? Or practical politics? Or advertising and salesmanship? Bring them all together and you have a sort of rule-of-thumb technology of vast power. No, Mr. Castle, the science is there for the asking. But its techniques and methods are in the wrong hands—they are used for personal aggrandizement in a competitive world or, in the case of the psychologist, to take up and wield the science of behavior for the good of mankind? You answer that you would dump it in the ocean! (pp. 256–257). ·

The protagonist in Skinner's book was maintaining that operant conditioning is not something that we have a choice in applying. It is, always has been, and always will be prevalent in all forms of social organizations and interactions. Operant conditioning is no more than the scientific application of the laws of human behavior. The laws *are*. They are not created by practitioners. Practitioners can use them for good or for evil. The members of the society in the novel presented a compelling argument for using them for good.

Right Behavior Without Rewards. The popular concept that one should engage in activities without wanting to be rewarded concerned Kanfer (1968). He believed that the destructive notion that one should do the *right* thing without the hope of being rewarded stemmed from an underlying value of our society and government. Kanfer maintained that our societal structure is based on the use of coercion, not reinforcement, for maintaining order. Coercion is in the form of adverse contingencies for noncompliance or nonperformance. For example, laws are created to specify what actions need to be taken to avoid a punishment. If you do not stop when the traffic light turns red, you will receive a ticket and must pay $100; if you commit a violent crime, you will go to jail if caught; if you do not pay your taxes by April 15, you will pay a fine and may go to jail. In *Walden Two* the visitor receives a lesson on the use of positive reinforcement rather than punishment (Skinner, 1948):

> We are gradually discovering—at an untold cost in human suffering—that in the long run punishment doesn't reduce the probability that an act will occur. We have been so preoccupied with the contrary that we always take force to mean punishment. We don't say we're using force when we send shiploads of food into a starving country, though we're displaying quite as much power as if we were sending troops and guns. (p. 260)

The notion of not reinforcing children for *good* behavior is illogical. It is unreasonable to expect children to do certain behaviors when nothing is rewarding about the behavior or its completion. If you are a college student you are reading this book with the hope of being reinforced. Either the material is sufficiently interesting that you are reading it for the sheer joy of accumulating knowledge, or you are anticipating eventually applying the techniques presented, or you will be tested on its contents and receive a grade related to the information you have acquired. If you are a practicing clinician, you hope that the material in this book will enable you to fine tune your therapy resulting in the delivery of a better product for your clients. If none of the above reinforcements are present, it is doubtful if you would have even purchased this book. And if the material contained to this point had not been reinforcing, the likelihood that the book would be completely read is minimal. Why should children be different than readers of this book? Learning must be reinforcing or it will not continue.

Unethical and Incompetent Applications. One may reasonably conclude that the negative image of operant conditioning developed from incompetent applications through the 1960s and 1970s. Initially, practitioners expected too much of the procedure. Instead of viewing it as a technique that could result in the efficient application of content knowledge, it became its substitute. Poorly trained individuals applied the techniques without really understanding the technical complexities of operant conditioning and its limitations. An inappropriate application of a principle is not sufficient evidence to damn it. If, for example, a mentally deranged individual was seen attacking another person with a teaspoon, it would be ludicrous to label spoons as weapons that should be banned. Few people would be so incensed as to form a "Citizens Against Spoons" movement. Yet, this is exactly what happened in the 1960s with operant conditioning.

The argument has also been made that it is not sufficient to blame just the practitioners of a procedure, the whole procedure needs to be indicted. After all, was this not the line of reasoning so popular during World War II? "I only make the rockets go up. There is nothing wrong with that. Punish the people who are responsible for making them go down; they are the evil ones." If operant conditioners were similar to the "up-rocket" men, the argument could be valid. However, the opposite is true. Individuals who clearly understand operant procedures and appropriately apply them believe in the very positive ethical values associated with operant conditioning. The use of positive reinforcement to establish new behaviors is a good example. What better, more humane way is there to establish new behaviors than by providing individuals with strokes for their accomplishments? What is immoral or unethical about using successive approximations to give people the feeling that they can succeed? Is it immoral to use aversive stimuli to stop the physically self-destructive behaviors of an autistic child?

The End Justifies the Means. Even if one accepts the ethical nature of the goals of operant conditioning, many people are still uncomfortable with the methods that are employed to achieve those goals (Baroff, 1976; Koocher, 1976,). The "end justifies the means" principle is the most common ethical criticism encountered by operant conditioners. Simply put, it states that in behavior modification any degree of punishment or unethical behavior is appropriate if the end goal is sufficiently important. The underlying assumption is that aversive stimuli will usually be the "means." In fact a competent operant conditioner will initially try to use positive reinforcement to teach a new behavior or eliminate a maladaptive one. Under no conditions would punishment be used to develop a new behavior, since research has shown that it is not effective. However, the application of aversive stimuli is effective in eliminating some behaviors. Since the operant conditioner must continually face the dilemma of when to use aversive stimuli, the decision is not made lightly. One principle is to use the lowest possible strength of an aversive stimulus to change the behavior. The strength of an aversive stimulus may need to be increased if the behavior is interfering with the acquisition of a new, desirable behavior.

Although the "end justifies the means" argument is an important one, it should not be made in a vacuum. The disorder, parental feelings, and societal norms are all considered in the decision to use aversive stimuli. The problem of weighting the means and ends of therapy is one that is constantly present, regardless of the clinician's orientation. By continually facing it, the operant conditioner may in fact be acting more ethically and in the better interest of the client than the supposedly more "humane" practitioner who refuses to deal with the issue.

Operant conditioning is a very positive helping approach. It views the individual as responding better to positive reinforcement than to punishment. It tries to develop procedures that allow even the most severely involved individual to experience feelings of success. Operant conditioning is not the incursion of experimentally contrived procedures for controlling human behavior. It is the application of techniques that are directly related to how human beings function regardless of what is or is not done in the laboratory (Wilson, 1984). Operant conditioning is simply an understanding of the laws of human behavior. The decision not to use operant procedures is really a choice to ignore the reasons we behave as we do. To ignore information that can be helpful in allowing our clients to achieve their greatest potential is unethical. It is not the operant conditioner who faces the greatest moral dilemma, but rather humanitarians who prevent their clients from achieving their maximum potential.

Basic Concepts and Procedures

One must understand a set of basic definitions and concepts if effective operant programs are to be developed for the remediation of speech and language disorders. That will be the purpose of this section. Terms are precise and refer to specific events or objects that are operationally defined. For each definition or concept an example will be provided. Table 4–16 lists various uses of these basic concepts and procedures.

Reflexive Behavior. A reflexive behavior occurs as a result of the contraction of smooth muscles and does not involve any volitional action. An example would be the involuntary leg movement that occurs when a physician taps a knee. Although reflexive behaviors do not involve any learning, the behavior can be conditioned through association with a stimulus. The classic example is Pavlov's experiment in which a bell elicited the response of salivation in a dog. Some theorists believe that stuttering involves conditioned reflexive behavior. Brutten and Shoemaker (1967) maintained that primary stuttering results when the speech mechanism physically breaks down under stress. It involves no learning and is therefore a reflexive behavior. However, associating specific people or situations with stress does involve learning. After a sufficient number of pairings, the mere presence of certain people or situations can create the stress, which causes the speech mechanism breakdown to occur. If one adhered to Brutten and Shoemaker's position, therapy would involve deconditioning the learned reflexive behavior (primary stuttering) by changing the eliciting stimulus to a neutral stimulus.

One method of doing this is called *systematic desensitization*. It involves reducing the eliciting stress of the stimulus through initially presenting the stimulus at a very low level of eliciting power and gradually increasing it. For example, if it was determined that a client became very disfluent when he had to speak in front of the group of strangers, we might have him practice speaking in the following situations, in the order that they are listed.

1. Speaking alone in a room
2. Speaking alone in a room with a friend outside the door
3. Speaking with a friend in a room
4. Speaking with two friends in a room
5. Speaking with two friends in a room and a stranger outside the door
6. Speaking in a room with two friends who can hear you and a stranger who has his ears covered
7. Speaking with two friends and one stranger in a room
8. Speaking with one friend and one stranger in a room
9. Speaking with one stranger in a room
10. Speaking with two strangers in a room
11. Speaking with three strangers in a room
12. Speaking with four, five, six (and so on) strangers in a room

As you can see, the process involves many small steps. By increasing the strength of the stimulus only slightly when the client has become accustomed to the preceding stimuli, the eliciting power of the stimulus is reduced or eliminated. Approaches of this type also have been used in voice therapy for spastic dysphonia (Boone, 1983).

Another method of deconditioning reflexive behavior is *relaxation therapy*. Clients are usually asked to assume a prone position with their eyes closed. The clinician then suggests that various parts of their body are becoming relaxed. When the client is in a state of physical relax-

TABLE 4–16
Operant Conditioning Concepts and Procedures

Concept/Term	Explanation	Example
Conditioned Reflexive Behavior	Conditioning the autonomic nervous system.	Relaxation therapy, systematic desensitization; reducing the level of arousal in stutters in order that they can maintain control over speech
Positive Reinforcer	Something that is viewed as desirable by an individual.	A piece of fruit
Positive Reinforcement	An event involving the administration of a positive reinforcer which increases the likelihood that something will occur in the future; used to teach new behavior.	Providing a child with a piece of fruit if a desired response occurs.
Aversive Stimuli	Something that is viewed as negative by an individual.	Yelling something negative.
Punishment	The (1) administration of an aversive stimuli, or (2) the removal of a positive reinforcer which increases the likelihood that a behavior will not occur in the future; used to eliminate maladaptive behaviors.	(1) saying "sit down" using negative intonation patterns when a child leaves her seat. (2) removing a token whenever a child leaves his seat.
Response Cost	Removal of a token that was received for a desired behavior, contingent upon an undesirable behavior occurring.	Taking one token away that was received for producing a desired response, whenever the child does not attend to the activity.
Instrinisic Reinforcement	To teach new behaviors	When the act itself is reinforcing, e.g., speaking fluently for a stutterer.
Extrinsic Reinforcement	To teach new behaviors	When the completion of the act is reinforcing, e.g., receiving whatever an utterance refers to ("give milk").
Extraneous Reinforcement	To teach new behaviors	When the reinforcer has nothing to do with the act or its completion, e.g., money. *(continued)*

TABLE 4–16 *(continued)*

Concept/Term	Explanation	Example
Criteria for Advancement	A specific number or percentage of correct responses, or number of minutes an activity must occur, before it is thought to be learned.	If the child can produce /r/ in isolation 85% of the time correctly, it is assessed as learned, and the next step can begin.
Ratio Schedule of Reinforcement	When a reinforcer is provided (1) after a specific number of responses are provided (fixed), or (2) after a varying number of responses are provided (variable). Fixed ratio schedule easiest to administer for correct responses.	(1) After producing 5 correct responses, the child receives 1 token (5:1 fixed ratio schedule).

(2) After producing 5, 3, 2, 6, etc. responses, the child receives 1 token (variable ratio schedule). |
| Interval Schedule of Reinforcement | When a reinforcer is provided (1) after a specific amount of time transpires, or (2) after a varying amount of time. Variable interval schedule is best for eliminating maladaptive behaviors. | (1) If the child remains in her seat for 2 minutes she will receive a token.

(2) If a child is in seat when egg timer goes off at 2, 4, 3, 7, 5, etc. minutes, she will receive a token. |

ation, the eliciting stimulus is reduced and hopefully eliminated. This approach has been limited to certain forms of stuttering (Brutten & Shoemaker, 1967) and voice therapy (Andrews, 1995).

Operant Behaviors. Operant behaviors are behaviors whose rates of occurrence can be controlled by the consequences of the behaviors. This definition will become clearer in the example that follows. Operant behavior differs from reflexive behavior in terms of volitional action. In other words, operant behavior involves decisions. Also the order of events is different. When conditioning reflexive behavior, a stimulus is presented first, and then the response occurs. In operant conditioning, a response appears first, and then a reinforcing stimulus is presented. According to Bandura (1969),

In most real life circumstances the cues which designate probable consequences usually appear as part of a bewildering variety of irrelevant events. One must, therefore, abstract the critical feature common to a variety of situations. Behavior can be brought under control of abstract stimulus properties if responses to situations containing the critical element are reinforced, whereas responses to all other stimulus patterns lacking the essential elements go unreinforced. (p. 24)

Positive and Aversive Stimuli. New clinicians often are confused about the differences that exist between positive reinforcers, positive reinforcement, negative reinforcement, aversive stimuli, and punishment. Table 4–17 is a grid that can make the distinctions among these terms

TABLE 4–17
Reinforcement and Punishment Matrix

	Aversive Stimuli	**Positive Stimuli**
Presentation	Punishment	Positive Stimuli
Withdrawal	Negative Reinforcement	Punishment (Response Cost)

more obvious. There are two rows and two columns. The rows represent what one can do with a stimulus. One can present it or withdraw it. The columns represent a positive or a negative stimulus. With a 2 × 2 grid, four combinations are possible. If one presents a positive stimulus it is called *positive reinforcement*. If one presents an aversive stimulus, this is known as *punishment*. If one withdraws a positive stimulus it is called *punishment* or *response cost*. If an aversive stimulus is withdrawn, it is called *negative reinforcement*. A positive reinforcer is a specific stimulus, such as a piece of fruit, a token, a toy, or a specific number of minutes at a pleasurable activity. A positive reinforcer is simply *something* that a person receives for doing a desired behavior. If the stimulus increases the likelihood that the desired behavior will occur again, it is a positive reinforcer. If it does not increase the likelihood that it will occur again, we call it a *neutral stimulus*. Therefore, our definition of what is a positive reinforcer depends on the effect it has on the client.

Reinforcement refers to the entire *event* during which a positive reinforcer was given or an aversive stimuli is withdrawn. For example, a child is asked to produce the phoneme /s/ when the clinician raises her hand. If the child produces it correctly, the clinician gives him a small piece of an apple. The positive reinforcer is the apple. The reinforcement would be the presentation of the apple contingent on the production of a correct response. There are many

ways of classifying reinforcers and reinforcements. The major classification appear in the following sections. Often it is possible for a positive reinforcer or positive reinforcement to be classified in more than one way.

Positive Reinforcement

Positive reinforcement should be an integral part of all therapy. When present it has been found to be correlated with effectiveness (Sriram et al., 1990; Swanson & Stillman, 1990; Vu, Barrows, Marcy, Verholst et al., 1992). When reinforcing client responses consideration should be given to the type of reinforcement provided and how it is administered. When providing social reinforcement (e.g., "good job"), it is advisable that the words chosen are appropriate for the client's age, are variable but mean the same thing (e.g., "good job," "that's great," "nice going," etc.), and are judiciously applied. In Table 4–18 65 different ways that can be used to convey to the client that the desired response was produced.

When designing intervention programs, the clinician should be concerned not only about providing a specific generalized reinforcer at the end of the activity, but also about the reinforcing qualities of the activity. The clinical activity can be divided into three units, each presenting an opportunity for the clinician to apply reinforcement procedures: (1) the activity itself for intrinsic reinforcement, (2) the completion of the

TABLE 4–18
Words That Can Be Used for Social Reinforcement

A+ job	Hurray for you	That's incredible
Awesome	I knew you could do it	That's correct
Beautiful sharing	I'm proud of you	That's the best
Beautiful work	Looking good	Way to go
Beautiful	Magnificent	Well done
Bingo	Marvelous	What a good listener
Bravo	Neat	Wow
Creative job	Nice work	You learned it right
Dynamite	Nice job	You tried hard
Excellent	Nothing can stop you now	You're a real trooper
Exceptional performance	Now you're flying	You're a winner
Fantastic	Now you've got it	You're spectacular
Fantastic job	Outstanding performance	You're sensational
Good job	Outstanding	You're beautiful
Good for you	Phenomenal	You're on top it
Good	Remarkable job	You're on your way
Great discovery	Remarkable	You're on target
Great	Spectacular	You're fantastic
Hip, hip, hurray	Super	You're incredible
Hot dog	Super job	You're catching on
How nice	Super work	You've discovered the secret
How smart	Terrific	

activity for extrinsic reinforcement, and (3) an event occurring after the activity is completed for extraneous reinforcement. Although these types of reinforcements were discussed in Chapter 2, it will be worthwhile to briefly review them again. In Tables 4–19 to 4–21 general suggestions for types of reinforcing activities for clients are listed. In Table 4–22, a simple check sheet is provided for analyzing specific activities.

Intrinsic Reinforcement. An activity can be intrinsically reinforcing. This means that the activity itself may be pleasurable enough so that the individual would engage in it just out of the sheer enjoyment the activity causes. Accomplished musicians may cry with pleasure as they play a passage in a violin concerto that is especially moving. Or the Saturday morning softball player may feel euphoric as she reaches high in the air to catch a ball. Everyone's life is hopefully filled with these types of activities—activities that are pleasurable in and of themselves. In a clinical setting, the clinician should always attempt to construct activities that are intrinsically reinforcing. This will be easier for some activities than for others. In some types of disorders, such as stuttering and language, the production of an appropriate speech or language behavior is intrinsically reinforcing. For most stutterers, speaking fluently is very rewarding. Not having to repeat or block on words can be more reinforcing than anything given to stutterers because they were fluent. At the other end of the continuum would be the young child with a minor articulation problem who does not find it reinforcing to produce /r/ rather than its substitute /w/. For this child, reinforcement needs to be structured in other ways.

TABLE 4–19
Reinforcing Activities for Children

DISORDER	INTRINSIC (activity itself)	EXTRINSIC (completion of the behavior)	EXTRANEOUS (nothing to do with the behavior)
Articulation/ Phonology	It is difficult to find anything intrinsically reinforcing about correctly producing a phoneme. Focus on extraneous forms of reinforcement.	It is difficult to find anything extrinsically reinforcing about correctly producing a phoneme. Focus on extraneous forms of reinforcement.	**Activity.** Incorporate critical features listed in Table 4–2 **Token System.** Use fixed ratio schedule of reinforcement. See Table 4–24 **Social.** Continually provide positive reinforcement for every correct response. See Table 4–18 for different ways of indicating correctness.
Language	The use of language can be intrinsically reinforcing to children, if the target behaviors involve concepts and constructions that are meaningful to the client Try to make all language activities intrinsically reinforcing.	All language therapy can be extrinsically reinforcing if the target behaviors involve some form of environmental manipulation (e.g., when learning the rule action + object, "give milk," results in the client receiving a glass of milk).	See above.
Stuttering	For a child who has difficulty consistently producing fluent utterances, the production of fluent speech is intrinsically reinforcing. Use whatever techniques are appropriate to immediately produce any form of fluency.	Initially use short periods of time (1 minute) or short units of language (sentence). The completion of either, through the use of fluent speech, will be reinforcing.	See above.
Voice	For a child who has a voice problem, the production of the target behavior will probably not be intrinsically reinforcing. Rely on extraneous reinforcement.	It is difficult to find anything extrinsically reinforcing about correctly producing appropriate voice quality. Focus on extraneous forms of reinforcement.	See above.

TABLE 4-20
Reinforcing Activities for Adolescents

DISORDER	INTRINSIC (activity itself)	EXTRINSIC (completion of the behavior)	EXTRANEOUS (nothing to do with the behavior)
Articulation/ Phonology	It is difficult to find anything intrinsically reinforcing about correctly producing a phoneme for adolescents who are unconcerned about their speech. If the client understands and accepts the value of correct articulation, the production may be intrinsically reinforcing.	For adolescents who are aware and concerned about their articulatory problems, playback on an audiotape of correct articulation may be reinforcing.	**Token System.** For older adolescents, the use of a token system will probably not be appropriate. **Social.** Continually provide positive reinforcement for every correct response. See Table 4-18 for different ways of indicating correctness.
Language	The use of language can be intrinsically reinforcing to adolescents, if the target behaviors involve concepts and constructions that are meaningful to the client. Try to make all language activities intrinsically reinforcing.	All language therapy can be extrinsically reinforcing if the target behaviors involve some form of environmental manipulation (e.g., when learning the rule action + object, "give milk," results in the client receiving a glass of milk) for more severely impaired clients or increased classroom abilities for less impaired clients.	See above.
Stuttering	For adolescents who have difficulty consistently producing fluent utterances, the production of fluent speech is intrinsically reinforcing. Use whatever techniques are appropriate to immediately produce any form of fluency.	Initially use short periods of time (1 minute) or short units of language (sentence). The completion of either, through the use of fluent speech, will be reinforcing.	See above.
Voice	For adolescents who have a voice problem, are aware of it, and are motivated to change it, the production of the target behavior will be intrinsically reinforcing.	For adolescents who are aware and concerned about their voice problems, playback on an audiotape of correct voicing may be reinforcing.	See above.

TABLE 4–21
Reinforcing Activities for Adults

DISORDER	INTRINSIC (activity itself)	EXTRINSIC (completion of the behavior)	EXTRANEOUS (nothing to do with the behavior)
Articulation/ Phonology	Adults who come to therapy understand and accept the value of correct articulation. Therefore the production will be intrinsically reinforcing.	Playback on an audiotape of correct articulation may be reinforcing.	**Token System.** For adults, the use of a token system is not appropriate. **Social.** Continually provide positive reinforcement for *every* correct response. See Table 4–18 for different ways of indicating correctness.
Language	The use of language will be intrinsically reinforcing to adults, if the target behaviors involve concepts and constructions that are meaningful to them. Language activities should focus on functional language.	All language therapy can be extrinsically reinforcing if the target behaviors involve some form of environmental manipulation (e.g., when re-learning the rule action + actor + object, "give me water," results in the client receiving a glass of water).	See above.
Stuttering	For adults who have difficulty consistently producing fluent utterances, the production of fluent speech is intrinsically reinforcing. Use whatever techniques are appropriate to immediately produce any form of fluency	Initially use short periods of time (1 minute) or short units of language (sentence). The completion of either through the use of fluent speech will be reinforcing.	See above.
Voice	Adults who come to therapy are aware of their voice problem and motivated to change. The production of the target behavior will be intrinsically reinforcing.	Playback on an audiotape of correct voicing may be reinforcing.	See above.

TABLE 4–22
Analysis of Reinforcement of Selected Activities

Description of the Activity	Date of Activity	Intrinsically Reinforcing Elements	Extrinsically Reinforcing Elements	Extraneously Reinforcing Elements

Extrinsic Reinforcement. When the completion of an activity is reinforcing, regardless of the reinforcing quality of the activity itself, the activity is extrinsically reinforcing. An example might be cleaning one's kitchen. A person may hate the drudgery involved in cleaning a kitchen following a party. If the cleaning depended on the reinforcing qualities of the activity itself, many kitchens would probably become breeding grounds for as yet unknown diseases. Why then should one engage in an unpleasant activity such as cleaning? Reinforcement lies in the completion of the activity. The extrinsic reinforcement in this example would be a clean kitchen. To have it, the person would be willing to engage in the activity of cleaning. In therapy, the client is often involved in similar situations. Hopefully, the activities are not aversive but merely neutral. For example, if a young child is being taught to combine single-word utterances to produce action + object constructions, she may not feel anything rewarding in the actual production of the phrase "push car." However, if at the completion of the utterance the clinician then pushes a car that the child wanted in her direction, the child is being extrinsically reinforced at the completion of the verbal production "push car," by having the car move.

Extraneous Reinforcers. If neither the activity nor its completion is reinforcing, an extraneous reinforcer is necessary for the person to continue to engage in the activity. An extraneous reinforcer is a reinforcer that has nothing to do with either the act or its completion. For example, an automobile worker may be responsible for the production of bumpers. To produce a bumper, a button must be pressed to engage a computerized operation. The worker finds nothing reinforcing about the pushing of the button. Nor does he get any pleasure from seeing hundreds of shiny bumpers made every day. Why then should he continue working in the factory since there is nothing intrinsically or extrinsically reinforcing about his job? Because he is being extraneously reinforced. That is, he is receiving enough money every 2 weeks to make his job acceptable, even though he might hate it. In the clinic, two types of extraneous reinforcers can be used. One is verbal praise and the other involves a token system. In a study comparing the performance of subjects who received verbal praise and those who did not, it was found that subjects who received verbal praise performed significantly better than those who did not (Chang, 1994). The subjects in this study all had normal intelligence and appropriate social interaction patterns. However, not all of our clients meet these two criteria. Some clients have cognitive impairments and others have abnormal social interaction patterns. For these clients, the use of verbal praise may not be sufficient. In fact, many clients with both normal intelligence and social interaction patterns may not have any interest in producing the desired behaviors in order to receive the verbal praise of the clinician. Unfortunately, not all children believe that their clinician's praise is that important. For these children, a token system can be very effective, especially if the activities they are engaging in are neither intrinsically nor extrinsically reinforcing. Extraneous reinforcers are also generalized reinforcers. A *generalized reinforcer* is one that is effective regardless of the present condition of clients or their feelings toward the clinician. This is the prime advantage of extraneous reinforcers. They are not dependent on a current state of need. For example, although the child may not be interested in eating or playing a game while in therapy, tokens could be exchanged at a later date for the food or an activity.

Some researchers in psychology have raised the concern that the use of extraneous reinforcers may diminish the value of intrinsic and extrinsic reinforcing activities (Flora, 1990). However, studies have shown that any reduction of the reinforcing properties of the intrinsic and extrinsic reinforcers is only temporary, and their importance in controlling behaviors quickly resumes (Dickinson, 1989). It should be noted that the research in this area may use different terminology to identify reinforcing events than what is used in this book. Some researchers make no distinction between intrinsic and extraneous reinforcement and identify both as "intrinsic reinforcement" or extraneous reinforcement as "extrinsic reinforcement" (Dickinson, 1989; Flora, 1990) while other researchers use the term "extraneous reinforcement" in a manner similar to the way it is used in this book. Regardless of how the terms are used, the conclusion is that the use of extraneous reinforcers does not diminish the value or strength of either intrinsic or extrinsic reinforcers.

The term *contingency* refers to the process of providing an extraneous reinforcer to the client. A reinforcer is provided to the client *contingent* on the production of a correct response. This is a timing issue. If a client is provided with a reinforcer prior to performing the required behavior, the motivation to produce the correct response may be diminished. A very common example occurs in the playing of many board games requiring the client to spin a wheel in order to determine how many steps to move a board piece. Often the client will spin the wheel, move the required number of spaces, and then be asked to produce the behavior. In this case, the reinforcement (moving the pieces) occurs prior to the initiation of the behavior. Since reinforcement is occurring prior to the behavior, it has no effect on the production of correct responses. Not only is this an inappropriate operant procedure, but it also conveys a message to the client that there will be no consequences for incorrect behaviors.

An equally inappropriate timing decision is reinforcing long after the desired behavior is exhibited. For example, a sticker is provided to the child at the end of the session for "doing well today." Since the session probably consisted of correct and incorrect productions, the client may not have any idea why the reinforcement is being provided, or may assume that reinforcement is being provided for any response, both correct and incorrect. Conversely, if a reinforcer is not provided at the end of therapy, the client may not know why the sticker was not received.

When one thinks about reinforcement, more often than not it is extraneous reinforcement that receives the attention and criticism. This should be the last form of reinforcement on which the clinician should concentrate. First design an intervention program that is intrinsically reinforcing. Then have the completion of the activity be extrinsically reinforcing. Finally, have an extraneous reinforcer available if all else fails. Although desired behaviors may be elicited merely by having the child engage in an intrinsically reinforcing activity, it is often not sufficient. The most powerful intervention program involves intrinsic, extrinsic, and extraneous reinforcers. By incorporating all three into an intervention program, a loss of motivating strength of one or even two still will not affect the ability of the program to produce the desired behaviors.

Criteria for Advancement

A criterion for advancement is an objective method for determining if clients have mastered a specific behavior. It is usually given in terms of percentage of correct responses, number of consecutive correct responses, a percentage of time, or an absolute amount of time for which a behavior must occur.

Percentage of Correct Responses. It is generally agreed that at a 90% criterion level, advancement is sufficient for guaranteeing that the client has mastered the task (Goldberg, 1993). Some research indicates that an 80 to 85% criterion level may be sufficient (Diedrich & Bangert, 1980). Until more research is available, it is advisable to use the 90% criterion level as a standard from which slight downward deviations can be made so that the client does not become bored with the activities through endless repetition. This is justified because not all errors are related to not mastering the task. Inattention may be present.

When expressing criterion levels, some clinicians refer only to a percentage figure. Although this does provide some information to the listener or reader, a significant element is missing: the number of items in each trial. Therefore, when specifying criterion levels, always refer to the number of items. For example, "Criterion for advancement in each stage of the program is 90% for trials containing 20 items."

A misuse of this criterion occurs when a client is expected to perform at a lower percentage of correct responses, with gradual increases in the level. For example, on a difficult task, the clinician may state that "the client will respond with 45% accuracy." The following day, the criterion level may be adjusted upward to 60%. This is an inappropriate use of a criterion level. If the expectation that a client can only be successful at a 45% level of accuracy, the task most likely is too difficult. Instead of lowering the criterion level, it is more efficient to reduce the complexity of the task and keep the criterion level at 90%. When the simplified task is mastered at the criterion level, it should then be made slightly more complex with the criterion level remaining constant. In Chapter 6, methods for structuring activities in this way will be discussed.

Number of Consecutive Correct Responses. Although some people use this as a criterion for advancement, it does not seem to be based on any objective standard. For example, why is it better to have five consecutive correct responses rather than four or seven or nine? There are no data to support using this type of criterion.

Percentage of Time. The use of this criterion is limited to general behaviors relating to attending. For example, the percentage of time a client initially remains in her seat during a learning task of 15 minutes duration was 30% or 5 minutes. To facilitate learning, the clinician has decided that in each session the criterion for sitting will be raised by 5%. The problems with using percentage of time and absolute amount of time are similar to those cited in the misuse of criteria. Simply increasing the percentage of time or the amount of time a client is required to attend does not address the precipitating reasons for inattention. Although progress may be made by gradually increasing the percentage of time or absolute amount of time, a more efficient method would involve modifying the activity in a way that addresses the causes of inattention.

Absolute Amount of Time. Problems with the use of this criterion were cited in the last section. However, determining the amount of time is more a practical manner, based on individual client characteristics rather than a standard to be used for everyone. For example, if a clinician wishes to increase the amount of attending behavior of a distractable child, she may decide to make the first criterion level 1 minute more than the amount of time the child has demonstrated the ability to attend during the last activity. With success, the criterion level could be moved upward.

Punishment

Punishment can involve either the administration of aversive stimuli or the withdrawal of positive reinforcers. Punishment has been inappropriately used to establish new behaviors and appropriately used to extinguish maladaptive ones. Situations for using punishment and considerations involved in its administration appear in Table 4–23.

Inappropriate Use of Punishment. The administration of an aversive stimulus should not be used to establish a new behavior for three reasons. First is that, when the aversive stimulus is eliminated, the behavior is likely to be extinguished (Skinner, 1953). Human conditions within prisons parallel the laboratory experiments conducted by Skinner and exemplify this point. In prisons there is little training of, nor reinforcement of, new, socially acceptable behaviors. The threat of continued aversive stimuli is effective in minimizing antisocial behavior only as long as the threat continues. With the removal of the aversive stimuli, the antisocial behavior reoccurs. This is evidenced by the very high recidivism rate associated with individuals who are incarcerated in prisons that are little more than holding cells for criminals. In clinical situations, it is not effective to use aversive stimuli to establish a behavior that the client does not know how to perform.

The second reason that aversive stimuli should be avoided is that the clinician must be committed to increasing the strength of the aversive stimulus when the client does not respond appropriately. By definition, something is not aversive unless it reduces or eliminates a behavior. People can and do adapt to the strength of an aversive stimulus. For example, an abused child who initially may have been terrified of a parent's slap across the face eventually learns to tolerate severe beat-

TABLE 4–23
Use of Aversive Control

GOAL	ADMINISTRATION OF AVERSIVE STIMULI	WITHDRAWAL OF POSITIVE REINFORCER
Teaching of New Behaviors	**Do Not Use.** The use of aversive stimuli to teach new behaviors is inappropriate. When the aversive stimuli is removed, the behavior disappears.	**Do Not Use.** Withdrawing of a positive behavior to teach new behaviors is inappropriate. Change the learning activity.
Elimination of Maladaptive Behaviors	**Escalation of Aversive Stimuli.** Administering aversive stimuli can be used to eliminate maladaptive behavior if clinicians are willing to escalate the strength of the stimuli if the maladaptive does not stop. **Ethical and Legal Issues.** Both ethnical and legal issues need to be thoroughly examined before using aversive stimuli. **Approval by Parent.** Do not administer any aversive stimuli until it has been discussed with the parents and has received their approval. **Negative Relationship.** The use of aversive stimuli may result in the development of a negative relationship between the client and the clinician. **Lack of Reinforcing Activities.** Maladaptive behaviors often result because the learning activities are neither intrinsically, extrinsically, or extraneously reinforcing. Elimination of the behaviors may not improve performance.	**Effectiveness.** If a token system is in use, the removal of a token when maladaptive behaviors occur can be very effective. **Sufficient Regular Productions.** The use of this procedure assumes that the client is capable of producing the desired behavior with sufficient regularity to warrant the removal of tokens. Nonperformance must be related to inattention, not difficulties in learning the behavior. **Lack of Reinforcing Activities.** Maladaptive behaviors often result because the learning activities are neither intrinsically, extrinsically, or extraneously reinforcing. Elimination of the behaviors may not improve performance.

ings. In a clinical situation a clinician may decide to say "no" in an angry tone whenever the child does not respond correctly during an imitative vocal activity. If the aversive quality of "no" is effective in increasing vocal imitation, then the clinician can feel comfortable in the decision to use aversive stimuli. But what happens if the utterance has no effect or loses its effect after a few presentations? The clinician who is committed to using aversive stimuli must now increase the strength of the stimulus. What would be more aversive: talking firmly, yelling, or hitting the child's arm? Possibly all would have to be tried as each in turn loses its punishing effects.

The third reason that aversive stimuli should not be used to teach a new behavior is that their use presents a model of teaching that is antithetical to the values of our profession. If we are committed to the humane development of a person's maximum potential, it is inappropriate to rely on punishment to accomplish it. The clinical setting becomes a place to which the client no longer enjoys coming; it is transformed to a place where punishment will be applied if the client cannot perform adequately. The use of punishment in animal societies by its members results in many tangential consequences, most of which are applicable to clinical settings. It was found that in societies were punishment was commonly practiced, domineering relationships prevailed in which negative reciprocity and retaliatory aggression were common (Clutton, Brock, & Parker, 1995). In the clinic this translates into modeling dominant-submissive behavioral relationships for clients that are based on who has the most power, or with children, who is older and bigger.

Appropriate Use of Aversive Control.

If aversive stimuli should not be used to teach a new behavior, do their use have a place in clinical practice? Yes. Aversive stimuli can be used to reduce or eliminate maladaptive behaviors. In eliminating maladaptive behaviors, the clinician is not teaching the client a new behavior but rather is suppressing an old one, thereby allowing clients to substitute one they already know how to do. Inattention, excessive physical movement, and abusive and aggressive behaviors are types of behaviors that respond favorably to punishment. Although it is appropriate to use aversive control to reduce or eliminate maladaptive behaviors, its use may prevent the clinician from examining the nature and structure of the instructional activity. If clients are not willing to engage in clinical activities, it may be because nothing reinforcing is occurring. By instituting methods of reducing maladaptive behaviors, the poor construction of the activity is not questioned. A good rule of thumb is to assume initially that, if clients are exhibiting maladaptive behaviors, the fault is that there is nothing reinforcing about the activity, and only after the activity has been modified, should aversive controls be used to minimize or eliminate the maladaptive behaviors.

Administration of an Aversive Stimulus.

If the clinician decides to administer an aversive stimulus, all of the problems associated with adapting to punishing situations are again encountered. In severely disturbed children or children with significant cognitive deficits, the clinician may find few consequences as effective as the presentation of aversive stimuli to eliminate maladaptive and self-destructive behaviors. In studies done by Lovass and his associates (Lovaas, Freitag, Gold, & Kassorla 1965), administering aversive stimuli was the most effective way of rapidly eliminating the self-destructive behaviors of psychotic children. Unfortunately, it may be too effective. Often the use of bizarre or socially inappropriate behaviors by severely communicatively impaired children appears to be correlated with difficulties in communicating. For example, one autistic child only hit her head and bit her hand during situations were she was unable to communicate her needs. Although these are unacceptable behaviors in any circumstance, if they were eliminated prior to the clinician understanding the correlation, an important clue for identifying the reason why the behaviors were occurring would not be known. With the knowledge, the clinician was able to develop a self-help program that not only eliminated the self-destructive behaviors, but replaced them with socially appropriate ones.

Removal of a Positive Reinforcer.
Instead of administering an aversive stimulus, punishment may involve the removal of a positive reinforcer. This is usually done through two clinical procedures: time-out and response cost. Time-out is a procedure that was developed by Ferster (1957) and refers to the removal of a child from a reinforcing setting to one that contains no reinforcers. Typically, a child who was acting out was placed in a bare, windowless room or small enclosure, often with the lights turned off. The assumption was that this form of punishment not only was more humane than the administration of aversive stimuli, but also was easy for parents and trainers to use. Time-out is effective only if it is viewed by the child as removal from a reinforcing situation. Unfortunately, being moved from a therapy room that the child views as aversive to a setting where no demands are made is not punishing, but rather reinforcing. Instead of the clinician conditioning the children, the children condition the clinician. Whenever the situation becomes too demanding or too unpleasant, the children know that if they act out, they will be placed in the calmer, less demanding room, where they can rest or be entertained by their own fantasies. Time-out can also be very inefficient. During that period of time when the child is isolated, no learning of new behaviors can take place. With some children time-out

may need to last an extensive amount of time to be effective.

The use of response-cost in many situations may be more effective than time-out to eliminate maladaptive behaviors, because the procedure is coupled with a schedule of positive reinforcement. Typically, a token or positive reinforcer is removed whenever the child either does a maladaptive behavior or responds inappropriately. The relationship between response-cost and positive reinforcement is exemplified by the following example.

A child is given a token for every five correct productions of the phoneme /r/. If at the end of the session he has accumulated 10 tokens, he can cash them in for a very desirable prize. With 15 minutes left in the session, the child has accumulated nine tokens. With five additional correct responses, the prize is his. However, he realized that with 15 minutes left, he can be inattentive, produce a large number of incorrect responses and still have time to receive the tokens. Worse, he can even act out, deliberately ignoring the clinician for a good portion of the 15 minutes.

The clinician now faces a dilemma. She realizes the importance of honoring her commitment to reinforce correct productions, regardless of the number of incorrect productions. But she also knows that the child is using this fact to manipulate her behavior. If she decides to administer aversive stimuli or institute a time-out procedure, the consequences of the punishment may not be effective since the child is so close to receiving the positive reinforcer for the acceptable behavior he already displayed. In this case, punishment may not be effective in increasing the likelihood that appropriate behaviors will result. The child may stop the maladaptive behaviors even with no punishment in order to have enough time to produce just the right amount of responses to receive the positive reinforcer.

The situation is changed dramatically if a response-cost is introduced. The clinician may explain to the child that, since the child knows how to produce the /r/ phoneme, he not only will get a token for every correct response but also will lose one for incorrect responses or inattention. When response-costs are introduced, the effects on maladaptive behaviors are quite dramatic if the client views the positive reinforcer as something that is very desirable. The clinician must be careful, however, in coupling incorrect responses with a response cost. This could be equivalent to using aversive stimuli to teach a new behavior if the child did not already know how to perform the behavior. Response-costs for incorrect behaviors are appropriate only if the clinician believes that the incorrect behaviors are the result of inattention or contrivance rather than of not knowing the specifics involved in correctly producing the behavior. In a study on treatment acceptability, it was found that parents prefer response-costs as a method of eliminating maladaptive behaviors to other forms of punishment (Miller & Kelly, 1992).

Extraneous Reinforcement Schedules

The reinforcement of desired behaviors can occur after a specific number of responses or after a specified amount of time. Certain types of behavior are best reinforced using a ratio schedule (number of responses), while others require interval schedules (time). Both types of reinforcement schedules can be either fixed or variable. A 2 × 2 matrix with a description of their uses appears in Table 4–24.

Ratio Schedules of Reinforcement.
Reinforcement schedules that are related to the number of correct responses are called *ratio schedules* of reinforcement. If the client is reinforced after every response, a 1:1 or continuous schedule of re-

inforcement is used. A 1:1 schedule of reinforcement may be necessary to establish a reinforcing paradigm with children who are severely cognitively or emotionally impaired. After the association is made between the behavior and the reinforcer, the schedule of reinforcement is changed, requiring additional amounts of correct behaviors to be exhibited before a reinforcer is given. If the reinforcer is given after a specific number of correct behaviors, such as 3 or 5, then the reinforcement schedule is a fixed ratio schedule of reinforcement. In these cases it would be a 3:1 or 5:1 fixed ratio schedule. Technically, you could vary the schedule during an activity. This would be a *variable ratio* schedule. For example, you might go from 1:1 to 4:1 to 2:1 and then finally 3:1. Although technically possible, there is no evidence to suggest that the variability is efficacious. Some clinicians call a variable ratio schedule one that systematically advances from a lower ratio to a higher one. For example the number of responses required could move from 2 to 3 to 4 to 8. The use of this type of variable ratio schedule has been shown to be more effective than fixed ratio schedules in terms of resulting in higher percentage of correct responses (deLuca and Holborn, 1992). The way in which this would occur in a clinical situation is that a low ratio schedule of reinforcement would initially be used, such as 2:1. After reaching criteria, the ratio would be increased to 3:1 and then continue on until arrival at the last ratio schedule. The shifts in ratio should be systematic and proceeded by complete explanations to the client, such as "you are doing these so well, let's see if we can make it a little harder for you." Although identified as a variable ratio schedule by some, others would maintain that they constitute a series of different fixed ratio schedules. Regardless of how one labels them, the systematic increase of ratios in reinforcement schedules increases the percentage of correct responses.

TABLE 4–24
Schedules of Reinforcement

	RATIO (per behavior)	TIME (time)
FIXED (Unchanging)	**1:1/Continuous.** Use continuous reinforcement for clients who are not under stimulus control (e.g., severely impaired clients). **Specific Responses.** Use ratio schedules when target behavior is discrete (e.g., identification of concepts). **Satiation.** If reinforcement involves food or drink, use very small amounts during continuous reinforcement. Gradually switch to increased ratios (e.g., 2:1, 3:1, 4:1). **Token System.** Easiest method of constructing a fixed ratio schedule of reinforcement. Token is received for each correct response. Exchange specific amount of tokens for a designated reinforcement.	**Elimination of Maladaptive Behaviors—Total Time.** Client can be reinforced for attending or sitting for a specific amount of time.
VARIABLE (Changing)	Not Appropriate.	**Elimination of Maladaptive Behaviors— At Time Specific.** Client is reinforced for attending or sitting when a signal occurs (e.g., bell on an egg timer). Variable schedule more effective than fixed schedule.

Interval Schedules of Reinforcement. Interval schedules of reinforcement involve the administration of a positive reinforcer after a specified amount of time. It is not related to the number of correct behaviors. If the reinforcer is given after a specific amount of time, the client is on a fixed interval schedule or reinforcement. If the amount of time varies, the client is on a variable interval schedule of reinforcement. As was the case with the variable ratio schedule, variable interval schedules can be determined prior to the clinical interaction or can be random. Interval schedules are less effective in teaching new behaviors than are ratio schedules because they do not provide feedback on the correctness of a behavior immediately after it occurs. However, they can be very effective in eliminating maladaptive behaviors. For example, a child is told that after he sits quietly for 5 minutes he will receive a token. This would be a 5:1 fixed interval schedule of reinforcement. If the amount of time is variable, then the child would be on a variable interval schedule of reinforcement.

Mixed Schedules of Reinforcement.

In a clinical session, it is possible to use multiple reinforcement schedules to achieve various results. For example, a clinician could use a 5:1 fixed ratio schedule of reinforcement for correct productions of personal pronouns in sentences, 2:1 fixed ratio schedule if the sentence had at least five words, 3:1 fixed ratio schedule if the sentence dealt with future relationships, and a variable interval schedule that reinforced quiet sitting. By using multiple schedules, various behaviors can be simultaneously reinforced. However, the clinician should not make the situation so complex that the client's ability to focus on the production of target behaviors becomes diluted.

PLANNING ACTIVITIES

Effective activities tend to be those that have been planned in advance of the session and are structured so that a sequence of events is apparent. Activities that have a structure and have been planned in advance tend to produce more positive results than those that are unplanned and lack a sequential structure (Meredith, 1985). Sequenced activities have distinct parts, with the production of one based on the acquisition of a previous one. While a lack of planning may not result in young clients perceiving the clinician as disorganized, that perception is more likely to develop with adult clients (Morris, 1991). The planning of a session may involve variables of time, materials, stimulus configurations,

and objectives. Tables 4–25 to 4–27 include comprehensive checklists of activities that should be planned in advance of the session.

Time

When planning a therapy session, clinicians should think of three time frames: (1) immediate, (2) intermediate, and (3) long term.

Immediate. Every session has specific components, each of which takes planning. The first and overriding component is the *goals* of the session. These are specific objectives the clinician wishes to achieve with the client. They may involve teaching behaviors, redirecting attitudes, learning of strategies, or gaining information. Regardless of the purpose, each will require a *method* or series of methods for the goal to be achieved. With the method specified, it becomes possible to then select the *materials* that will be used to achieve the goal. With a plan for achieving a goal, some means for determining if the goal has been achieved must be used. The standard is referred to as the *criterion for advancement*. It can be expressed as the number of times a behavior must be exhibited, a percentage of correct responses, or an acceptance or acknowledgment on the part of the client of an attitude, belief, or commitment. Regardless of the form the criterion takes, it has a certain degree of objectivity. In other words, something very specific must occur by the end of the session or activity if the clinician is to be assured that the goal has been met.

Intermediate. It is very easy to be so involved with the goals of a single session that its relationship to longer term goals is ignored. It is important that there is a continuity of activity that transcends more than a few sessions. One approach to designing intervention programs that suc-

TABLE 4–25
Planning Activities for Children

Below you will find various categories that should be considered when planning any activity. Check off the boxes where the category applies, then fill in the space provided.

BEHAVIORAL OBJECTIVE _____

**DESCRIPTION OF ACTIVITY
TO ACHIEVE OBJECTIVE** _____

**RELATIONSHIP OF ACTIVITY
TO INTERMEDIATE AND
LONG RANGE GOALS**

	Activity	*Intermediate Goal*	*Long Range Goal*
	_____	_____	_____

PLANNING CATEGORY	SPECIFIC COMPONENTS	
Advance Organization Statements	❏ What _____ _____ ❏ How _____ _____ ❏ Why _____ _____	
Sources of Information For Activity	❏ Family ❏ Job ❏ Hobbies ❏ Books ❏ TV/Movies	❏ Current Events ❏ School sports ❏ School Activities/Clubs ❏ School Social Events ❏ Rival School Activities
Critical Activity Features	❏ Mobility _____ ❏ Construction _____ ❏ Destruction _____ ❏ Movement_____ ❏ Completion _____ ❏ Flexibility _____ ❏ Surprise _____ ❏ Competition _____	
Generalizable Features of Activities	❏ Family_____ ❏ School_____ ❏ Sports/Leisure _____ ❏ Social/etc. _____	
Reinforcement	❏ Intrinsic _____ ❏ Extrinsic _____ ❏ Extraneous _____	
Schedules of Reinforcement	❏ Fixed Ratio _____ ❏ Fixed Interval _____ ❏ Variable Interval _____	

(continued)

PLANNING CATEGORY	SPECIFIC COMPONENTS
Aversive Control	❑ Administration of Aversive Stimuli _____ ❑ Withdrawal of Positive Reinforcer _____
Cultural Considerations	❑ Ethnicity/National Origin _____ ❑ Religion _____ ❑ Gender/Sexual Orientation _____ ❑ Exceptionality _____ ❑ Urban-Suburban-Rural _____ ❑ Geographic Region _____ ❑ Socioeconomic Class _____

TABLE 4–26
Planning Activities for Adolescents

Below you will find various categories that should be considered when planning any activity. Check off the boxes where the category applies, then fill in the space provided.

BEHAVIORAL OBJECTIVE _____

DESCRIPTION OF ACTIVITY
TO ACHIEVE OBJECTIVE _____

RELATIONSHIP OF ACTIVITY
TO INTERMEDIATE AND
LONG RANGE GOALS

Activity	*Intermediate Goal*	*Long Range Goal*
_____	_____	_____

PLANNING CATEGORY	SPECIFIC COMPONENTS		
Advance Organization Statements	❑ What _____ _____ ❑ How _____ _____ ❑ Why _____ _____		
Sources of Information For Activity	❑ Family ❑ Adults ❑ Hobbies ❑ Books ❑ TV/Movies	❑ Music ❑ School Sports ❑ School Activities/Clubs ❑ School Social Events ❑ Rival School Activities	❑ Dance Clubs ❑ Cars ❑ Communicative Disorder
Critical Activity Features	❑ Mobility _____ ❑ Construction _____ ❑ Destruction _____ ❑ Movement _____ ❑ Completion _____ ❑ Flexibility _____ ❑ Surprise _____ ❑ Competition _____		

(continued)

TABLE 4–26 *(continued)*

PLANNING CATEGORY	SPECIFIC COMPONENTS
Generalizable Features of Activities	❐ Family _____ ❐ School _____ ❐ Sports/Leisure _____ ❐ Social/etc. _____
Reinforcement	❐ Intrinsic _____ ❐ Extrinsic _____ ❐ Extraneous _____
Schedules of Reinforcement	❐ Fixed Ratio _____ ❐ Fixed Interval _____ ❐ Variable Interval _____
Aversive Control	❐ Administration of Aversive Stimuli _____ ❐ Withdrawal of Positive Reinforcer _____
Cultural Considerations	❐ Ethnicity/National Origin _____ ❐ Religion _____ ❐ Gender/Sexual Orientation _____ ❐ Exceptionality _____ ❐ Urban-Suburban-Rural _____ ❐ Geographic Region _____ ❐ Socioeconomic Class _____

cessfully deal with this problem is the *Competency Based Clinical Intervention Format* (CBCIF) (Goldberg, 1993). The CB-CIF incorporates successive approximations throughout the program and contains four structural levels: (1) terminal competency, (2) specific competencies, (3) instructional objectives, and (4) learning activities. The program is fully explained in Chapter 6 in the Successive Approximations section.

Long Range. Often when planning therapy, clinicians can be short-sighted, even if an intermediate instructional format is used. The purpose of therapy is not just to correct specific communicative problems. Rather it is to enable clients to develop and use communication as normally as possible to maximize their potential as human beings. For the adult aphasic this means not merely learning specific grammatical structures or retrieving names of objects, but also regaining the means to communicate. For stutterers, it means not just teaching them how to use fluent speech, but also enabling them to adjust to the changes that will occur in their lives when fluency is developed. For Down syndrome children, it means not just learning increasingly complex grammatical structures, but also developing language that will enable them in adulthood to lead as normal and independent a life as possible.

Organization

Activities can be organized either categorically or sequentially. Each type of organizational strategy fulfills a distinct purpose and adds to the client's ability to acquire the information and retrieve it (Frank & Keene, 1993).

TABLE 4–27
Planning Activities for Children

Below you will find various categories that should be considered when planning any activity. Check off the boxes where the category applies, then fill in the space provided.

BEHAVIORAL OBJECTIVE _____

DESCRIPTION OF ACTIVITY TO ACHIEVE OBJECTIVE _____

RELATIONSHIP OF ACTIVITY TO INTERMEDIATE AND LONG RANGE GOALS

| | *Activity* | *Intermediate Goal* | *Long Range Goal* |
| | _____ | _____ | _____ |

PLANNING CATEGORY	SPECIFIC COMPONENTS
Advance Organization Statements	❏ What _____ ❏ How _____ ❏ Why _____
Sources of Information For Activity	❏ Family ❏ Communicative Disorder ❏ Work ❏ Politics ❏ Hobbies ❏ Sports ❏ Books ❏ Current Events ❏ TV/Movies _____ ❏ Leisure Activities _____
Generalizable Features of Activities	❏ Family_____ ❏ School_____ ❏ Sports/Leisure _____ ❏ Social/etc. _____
Reinforcement	❏ Intrinsic _____ ❏ Extrinsic _____
Cultural Considerations	❏ Ethnicity/National Origin _____ ❏ Religion _____ ❏ Gender/Sexual Orientation _____ ❏ Exceptionality _____ ❏ Urban-Suburban-Rural _____ ❏ Geographic Region _____ ❏ Socioeconomic Class _____

Categorical. Categorical organization allows the learner to link various objects, behaviors, activities or concepts. Take, for example, a child who is being taught the following new vocabulary words: "dog," "hammer," "cup," and "car." They have no apparent relationship other than all being nouns. Lacking any interconnectness, the child will have difficulty developing a strategy for learning them. Contrast the above example with the following list: "cup," "plate," "glass," "bowl." In this example the interrelationship of words is obvious, all hold things that can be ingested. When activities are organized with the notion of interconnectedness, individuals learn more efficiently and can retrieve the information better.

Sequential. Certain activities are better organized sequentially. For example, in order for an aphasic client to go from her house to the clinic, she may need to (1) know the day for her appointment, (2) remember to take the exact amount of change for her bus fare, (3) be able to read the route designation on the bus and, (4) be able to read the number on the elevator in the clinic building. An appropriate way to organize the clinical activities with this client would be start with calender reading and end with elevator numbers.

Clinical Materials/Activities

Clinical materials and activities are the means by which learning takes place. For example, when practicing the production of a target phoneme, the client may be involved in a game. The game is the clinical material since it is not directly related to learning how to say the sound. The game may be an extraneous reinforcer or just a neutral vehicle for moving a learning activity along to its final goal. In selecting materials for a session, a number of considerations should be made. These involve interest, motivation, ease of generalization, efficiency, safety, and expense. In previous sections the first four considerations were explained. In this section, the safety and expense of materials will be discussed.

Safety. In terms of safety, the old adage that "if it can happen, it will happen" is an excellent guiding principle. Sharp objects

cut. Hard objects break. Unbalanced objects fall. Objects that should not be placed in the mouth are inevitably placed in the mouth. The selection of safe objects seems to be second nature to new clinicians who have children of their own or who have had extensive experience with children. For others with little experience, the hidden dangers of many objects are unseen. Often clients who will be using the materials have impaired cognitive abilities and may not be able to assess how materials can be safely used. Continually refer to the above adage as your guiding principle. Some consumer groups publish lists of objects and materials to avoid when working with children of various ages.

Expense. Materials should involve a minimum of expense. Usually the more expensive the materials, the more elaborate their configuration and the less flexible they are. Materials should not be the main focus of the therapeutic activity. They are merely the means by which strategies are taught. The more elaborate and expensive the materials, the more likely is that their use will overshadow the purpose of therapy. Keep materials simple and inexpensive.

Stimulus Configurations

Stimulus configuration is a term that refers to everything that is presented to a client and will be used to learn a new strategy, concept, or behavior. Its design may be the critical component in whether or not a client will be successful. In choosing or designing the stimulus configurations, a number of considerations need to be made. These are (1) simplification, (2) rate, (3) variation of configurations, (4) visualness, (5) redundancy, (6) task complexity, (7) context, and (8) figure-ground comparison.

Simplification. When designing a stimulus configuration there is a tendency to make it too complicated. Instead of using a simple method of teaching the client where to place his or her tongue in the production of a phoneme, an elaborate diagram will be drawn accompanied by arrows, charts, and words. Or instead of identifying one component necessary for the production of fluent speech, clients may be asked to focus on three or more behaviors. Clinical studies have shown that, as the stimulus configuration presented to subjects becomes more complex, it takes longer for them to learn the required task (Gillan & Lewis, 1994; Greenfield et al., 1994). Not only do simplified stimulus configurations result in quicker learning, but they are preferred by learners (Ramsay & Oatley, 1992). In the movie *City Slickers,* the cowboy eventually shares his secret of life with the main character. He holds up one finger and says, "one thing, that's the secret of life." Throughout the movie, the main character ponders the cowboy's philosophy until he comes to realize that the focus of life should be on one thing. It has direct applicability to the selection and creation of stimulus configurations. Never forget the purpose of the configuration. First identify it, then magnify that element so that everything else has less relevance. Table 4–28 provides a check sheet for analyzing stimulus configurations.

Rate of Presentation. Stimulus configurations can be presented for different lengths of time. For example, when demonstrating the position of articulators for the production of a sound, the clinician could momentary hold her tongue in place or keep it there for 10 seconds. When working with an aphasic client, a graphic representation of a strategy can be shown for a few seconds or for 30 seconds. Studies have shown that rate and length of presentation have a bearing on short-term memory (Frensch & Miner, 1994). The shorter the presentation, the more likely there will be problems in retrieving the stimulus configuration. Unfortunately, there are no standard times that are effective for every

client. Factors such as age, cognitive ability, and complexity of the stimulus make this impossible. Clinicians should use these findings in the French and Miner study as a general guideline for how long to allow the stimulus configuration to remain before expecting clients to retain it in their short-term memory. If clients are having difficulty in retaining information for short-term tasks, increase the amount of time the stimulus configuration remains visually or aurally observable. Experimentation is the key to determining the appropriate amount of time.

Often, clients are asked to do sequential tasks. That is to say, they contain more than one part. For example, when young clients have final consonant deletion problems, clinicians will often teach them how to say the word by chaining each of the syllables together (Bleile, 1995; Crary, 1993). In tasks that are sequential, the amount of time between the first response and the beginning of the second stimulus presentation should be as short as possible. Studies have shown that reducing the time between steps increases the probability that the task will be successfully completed (Frensch, Buchner, & Lin, 1994). To illustrate this we might use the example of the child with a final consonant deletion error. A clinician could ask the child to say "cu" (/ka/) a number of times to establish a consistent response pattern. Then have the child produce /p/. Finally, work on the production of "cup" (/kap/), with a delay of a few seconds between the stimulus for /ka/ and the stimulus for /p/. This would be an example of extending the amount of time between the production of the first part of the response and the presentation of the stimulus for the second part. In some approaches to teaching phonological rules, there is a minimal amount of time between these two events. An example of this occurs in Hodson and Paden's therapy program (1991). The stimulus for the first part of the utterance is a downward movement of the finger on the child's arm. With the pro-

TABLE 4–28
Stimulus Configuration

Use this form to analyze and modify one stimulus configuration. Version 1 should be the original configuration. Each of the subsequent versions should be the modifications you made in order to make it more effective. By systematically changing specific elements of your configuration, you will be able to see how each affects the performance of your client.

	VERSION 1	VERSION 2	VERSION 3
Simplicity Specify reductions of configurations.			
Rate of Presentation Length of time presentation will be present.			
Visualness Describe the most obvious visual components of the configuration.			
Redundancy List redundant stimulus configurations.			
Task Complexity For simple task, list obvious components. For more complex tasks, list less obvious oomponents (e.g., relational ones such as rules)			
Figure/Ground List both figure and ground elements	Figure Ground	Figure Ground	Figure Ground
Context Indicate the context in which the stimulus configuration will be taught and acknowledgment that the client is familiar with it.	Context Familiarity	Context Familiarity	Context Familiarity
Strategy List any categorization strategy that is used.			

duction of /ka/ the clinician's finger abruptly stops and taps the child's arm as the sound /p/ is presented by the clinician for the child to model. By reducing the amount of time between the first and second behavior, the likelihood of the child successfully completing the task is enhanced.

Variations in Stimulus Configurations. There may be times when it will be necessary to change stimulus configurations during a single learning task. For example, voice disordered clients who have both a gravelly and monotone voice may need to use two different strategies to learn how to improve their overall vocal quality (Andrews, 1995). This may require that during acquisition exercises both strategies need to be used. If clients are informed before the exercise begins that more than one strategy will be necessary and what the strategies should be, the likelihood that the exercise will be successfully completed will be increased (Cave, Pinker, Giorgi, Thomas et al., 1994).

Visualness of Stimulus Configurations. Many of the stimulus configurations presented to clients are auditory. Clinicians ask clients to perform certain tasks, and oral models are provided or strategies are described orally. Although it is necessary that speech is used to present these configurations, there is evidence that the presence of visual stimuli can increase the client's attention to the stimuli (Broadbent, 1992; Livesay & Porter, 1994). Not only is attention enhanced, but material is better retained, retrieved in controlled settings, and used more frequently in nontest and nonclinical settings (Dortch & Trombly, 1990). For example, if clients are being taught to expand two-word utterances into three-word utterances, the use of three blocks or even three pieces of paper to represent the new strategy may greatly increase the client's attention to the task. Some studies have shown that the use of visual configurations increases

attention, perceptions of the relevance of the configuration, confidence of the learner, and satisfaction with the learning experience (Klein & Freitag, 1991). There is evidence that the use of only visual configurations without verbalizations may reduce performance if the visual stimulus does not adequately represent the complexity of the task (DeeLucas & Larkin, 1991).

Other studies have investigated the relationship between the modality in which the configuration is presented and the modality in which the response is to be given. Ward (1994) found that visual configurations positively affected both graphic and vocalic responses in terms of accuracy and time required to emit the response. Auditory configurations, however, positively affected vocalic responses only. There are other advantages to using visual stimuli. Some studies have found that, when an individual is attempting to learn how a system with component parts works, the learning of the function of each component part is improved if the entire system is graphically displayed (Hegarty & Just, 1993; Kulhavy, Stock, & Kealy, 1993). For example, in teaching the concepts of time to cognitively disabled children, the concept of *past* should be graphically depicted in relationship to *present* and *future*. As another example, in producing all the phonemes within multisyllabic words with phonologically disordered children, each sound could be graphically depicted in multisyllabic words, with the target sound (the one that is omitted) highlighted in some way. Some studies have demonstrated that by constructing learning activities that focus on the relationship which exists between components and the whole, acquisition of component parts is improved (Oakhill, 1993).

Redundancy. It is a common practice to present only one stimulus configuration for a specific task that is to be learned. For example, when the clinician wishes to teach a client a new concept such as *ball,* only one ball may be presented. The hope is that by having a simple configuration the client will be able to acquire the concept of *ball-ness,* that is, objects that are symmetrical, have no corners, and bounce when dropped onto the floor. However, there is some evidence to suggest that concepts can be learned more quickly if there is a redundancy of complementary stimulus configurations (Sweller & Chandler, 1994). In this example, instead of presenting only one ball, several balls could be presented, each differing from the other in some form, such as size and color, yet all retaining the nature of *ballness.*

Task Complexity. The complexity of what clients are asked to learn ranges from the simplicity of placing the tongue on the alveolar ridge to the difficulty of understanding the rules for using relative clauses. There is evidence to suggest that what is remembered about the stimulus configuration may be related to the complexity of the task (Goolkasian, Van Wallendael, and Terry, 1991). Researchers found that, when tasks were less complex, subjects tended to use the more superficial parts of the configuration for solving problems. However, when the tasks were more difficult, success was related to how well they retained the more complex aspects of the configuration. Of importance to speech-language clinicians is an understanding that the stimulus configuration they will be presenting to clients will usually have many components. If the task is simple, the stimulus configuration should stress fairly obvious components. However, if the task is difficult, the more complex elements of the configuration should be stressed. In a study involving the retrieval of complex information requiring the integration of reading material, emphasizing simple configurations diminished the learners' ability to draw inferences from the material (Peterson, 1992). Components were emphasized in the study by highlighting parts

of written material with a highlighting pen. In speech-language therapy, take for example the correct placement of the tongue and lips to produce /p/. There is nothing very complicated about demonstrating lip closure. Clinicians may demonstrate by closing their lips with their fingers and/or using a picture depicting two lips meeting each other. However, understanding the correct use of relative clauses is significantly more complicated. In teaching relative clauses the configuration must stress the rules for their usage. This may involve highlighting both verbally and visually the conditions necessary for their use to be acceptable.

Figure-Ground. The term figure-ground refers to methods for causing one thing in a perceptual field to stand out from everything else (Piaget, 1963). For example, in advertising, a poster will feature some aspect of the picture to which the advertiser would like to direct the reader's attention. When looking at an advertisement of a vacation resort in an outdoor magazine, views of the resort's magnificent trout-inhabited river might appear in the foreground, with other activities appearing smaller in the background. The same resort advertising in a golf magazine would feature their golf course in the front of the advertisement, with a distant shot of the river in the background. By highlighting, or making one aspect of a stimulus configuration stand out from everything else, not only is the viewer's perceptual field manipulated, but changes also occur at the conceptual level. Highlighting gives things an added sense of importance. When this procedure is used in therapy, features of a stimulus which may be more critical for learning become the focal point of attention. By manipulating the stimulus configuration so that its most critical aspects are highlighted, learning is enhanced (Gopher, Weil, & Siegel, 1989). Take for example, teaching the use of articles to a child who frequently omits them. Normally, when asked to say "the boy runs fast," a cognitively impaired child responds with "boy runs fast." To teach the child to use articles, the clinician might decide to use a four card system where each card represents one unit of the utterance. On each card a symbol is used to present the word. The cards might look like the following.

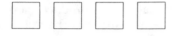

Although each item in the utterance is noted, there is nothing to indicate that the article in the first position is the focus of the activity. By minimally changing the stimulus configuration, it becomes very obvious where the focus of attention should be directed.

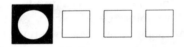

The same activity is presented, but with the modified cards the client's attention is focused more on the first unit because it is larger and has a different color. In presenting almost any kind of stimulus configuration, a similar modification can be made to involve increased vocalization, colors, shapes, textures, or other characteristics that enhance figure-ground differences. Another method for highlighting features is the use of intonation patterns. Recall is enhanced when an intonation pattern is used that either accents what is to be focused on, or an abrupt pitch change occurs on what is important (Frankish, 1995). In the above example of the child with the article problem, clinicians might want to vocally accent the article in their presentation.

Another important reason for producing large figure-ground distinctions is that, over a period of time, the distinguishing features of a stimulus configuration diminish (Riccio, Ackil, & Burch-Vernon, 1992). What this means is that over time the power of aspects of the configuration that originally were important in learning a behavior lose their distinctiveness. Therefore, it would seem that the more distinctive the feature is, the more resistant it is to decay.

Context. Much of the "whole language" movement is predicated on the concept that by incorporating language concepts within a broader context, children will learn significantly better (Naremore, Densmore, & Harman, 1995). Many research studies have justified the use of this approach for children with average or above average reading abilities (Umbach, Darch, & Halpin, 1989; Zabrucky & Commander, 1993). The whole language movement has been incorporated into speech-language therapy when teaching linguistic concepts to children with language disabilities. One of the basic tenets of the approach is that the language concept is always taught in meaningful contexts. Although the movement has much to offer, clinicians need to be aware of how cognition affects the clients' ability to use context for learning. An important study showed that subjects' ability to use context to learn new concepts varied with the context's familiarity (Shefelbine, 1990). The less familiar they were with the context, the poorer they performed when learning new language concepts. These findings can be directly translated into suggestions for using context as a teaching variable for clients with communicative disorders. Unless you are sure that the context in which you present your stimulus configuration is known and familiar to the client, the use of context may act as an interfering variable in the acquisition of new behaviors, rather than as a facilitative one. For example, a clinician may wish to teach the concepts of *bear, tiger,* and *elephant* to a child with limited productive language abilities. To facilitate the acquisition of the task, the clinician constructs an elaborate activity involving the creation of a zoo game. Unless the client is familiar with what a zoo is, the context may be confusing and result in poorer learning of the animal concepts than if no context was used. When the context is familiar to the client, it can significantly assist in enhancing retention. The most appropriate procedure would be for clinicians to orally or visually elaborate on what is to be retained. The elaboration becomes the context. It is a mistake to believe that clients will spontaneously perform this type of elaboration. In comparisons between instructor-elaborated events and events where the instructor allowed subjects to perform their own elaborations, instructor-elaborated events resulted in significantly better memory scores (Wood, Needham, Williams, & Roberts, 1994).

Categorization. One of the strategies individuals can use to organize objects and events is categorization. Although there are many ways in which objects and events can be categorized (all of which will be presented in Chapter 9), two of the most basic ones used with children are color and shape (Macario, 1991). As early as 2 years of age, children recognize that color has predictive validity for membership in some categories. Color was also the preferred strategy for 3-year-olds in categorizing things to eat. Shape was used with novel items that the children thought were play objects. Clinicians may wish, therefore, to utilize shapes as categorization devices for objects, while using colors for classifying foods.

Objectives

Clinicians may wish to accomplish many objectives during a session. These may involve: (1) gaining information, (2) redirecting attitudes, (3) learning of strategies and teaching behaviors.

Gaining Information. Often, one purpose of a session is to gain information about clients, or to determine their ability to retrieve and use behaviors or strategies that were previously learned. We can gain information by asking specific types of questions in formats that have been designed to yield the desired results (Culatta & Goldberg, 1995). For example, open-ended questions tend to produce more inclusive and better answers than close-ended questions. Information also can be gained through both normative and nonstandardized means. Normative tests are evaluative instruments that have been standardized on large populations and provide clinicians with specific data points for determining the ability of clients to perform a large variety of behaviors. One example of a standardized test is the *Peabody Picture Vocabulary Test* (Dunn & Dunn, 1981). The test was normed on a large number of children at various ages. Based on the data from this population, we can determine the range of normal responses for clients between the ages of 2.5 and 40 years. Nonstandard means are methods that do not have standardized data to compare the clients' performance to, but still provide valuable information to clinicians. An example of a nonstandard method would be an analysis of a conversation into its component grammatical and semantical units. The gathering of information is also called *assessment* or *diagnostic* evaluation. Regardless of the words used, they refer to the gathering of information, not intervention. What may appear to be therapy is often evaluation. The distinction between therapy and evaluation will be made in Chapter 8.

Redirecting Attitudes. The attitudes clients and their families have about certain behaviors and aspects of therapy may have a direct bearing on progress. For example, the mother of a Down syndrome child who believes that her child must continually be protected from society may unwittingly prevent her child from gaining the ability to experience failures that are necessary for developing independent living skills. The stutterer who believes that she cannot exert any control over her fluency will never get beyond minimally modifying the stuttering response. The child with vocal nodules who sees no correlation between his screaming and the development of the pathology will have the condition recur in spite of the nodules' surgical removal. In all of these examples, a precursor to changing the desired behavior is the changing of an attitude that has negative effects on the therapeutic progress. In all of these cases, one immediate goal should be the redirecting of attitudes. In Chapter 9, methods for changing attitudes are discussed.

Learning Strategies. Clients come to therapy because they have been unable to learn how to produce a group of behaviors, rarely because they cannot produce only a single behavior. Even with misarticulations, children usually do not misarticulate only a single sound in only one word. The error will probably be pervasive in most words containing that sound in the child's language. For example a 4-year-old, who is still using single-and two-word utterances to express needs is not brought to the clinic to learn new unrelated two- to five-word utterances. Rather, she has been unable to learn the rules for combining words that result in the production of two- to five-word utterances. If therapy focuses on merely teaching each new utterance as if it was unrelated, progress would be painstakingly slow. Effective therapy in this example would involve teaching the child the rule for producing utterances of specific lengths. The rule becomes a strategy that the child will use to produce unique structures she has not been taught. Virtually all therapy should involve the teaching of strategies, whether that means the rules for producing three-word utterances, a strategy for retrieving the units of mea-

surement in money, methods for remembering to include the final syllables of words, or retrieval of cues for producing fluent speech. In Chapter 9 the methods for structuring strategies will be discussed.

Teaching Specific Behaviors. There will be times when a very specific behavior will need to be taught to the client. It may involve learning the correct placement of the tongue to produce a phoneme or learning the rate of speech to use in order for fluency to occur. Even when the behavior appears to be incredibly small and well defined, a strategy can usually be found to facilitate its production. For example, the correct placement of the tongue may involve the use of a visual cuing system that will enable the client to achieve the correct placement, rather than merely modeling the placement.

MODELING

Modeling is a clinical procedure where an exact or similar representation of a behavior that is desired is presented to the client. It is widely used and thought to be an appropriate method of acquiring knowledge. Often it is the only procedure that will work with clients, especially individuals who have severe cognitive impairments, are young, or are attempting to develop a complex behavior whose description may defy words. As important as the procedure is, it does have a negative consequence. When clients are presented with a model to emulate, they forgo what Kendall (1984) calls "creative discovery." This term aptly describes the cognitive discovery process that individuals experience when problems are solved through the use of their own efforts. There is some concern that when modeling is used instead of creative discovery, the learning process may be short-circuited. Some studies have shown that the observation of target behaviors as a learning technique is effective with simple behaviors, but not necessarily with more complicated ones (Berry, 1991)

When there is no alternative to modeling, it should be done by the clinician or another individual. When using models, clinicians should consider (1) how the model will be presented, (2) the type of model to be used, and (3) the sequence of model presentation.

Presentation of the Model

It is preferable that the model is presented by someone other than the clinician when the client has a cognitive impairment. The reason for this is to avoid confusion on the part of the client. If the clinician models the behavior, it may be possible for the client to confuse the roles of the person asking for responses and individual asked to respond.

Types of Models

Modeling behaviors is very effective in presenting appropriate motor targets or simple responses for clients to emulate (Dworkin, 1991). Modeling can take many forms, from visual presentations by the clinician to recorded videotapes. Although modeling can be effective for demonstrating more complex behaviors such as grammatical structures, it should be used with caution. The purpose of modeling is to enable the client to imitate a response. If complex behaviors are imitated, the client may short-circuit the process of learning the rules necessary to acquire the behavior. Take for example a situation where a clinician wishes to teach a client to produce a three-word utterance such as "blue car goes." If she just uses the model "blue car goes," and asks the client to say what she says, the probability that the client will learn the rule "attribute + object + action" is significantly reduced. Evidence of this problem usually occurs when utterances such as "big car stops" and "little boy runs" also must be modeled. When more complex

behaviors cannot be mastered even when the therapy process has been restructured, modeling can be used, but what should be modeled is the strategy for producing the correct response, not the response itself.

Sequence for Presentation and Withdrawal

Regardless of the form the model takes, it should be presented in the following sequence: (1) the clinician provides the model with the client watching and listening, (2) while the modeled behavior is presented, the client emulates it, and (3) the client emulates the behavior without the model being present.

Provide Model with Client Watching and Listening. During the first presentation of the model, the client is required only to watch and listen. The model can be presented more than once. Before moving on to the next stage, clinicians should be reasonably certain that the client was attending and the components of the model were understood. For some clients this might require multiple presentations, extending the length of time necessary to present the model, or highlighting each of its components. For example, when demonstrating extensive prolongation to a client, clinicians may want to decrease the rate of speech even slower than the target rate to emphasize the importance of slowing down. They may even move their hands in an exaggerated slow manner to visually represent the importance of slowing the rate on every syllable.

Client Emulates Behavior with Model Present. After clients have had sufficient time to observe and understand the model, clinicians should ask clients to produce the model with them in unison. Often this takes the form of the request, "Now watch me and do what I do." The only problem with the structure of the activity is that it may be difficult for clients to model the clinicians' behavior without directly comparing them. Clients who are asked to match the placement of articulators by observing the clinicians and kinesically determining whether their tongue placement is identical are at a disadvantage. They are trying to match a model using different modalities: visual presentation by the clinicians, kinesic response by the clients. Modalities used for presentation of the model should be the same modalities used by the clients for responding. There is evidence to suggest that a mismatching of model and response modalities results in poorer performance then when the two are matched (Glenberg & Langston, 1992; Norris, 1994). In the above example, this simply would mean having both the clinician and the client look into a mirror when the model is presented. When modeling strategies, both the clinician and client should use the graphic representation of the strategy together. For example, in teaching a client to produce three-word utterances with the use of cards, the clinician may take the client's hand and together they would touch each card as a word is produced.

Performing Behavior Without Model Being Present. The final activity in modeling procedures is the removal of the model. For some clients this may occur after only one joint production of the behavior. For other clients with more severe cognitive deficits, or when more complex behavioral responses are requested, several joint productions may be necessary. The elimination of the model may also require a gradual reduction of its components rather than the abrupt termination of it. With clients with apraxia, for example, modeling of a word may start with the entire word, then progress to modeling only the final phoneme, and eventually phasing out the model completely.

CONSISTENCY

A recurring theme of most good therapy is consistency. Consistency should not be confused with rigidity. Consistency refers to the recurring application of a specific skill with minimal differences.

Areas of Importance

Although it is important to be consistent in all areas of therapy, three areas may be more important than others: (1) interaction styles, (2) skills application, and (3) consequences for behaviors.

Interaction Style. Clients rely on consistency in their clinicians. In most cases, clients look to clinicians for direction and guidance. Suggestions are taken and actualized either into behaviors or new attitudes. As teachers, mentors, and supportive individuals, clinicians need to be consistent in their own behaviors. What is deemed appropriate today, should be so next week. What is reinforced in one session should be reinforced in subsequent sessions. What is unacceptable in one session should be unacceptable in all sessions.

Skills. Consistency in the application of skills seems to be one critical distinction between master clinicians and less experienced clinicians. In the process of identifying skills for this book, the clinical behaviors of master clinicians and advanced graduate students were compared. Although virtually all of the skills were present in the therapy of the students, very few were applied consistently. The master clinicians, however, consistently and appropriately applied all of the clinical skills they used. It appears that the consistent application of skills may be related not only to their knowledge, but also to experience.

Consequences. Few things can alienate and confuse children as much as the inconsistent application of consequences. Children look for and need consistency in adults, especially their clinicians. It is important that there are no gray areas. When clinicians tell their clients what the consequences will be for certain behaviors, it is crucial that they occur. This applies to both positive reinforcement and punishment.

If a positive reinforcer does not occur when one was supposed to, the child may believe that the behavior either was not correct or is no longer desirable. For example, in working with a cognitively impaired blind child, a clinician was attempting to establish imitative vocal behavior. The child was able to consistently imitate the clinician's production of sound sequences containing two, three, and four repetitions of the sound. After each correct sequence, the clinician would reinforce the child by hugging her and using verbal and vocal patterns that in the past had been shown to be reinforcing. After the fifth alternation of sequences, the clinician forgot to reinforce the child. For the next request, the client produced an incorrect sequence that she had produced correctly earlier in the session. After four attempts she produced it correctly and was reinforced. During the remainder of the session, she correctly produced various sequences and the clinician was more diligent at reinforcing every one of them.

If clinicians use the threat of punishment for inappropriate behavior, it is crucial that it is applied. This usually takes the form of threatening the child that, if a behavior occurs, such as acting out or going off task, certain desirable activities will not occur. Although the threat may be effective with many children, with others it will not be until they test the clinician. Tests sometimes are subtle. If a child is told that he will not be allowed to participate in an activity if he gets out of his chair, he may stand up but hold on to the top of the chair to see if the clinician will really institute the threat. If none if forthcoming, the next test may be to actually leave the chair.

When using punishment, it is important that the parameters are very clearly and unambiguously explained to children, and then consistently and rigorously applied.

Effects

Theoretically one can easily see why it would be important to be consistent in therapy. On a practical level, the effects of consistent clinical practice have been amply documented (Oliver, Lightfoot, Searight, & Katz, 1990). Consistency in therapy has been found to be correlated with therapy duration and participation. The more consistent the clinician, the more likely it is that therapy will not be prematurely terminated, and the client will take an active position in the clinical process. A lack of consistency can produce different results in different age groups. With adults, inconsistent practice results in less favorable opinions of clinicians, but no negative opinions result on the part of adolescents (Morris, 1991). The inconsistent use of skills with children results in more direct effects in therapy. Children, by nature, are constantly seeking to find the limits of acceptable behavior, regularities, and rules of interaction, and the consequences of both acceptable and unacceptable behaviors. Clinicians whose behaviors are inconsistent create tremendous problems for children who are attempting to understand the adult world in which they are forced to live. What may have been acceptable during the first 15 minutes of the session is no longer acceptable 15 minutes later, and may now result in a negative consequence. A behavior that produced adulation from the clinician 10 minutes ago, is now virtually ignored. Children become confused, irritated, and noncompliant when they think that the rules of the interaction are subject to the whims of the clinician. In situations like these, therapy tends to become a negative, nonproductive, or at best, an inconsistent experience for the child.

PROFESSIONAL TERMINOLOGY AND STYLE

For new students, one of the most difficult adjustments to make is in their writing style. What was reinforced in college classes in creative writing is now devalued. The ability to use flourishes, imagery, and intriguing ambiguities has no place in a clinical report. Reports require precise terminology, tight grammatical structures, clarity of thought, and a painstaking emphasis on justifications.

The emphasis on objectivity and clarity of thought is not based on a need to appear scientific. Rather, there are very practical reasons for the clinical format and style. The primary purpose of reports is not to provide the present clinician with a summary of events. Rather, it is to provide individuals who have no prior knowledge of either the client or clinician with information that will allow them to have a firm grasp of the clients' capabilities and problems.

Terminology

Although each clinical and school setting has its own report writing format, appropriate terminology is not dependent on the setting. What is acceptable terminology in university clinics, hospital settings, public schools, private practices, and clinical research facilities should be identical.

Descriptions of Behaviors and Events.

Many people see but very few observe. This was the view of the German photographer Renger-Patzsch who believed that life was so visually complex, that most people had difficulty really observing what was happening in front of them (Dooly, 1996). In all of his photography, he emphasized the intrinsic beauty of common objects that were always seen but rarely observed. Through his photographs the commonalty of things such as the ascending lines of a smoke stack and the inside of the foxglove plant were transformed into images of visual beauty that have been admired as classics for over 70 years. It was Goethe who said that the hardest thing to see is that which is before our eyes (Lowith, 1964). When verbally describing behaviors and events, clinicians need to be as exacting as the photographs created by Renger-Patzsch. Examples of appropriate and inappropriate descriptive terms can be found in Table 4–29. Terms that are identified as inappropriate have that designation because they are either too vague or convey a description that is subjective, evaluative, or nonverifiable. To the right of each term is a better way of describing what the clinician is attempting to convey.

Historical. The terminology used to identify ethnicity, disorders, and professional practice has changed throughout the history of our field. Even the name of our field has continued to undergo changes. Regardless of one's feeling about the terms used, it is appropriate to use currently acceptable terminology, not because it is the "politically correct" thing to do, but rather because of two other reasons. The first reason is that changes in terminology often are initiated by those to whom it refers. It is right and proper for individuals who will have terms referring to themselves to choose what those terms should be. The second reason is that, if the primary focus of clinical practice is to facilitate the development of new behaviors, it is important to minimize variables that may interfere with the process. Identifying a client by a term that is unacceptable to him or her can significantly interfere with the clinical process. Table 4–30 lists terms that have undergone changes throughout the years.

Justification

When writing a report, you should assume that the person who will be reading it does not know either you or your client. Therefore, no assumptions should be made

TABLE 4–29
Descriptive Terminology

INAPPROPRIATE	BETTER
___ %	give % of what
angry	qualify with specific behaviors
bad	?
believes	all right if in direct quote (e.g., the client said he believes...); not appropriate for clinician, describe behaviors, events
better	provide numbers/reference
consistent	provide numbers as ratio
cooperative	describe specific events
cute	describe features
distrusts	describe client's statements, behaviors that indicate distrust exists
fast	provide numbers
feels	all right if in direct quote (e.g., the client said he feels...); not appropriate for clinician, describe behaviors, events
good	?
happy	qualify with specific behaviors
hopes	all right if in direct quote (e.g., the client said he hopes...); not appropriate for clinician, describe behaviors, events
inconsistent	provide numbers as ratio
maybe	explain why qualification is necessary
mild	provide quantitative reference point
moderate	provide quantitative reference point
nice	describe behavior/object
OK	not professional
pretty	describe features and/or clothes
resistive	provide specific behaviors
sad	qualify with specific behaviors
severe	?
slow	provide numbers
sometimes	give number
strongly	describe behaviors
tried really hard	describe manner of attempt
trusts	describe client's statements, behaviors that indicate trust exists
uncooperative	describe specific events
very	if referring to quantity, describe in numbers; if quality, describe behaviors
worse	provide numbers/reference

TABLE 4–30
Historical Changes in Terminology

EARLY USAGE	INTERMEDIATE USAGE	CURRENT USAGE
Speech Therapist	Speech-Language Therapist	Speech-Language Clinician
Speech Correction	Speech Therapy	Speech-Language Therapy
Crippled	Handicapped	Disabled (appropriate) Challenged (inappropriate) [a]
Oriental	Asian	Asian/Pacific Islander [b]
Negro	Black	African American [b]
Mexican	Mexican-American	
Chicano	Hispanic [b]	
Indian	American Indian	Native American [b]
American Speech and Hearing Association	American Speech-Language-Hearing Association	American Association of Speech-Language Pathologists and Audiologists

[a] The use of the term *challenged* when referring to someone with a physical, medical, or cognitive disorder is an inappropriate and often cruel use of the term. Many disabled individuals are disturbed by its use.

[b] These terms are used by the federal government when identifying various ethnic groups. The use of more specific ethnic labels is appropriate (e.g., under Hispanic there can be Mexicans, Mexican Americans, Salvadorans, etc.).

regarding either knowledge of the client or the intent of your words. There are four questions you should consider when writing a report: (1) Can the statement in principle be justified? (2) If it can be justified, can the justification appear in the statement? (3) If the statement can be justified, but the justification does not appear in the statement, does it appear in the following statement? And (4) If the statement cannot be justified, why does it appear in the report?

Justification in Principle. One of the abiding rules of science is that all assertions must in principle be disprovable (Hempel, 1965). An example adhering to this principle would be the assertion that reducing the rate of a stutterer's speech will result in fluency. The statement is in

principle disprovable because the stutterer's rate can be slowed and the results documented. If the practice of speech-language pathology holds itself to be a clinical science, the above principle must not be violated. The extension of this principle is that descriptions of objects, people, behaviors, and events should be in terms that are in principle disprovable. An example of a disprovable event would be:

> The 11- year old-child came to the clinic wearing a white lace dress whose front was covered with peanut butter and whose back had what appeared to be smudges of dried red, green, and yellow paint.

Every word contained in the above description is in principle disprovable and also immediately understandable to the reader. If another individual was present when the girl entered the clinic, every description contained in the statement could be verified or disproved. Compare it with a description of the same event, using terminology which in principle is not disprovable.

> A charming 11- year old child came into the clinic wearing an adorable white lace dress which unfortunately was very dirty.

The terms "charming," "adorable," "unfortunately," and "very dirty" are all evaluative terms whose meaning is dependent on the observer's cultural values. Additionally, none are sufficiently precise to provide an observer who was not present and was not intimately knowledgeable of the writer's cultural values with an objective understanding of the events. The second reader is forced to intuit the events from a written description that was based on a subjective evaluation.This is not good science and not good therapy.

Immediate. As important as it may be to use purely objective terms when describing behaviors, events, objects, and people, there may be times when it is more practical to use a term or concept that is subjective. For example, when describing the vocal qualities of a client's voice, the term "harshness" conveys a specific qualitative nature regarding the client's voice that may not be evident in referring to the client (Andrews, 1995). In cases such as these, the term can be used if what immediately follows is a behavioral description containing objective measurements. Below is an example of an appropriate immediate justification for harshness.

> The client's voice could be described as "harsh," since pitch breaks occurred at the onset of phonation, and glottal fry occurred through the conversation.

Even if a reader of the report did not agree with the depiction of the voice as "harsh," by knowing the behavioral indicators of the judgment (pitch breaks and glottal fry), a reasonably accurate understanding of the client's voice is possible.

Delayed. For various stylistic reasons, it may not be possible to include the justification in the statement containing the subjective term. When that occurs, the justification should occur immediately in the next statement. It is not appropriate to place this justification in another section or delay it. When readers come to terms that are ambiguous or subjective, one of two things will occur. The first is that they will utilize their own frame of reference to understand what the term meant. In this case, unless their frame of reference is identical to that of the writer, there is a danger that the picture of clients' behavior may become distorted. If the description forms a basis of what will follow in the report, the distortion becomes magnified, affecting many aspects of an understanding of clients and their behaviors. The second thing that occurs when justifications do not follow subjective terms is that some readers may dismiss the observations since they are not in principle verifiable. This may lead to disregarding information that could be important in understanding clients and their problems.

No Justification. It is hard to imagine a reason for not being able to justify what is written in a report. Often the reason people give for not providing justification is that what they are presenting is more of an *impression* than a description. And by placing these statements in a section of the report called "Impressions," there is no obligation to provide justification. Wrong! Nothing in a clinical report is inconsequential. The report may be read by the client, the family, other clinicians, insurance agents, and professionals years after the writer can even remember doing the report. Reports have a life of their own, often conveying inappropriate information for many years. There is nothing wrong with providing impressions at the end of a clinical report. However, they should be clearly distinguished from observations and provide the reader with at least some behavioral observations that lend credence to the impressions. Impressions on clinical reports have far greater consequences than impressions one may have of a movie, novel, or painting. The consequences of inappropriate impressions in clinical reports may involve gross errors in the design of future intervention programs.

CHAPTER
5

Process Foundational Skills

*C*lients enter into a very special psychological place in therapy. It is a setting in which they are being asked to disregard all of their defenses, which have served them well, and place all of their faith in an individual whom they do not know, who has no a priori understanding of their life experiences, and whose professional experience, successes, and ethics are usually unknown. If clients willingly are to allow themselves to be vulnerable, they will need to perceive the clinician as a trusting, safe, and competent individual. Often the perception is based on the personal qualities displayed by the clinician. Most people acknowledge the importance of these clinician qualities in therapeutic settings. These include perceptions of clinician warmth, openness, compassion and empathy (Murphy, 1982; Rogers, 1965; Satir, 1967). Some feel that these qualities are innate and cannot be taught, while others believe that although the quality cannot be taught, behaviors that result in their perception by clients are teachable (Goldberg, 1993). Regardless of where one stands in this training issue, most agree

that when these characteristics are perceived by clients, it generally has a positive effect on therapy. Although clinical scientists may agree on their importance, most have expressed a difficulty with determining an appropriate way of measuring them. How does one measure the strength of *openness*, or *compassion*? It is difficult, if not impossible. Difficulties in measurement have led some clinical researchers to abandon the effort altogether (Ingham, 1984). Although difficult to measure, few would argue that they are not important. Instead of trying to assess the presence and strength of these qualities in clinicians, an alternative approach is to measure the effect of what these qualities are supposed to create. That is, *trust*. Trust is operationally defined here as a willingness on the part of the client or family to (1) provide the clinician with potentially damaging or embarrassing information or (2) willingly engage in behaviors that may be difficult or embarrassing, with the faith that through a discussion of requested experiences or by engaging in suggested behaviors, they will improve. Although difficult to establish, this clinical condition is the foundation upon which therapy is based. *Trust* as it is defined here relates to clients' willingness to do or say specific things because they have certain positive feelings about their clinician. It is an outcome measure, rather than a perception. What appears in this section are 11 categories of skills containing 58 techniques and behaviors. The application of these techniques and behaviors lead to perceptions of clinicians which will contribute to the development of trust.

RAPPORT

Rapport is important for developing a therapeutic relationship (Roberts & Bouchard, 1989). It is the establishment of a commonality of interest between two people or a mutual understanding of each other's values, beliefs, and experiences. Additionally, the interactions which occur between the interactants are viewed as positive (Tickle-Degnen & Rosenthal, 1990). Clinically, this would translate into a willingness on the part of the client to engage in activities because of the quality of the relationship which exists between the client and the clinician.

Benefits

Change is a threatening process. It requires individuals to examine the function of present behaviors, the commitment to establishing new behaviors, and possibly performing self-assessments that may be less then flattering. The natural reaction to any activity which is threatening is either to become defensive or to attack. In the clinic, a defensive posture results in the development of defensive reactions, and a hostile posture is usually exhibited through interpersonal conflicts. Although each behavior is distinct, they often are intertwined into a gestalt that can be difficult for clinicians to effectively defuse. It is

best to prevent them from occurring by using various skills, such as rapport.

Defensive Reactions. Defensive reactions usually take one of two different forms. The first is verbal statements constructed in the form of justifications to what is perceived as an accusation. Take for example, the following interaction that occurred between a clinician and a young adult.

Clinician: If you did not try your new voice at home, work, or at the party, then it seems to me that you aren't really that committed to change.

Client: No, that's not true. You have no idea how hard it is to concentrate on those things you told me to do when there's other things going on. What do you mean that I'm not committed? I haven't missed one session nor even been late. I really do want to change. Maybe the problem is with the things you told me to do.

Whether or not the clinician's statements are true, they are by their very nature threatening. By not having already established rapport with the client, the client response should have been expected. If rapport had been established, the response would have been far less defensive. The client may not have found it necessary to rationalize away his problem. The second form of a defensive reaction is what appears to be a "shut-down" of the person's ability to hear what is being said. He might be unresponsive to the clinician's statements or even attempt to change the topic completely. It is as if he has been encapsulated by something that prevents anything from penetrating his consciousness.

Interpersonal Conflicts. Not all clients will be defensive. Some choose to become verbally combative with their clinician. They meet every confrontative statement with a counter punch, in a style reminiscent of a welterweight boxing match. Some researchers have found that if rapport has been established with clients, interpersonal conflicts of this type are usually avoided (Cheng, 1973). Within the clinical context, there may be occasions when clinicians need to be confrontative with clients. It may involve confronting the clients' lack of responsibility, reluctance to accurately perceive their own behaviors or those of their children, or unwillingness to critically evaluate their own performance. In these and other difficult interactions, a normal reaction may be one of annoyance or even outright hostility, such as, "Who is this person who's telling me what to do or think!". If rapport has been previously established with clients, potential hostility-producing statements of clinicians will most likely be perceived as constructive and intended to help rather than chastise.

Methods

Three ways of establishing rapport are to create the perception of warmth, share a commonality of interest and values, and indicate a genuine concern for individuals and their problems.

Perceptions of Personal Warmth. Studies have shown that when the client perceives the clinician as a *warm* individual, the likelihood that rapport will be developed is enhanced (Jackson, 1985). It may be difficult to operationalize *warmth* into specific behaviors. Usually terms such as *open, understanding, genuine*, and *kind* are identified with individuals who are warm. These terms, just as is warm, are difficult to operationally define. They all appear to be related to a total, all encompassing perception of an individual. Possibly because of their global nature, opera-

tional definitions are difficult to create. We may be left with the Supreme Court judge's admonition about pornography. We may not be able to define warmth, but we can identify a warm individual when we see one.

Commonality of Interest. Having a commonality of interest does not necessarily mean that you and the client have similar knowledge of specific areas. Rather, the interest may be there regardless of the knowledge level. An example of this was a clinician whose client was an experienced sea kayaker. Although the clinician knew nothing about the sport, she was very interested in it. Since this was an area the client felt comfortable discussing, and was passionate about it, he welcomed the clinician's questions. It became the vehicle for establishing rapport. Unfortunately, it may not always be possible to find an area where both the client and clinician have similar interests. In cases such as those, by carefully constructing questions and following through on conversations, the perception of interest can be created. For example, an adult laryngectomized Japanese client who was a retired restaurant owner was assigned to a student clinician. She knew very little about Japanese culture and even less about the restaurant business. The client had been reluctant to use laryngectomized speech, possibly due to embarrassment or just because he had little to say. As the clinician began asking questions about the restaurant business, and appeared to be fascinated by his answers, the client's speech output increased substantially.

You can begin establishing a commonality of interest before the first session begins by reviewing the client's folder, if one is available. If that is not possible, a short conversation over the phone may be sufficient. In reviewing the information, you should think about categorizing it into various areas. Tables 5–1 to 5–3 are provided for your convenience. In the tables, you can

TABLE 5–1
Commonality of Interest
Children

CLINICIAN INTERESTS	CLIENT INTERESTS				
	Home	Sports/Leisure	School	Play	Television

identify specific areas of potential commonality and insert topics under each. For children and adults, conversations prior to the session are especially helpful.

Genuine Concern. Often when attempting to be *professional* or *scientific*, clinicians may be perceived as distant or *cold*. If the relationship between the clinician and client is a passive one, then the perception of concern may not be critical. For example, although it would be nice if the neurosurgeon could be perceived as concerned about her patient, it is irrelevant for the removal of a life-threatening tumor. However, the situation is quite different when the relationship between client and clinician is active. Communicatively disordered clients need to be ac-

tively involved in the development of their new communicative behaviors. The degree of their involvement may be directly related to their perception of the clinician. Clients who perceive their clinicians as genuinely concerned about their welfare are more likely to work cooperatively with them than those who are not perceived as concerned.

Limitations

Unfortunately, some people rely on rapport more than they should. Although critical for establishing a solid foundation for therapy, it is not a panacea on which one's laurels can rest. It is not sufficient for establishing trust, nor does it substitute for competence.

TABLE 5–2
Commonality of Interest
Adolescents

CLINICIAN INTERESTS	CLIENT INTERESTS					
	Home	Sports/Leisure	Music	Television	School	Other

Not Sufficient for Establishing Trust.

As important as rapport may be, it is not sufficient for the establishment of trust. Rapport refers to an interaction process that is not necessarily related to outcome. I may have a wonderful rapport with a individual I have known for many years, but I might be loathe to take his advice on child rearing if he has had no contact with children as an adult. In order to accept his advice, I would also need to trust his judgment about child rearing.

Not a Substitute For Competence.

Within the clinic, even excellent rapport with a client does not necessarily result in good therapy. Some would argue that although it can facilitate trust, it may not be a necessary component (Costello, 1980). Take for example the brilliant heart surgeon with a dismal bedside manner. You chose her to operate on you, not because you felt comfortable with her as a person or had anything in common with her, but rather you chose her because of your trust in her ability to increase your chances of survival after the operation. Rapport facilitates the development of trust, but is not sufficient to create it.

EMPATHY AND COMPASSION

The terms *empathy* and *compassion* are used interchangeably to describe a perception on the part of clients that clinicians are capable of understanding their feelings and emotions. In this text, *empathy*

TABLE 5–3
Commonality of Interest
Adults

CLINICIAN INTERESTS	CLIENT INTERESTS						
	Home	Sports/ Leisure	Television	Music	Current Events	Work	Other

will be used to describe this perception. As a perception, it may mirror reality or have nothing to do with it. For clinicians, it may be important that clients perceive them as empathetic, regardless of what they are feeling. The use of empathy in the helping sciences has been routinely accepted as an important part of the interaction process. In spite of its acceptance for over three decades, its efficacy in the clinical setting remains undocumented (Morse, Anderson, Bottorff, & Yonge, 1992). This has led some clinical educators to posit that empathy is a concept adapted from psychology that may not fit within the clinical reality of certain health care professions, such as nursing. Possibly the same is true for the area of speech-language pathology.

In spite of a lack of empirical data, most clinicians believe that empathy is an important component of therapy. Its value is best understood by examining its types and uses.

Types

The empathetic feeling that clinicians can have towards their clients can be of two different types: cognitive and emotional (Gross, 1994). While some may believe that emotional empathy is more genuine, it creates a variety of problems for clinicians that do not occur with cognitive empathy.

Emotional. Emotional empathy involves feelings clinicians experience by personally identifying with clients and their distress. On a very simplistic level, it is the equivalent of the current phrase "been there, done that." In the area of speech-language pathology the importance of emotional empathy has been extensively emphasized in treating only one disorder. In the 1930s there was a popular notion that only stuttering therapists should work with stuttering clients. The rationale was that only individuals who daily faced the problems of stuttering could render competent, compassionate service to clients who stuttered. The underlaying assumption was that the feelings one had as a stutterer were based on how the disorder affected one's life. Therefore, in order to understand the emotions of stutterers, it was necessary to experience the disorder directly. Because the number of stutterers requiring therapy far exceeded the number of therapists who stuttered, an instructional accommodation had to be made. This came in the form of requiring nonstuttering student clinicians to simulate stuttering in public places (Van Riper, 1939). The hope was that by personally experiencing the effects of the disorder, nonstutterers would be able to understand the humiliation and pain stutterers experienced whenever they spoke. Because of this belief, many of the early instructors in speech-language pathology would require their students to pretend to stutter with a stranger in a public place. Presumably, the experience would allow the student to empathize with stuttering clients on an emotional level. Although no longer widely practiced, some instructors still insist that their students go through the experience. Instructors hoped that once acquiring emotional empathy, services provided to stutterers would be more compassionate and effective. Through this period in our history, there was little or no emphasis upon remediating the problem. Rather, the emotional empathy that was now ex-perienced by clinicians led to approaches that stressed the acceptance of the problem (Bryngelson, 1939; Sheehan, 1978; Van Riper, 1971). Unfortunately, this belief did not result in better outcomes for stuttering clients. For many years, this belief resulted in the use of therapies that emphasized acceptance of the disorder, rather than finding ways of developing a more normal form of fluency (Culatta & Goldberg, 1995).

A second form of emotional empathy involves a personal commitment by the clinician to the client. It is all encompassing and may involve personal distress that leads to emotional exhaustion (Gross, 1994). Although it is only human to feel empathy for clients, a personal rather than a professional commitment reduces the clinician's ability to objectively assess the debilitating conditions of the disorder. Although most allied health care and health care providers recognize the need for compassion in the practice of their profession, there is a concern that compassion interferes with the maintenance of objectivity (Kahn & Steeves, 1988).

Cognitive. Cognitive empathy is defined as an understanding at an objective level of what the client is experiencing. To understand how clients may feel about the effects of a specific condition does not necessarily mean that clinicians have had to experience that communicative disorder. Emotions and feelings are not uniquely tied to specific communicative disorders. The feelings of humiliation that clients who stutter or have aphasia experience, when unable to effectively communicate, are probably no different than the feeling of humiliation an individual experiences when publicly berated by a supervisor for a poor performance. Cognitive empathy, therefore, does allow clinicians to understand the emotions individuals with communicative disorders experience, without having to directly experience the disorder.

Uses

As a Style of Communicating. It appears that the use of an empathic style of communication may be related to the comfort level of what is being said. In a study examining how physicians convey information to dying patients, it was found that, when physicians felt uncomfortable with the content of their message, empathic or compassionate communication was difficult to effect (Miyaji, 1993). Clinicians will not be comfortable discussing certain issues with clients. It may be difficult for a new young female clinician to listen and respond to an older adult aphasic's description of how he and his wife have lost the intimacy of their relationship after his stroke or the mother of a child with a severe cognitive disorder deals with how she cannot understand how a benevolent, loving God could have done this to her. Although it may be difficult expressing empathy for something that is not understood, clinicians should endeavor to find events in their own lives that resulted in similar feelings. This form of cognitive empathy is very useful when discussing emotions with clients.

Effects

There is limited research on the effects of compassion and empathy on therapy. Two studies involved perceptions of the clinician's ability to be compassionate in other settings and the effects of compassion on outcome results.

Generalization to Other Settings. Compassion is not necessarily generalizable. Clients do not necessarily believe that the compassion displayed by clinicians in one setting is transferable to other settings and behaviors. For example, although a teacher is understanding to a student who is having difficulty with an assignment in class, she might show no compassion for the problems the student may be experiencing at home. In a study conducted with minority and female students, teachers who were identified as compassionate were viewed as not having an understanding of what the students experienced outside of school (Van Galen, 1993).

On Outcome. When clients perceive clinicians as compassionate, they feel a greater degree of satisfaction with the therapeutic process (Silove, Parker, & Manicavasagar, 1990). Although being satisfied with the clinician's style of interaction is not necessarily correlated with progress, it does affect many other aspects of therapy such as willingness to discuss issues and engage in difficult behaviors (Morse, Anderson, Bottorff, Yonge et al., 1992; Redfern, Dancy, & Dryden, 1993). Although it is difficult to find any clinical studies that demonstrably can show that the use of empathy and compassion result in better results, the effects of this perception are pervasive. If clients perceive clinicians to be empathetic, they are more likely to discuss issues that have a direct bearing on the remediation of their communicative disorder. They also will be more likely to engage in activities that they would otherwise be reluctant to do.

SPEECH CHARACTERISTICS

The clinical experience for clients is a multidimensional one. They are being bombarded by a variety of experiences simultaneously. Not only are they being asked to engage in new and potentially embarrassing or difficult behaviors, but are continually aware of the clinicians' verbal and nonverbal behaviors. One area of nonverbal behaviors that clinicians can easily monitor and modify are their speech characteristics. Those that are most important are intonation patterns and characterizers. Table 5–4 provides suggestions for a self-analysis of both.

TABLE 5-4
Self-analysis of Speech Characteristics

Audiotape your therapy session for 15 minutes. Then analyze your speech in terms of the following five characteristics. After you have described each characteristic, determine if it was inappropriate or appropriate for the client and the context in which it was used. If inappropriate, propose how you would revise it.

SPEECH CHARACTERISTIC	DESCRIPTION	APPROPRIATE ✔	INAPPROPRIATE ✔	PROPOSED REVISION
Intonation Pattern	1. _____ 2. _____ 3. _____	☐ ☐ ☐	☐ ☐ ☐	1. _____ 2. _____ 3. _____
Amplitude (overall)	1. _____ 2. _____ 3. _____	☐ ☐ ☐	☐ ☐ ☐	1. _____ 2. _____ 3. _____
Intensity (for emphasis)	1. _____ 2. _____ 3. _____	☐ ☐ ☐	☐ ☐ ☐	1. _____ 2. _____ 3. _____
Identifiers	1. _____ 2. _____ 3. _____	☐ ☐ ☐	☐ ☐ ☐	1. _____ 2. _____ 3. _____
Characterizers	1. _____ 2. _____ 3. _____	☐ ☐ ☐	☐ ☐ ☐	1. _____ 2. _____ 3. _____

Intonation Patterns

The terms *intonation* and *prosody* are often used interchangeably. Regardless of which term is preferred, both refer to the qualities of intensity, pitch, register, tempo, duration, and tension. These behaviors serve important functions in understanding the communicative intent of verbal messages of both clients and clinicians. Attending to elements such as intensity, pitch breaks, and tension can provide information on the connotative aspects of a verbal communication. For example, a clinician noted that the only time abnormal tension and pitch breaks occurred in an adolescent client's speech was when he explained to the clinician that he was not bothered by people teasing him about his stuttering. The regularity of the association alerted the clinician that the client was probably considerably more upset than his verbal message indicated.

Just as it is important for clinicians to observe their clients' intonation patterns, so should they be attendant to their own. Clinicians tend to be products of their experiences. If one usually works with children, there is a tendency to continue similar interaction patterns with adults, and vice versa. Although the problem is usually minimized by the appropriate selection of words and activities, intonation patterns tend to resist change. Often, without realizing it, clinicians who use an intonation appropriate for one age group, may use it inappropriately for another. Intonation patterns can also be effectively used to reduce clients' defensive reactions. Finally, the ending intonation patterns of the clinicians' speech can affect the intent of their message.

Age Factors. With children, appropriate intonation may involve almost a singing pattern where certain words may be emphasized for effect, or words may be drawn out to highlight the importance of what is being said. The tone is also nurturing, with attempts made to present the image of an adult who is loving, caring, and nonthreatening. Although appropriate for children, it is completely out of place for adolescents and adults.

With adolescents, it is more appropriate to structure the intonation pattern of your speech to correspond more with one that would be used with peers. This may involve a normal speech pattern that would not be interpreted as formal or authoritarian. It probably would be described as *friendly* yet not condescending. It is difficult to define what the parameters of this type of speech would entail.

With adults, the intonation pattern should be more formal than with adolescents. Adults expect the relationship between themselves and clinicians to be professional, yet supportive. While avoiding patterns that convey authoritarianism, the pattern should be professional. Elders in institutions tend to be recipients of an inappropriate style of speech known as "baby talk," where there is a high pitch and exaggerated intonations. The use of this speech style results in the perception of the speaker as both disrespectful and incompetent (Ryan, Hamilton, & See, 1994).

Intensity and Amplitude. It is important for clinicians to conduct themselves in

a way that minimizes defensive reactions of clients. Although defensive reactions are basic survival responses, they have significant negative consequences in therapy. When clients become defensive they have difficulty accepting ideas or questions that may be perceived as threatening. Defensive reactions also can cause clients to erect rationales that have little relationship to reality. Although one can minimize defensive reactions through the choice of words (Shipley, 1992), another method involves the use of appropriate intonation patterns. There are two very specific behaviors clinicians can modify that can reduce the defensive reactions by clients (Gelinas-Chebat & Chebat, 1992).

The first is to lower the intensity of one's speech. This does not translate into reducing the personal characteristics of one's speech. Rather, it involves "taking off the sharp edges." As one speaks, there are various words and phrases which may receive more intonational stress than others. Although highlighting these components serves as important cues in learning parts of language, their highlighting feature can have negative consequences. Take for example the following statement: "Can you tell me why you decided not to do that activity at home?" Using the same words, the meaning of the statement can be changed just by shifting the focus of emphasis. With no words emphasized in the above example, the client may perceive the statement as just a neutral question asking for a factual explanation. However, by adding emphasis, an accusatory element may be perceived by the client. To understand the effect of emphasis, say each of the statements below to a different person. Then ask each to tell you what they thought you meant by the statement.

Can you tell me why **you** decided not to do that activity at home?

Can you tell me why you **decided** not to do that activity at home?

Can you tell me why you decided not to do that **activity** at home?

Can you tell me why you decided not to do that activity at **home**?

It may be difficult to be aware of intonation patterns as they are being produced. By audio taping a session and then analyzing the intonation patterns, clinicians may gain important insights into their own behaviors. A form for analysis is provided in Table 5–4. It can be used for intonation and intensity.

Intensity refers to loudness. In the observation of hostile or defensive interactions, what becomes apparent is that they tend to be accompanied by increases in vocal intensity. The more defensive or hostile a person becomes, the more likely their intensity will increase. Their behavior will usually trigger a similar response from the person with whom they are interacting. The vocal intensity of both parties may peak and plateau early, or it may escalate out of control. A very effective way for defusing the situation is when one of the interactants maintains a low level of intensity that remains consistent. The procedure is not only effective in hostile interactions, but in other types of interactions in which clients become defensive about what is said to them. Obviously, lower intensity levels may not be sufficient for reducing defensiveness, it is just one of many techniques that can be used in combination.

Intonation for Effect. Clinicians can manipulate their intonation patterns to convey various things to clients. Approval and disapproval are two of them. While its use for disapproval of the clients' behaviors and utterances can be easily discerned by clients, they find it more difficult to interpret approval from the clinician's speech (Hatfield, Hsee, Costello, Weisman et al., 1995). This does not mean that the voice should not be used to convey positive feelings to clients. Rather, because clients may have more difficulty discerning positive feelings from neutral and negative feelings just through intonation patterns, clinicians should use other nonverbal modalities, such as the face, and verbalizations to convey approval to clients.

Therapy need not be dull and humorless to be effective. The success of some very excellent clinicians relies on the use of various types of humor including slapstick, stand-up comedy routines, and sarcasm. Of the three, the use of sarcasm requires that greatest diligence in its application, because it relies primarily on divergent intonation patterns for its understanding. When the intonation cue is not comprehended, what the clinician wishes to convey as sarcasm can be misinterpreted by the client as literal. This is a problem found especially with children (Capeli, Nakagawa, & Madden, 1990) and adults who are unable to focus on intonation cues (Winner & Leekam, 1991). Sarcasm may be a clinical technique that requires a level of sophistication that is beyond many communicatively disordered clients.

Ending Intonation Patterns. The intonation pattern that occurs at the end of a statement can affect the statement's entire meaning. Of importance to clinicians is how it affects the client's perception of how committed the clinician is to the statement (Brennan & Williams, 1995). For example, when providing suggestions for what parents should be doing with their children, clinicians would not want to use a pattern that ends with a rising intonation. Patterns of this type have in the past indicated that the person issuing the statement has questions about its validity. Contrast the two statements below. Where the arrow appears, begin lowering or raising your intonation in the direction of the arrow.

Now, when he starts pointing to what

he wants, wait until he uses the target words.

Now, when he starts pointing to what

he wants, wait until he uses the target words.

The first sentence can only be interpreted as clearly declarative. The clinician is telling the parent what to do with her child. In the second sentence, a raising intonation pattern, which is usually associated with questions, can be interpreted in three different ways by the parent. First, it could convey to the parent that the clinician is not very committed to this course of action. If she was, why is a questioning format being used? Second, the clinician is asking for feedback on its appropriateness. Therefore, the parent is given permission to suggest alternative course of actions. Third, the clinician is unsure about the approach and is asking the parent to confirm its correctness.

Recently, in popular culture, rising intonation patterns are being attached to declarative statements. Not necessarily because their certitude is in question, but rather because a confirmation is requested from the listener. This pattern is developing as a matter of course with adolescents and even with young adults. Problems of misinterpretations can result when the clinician's and clients' frame of reference for rising intonation patterns differ. For example, one young clinician ended almost 60% of his statements in the clinic with a rising intonation pattern. With children and adolescents this did not cause any problems. Both populations used the same cultural frame of reference for interpreting the meaning of rising intonation patterns. However, when he worked with older aphasic clients, they interpreted it that he was not very certain of what he was saying, rather than just asking for confirmation from them.

Paralanguage

Parts of speech that are not identified as intonation features, and are not words, are called paralanguage. Paralanguage can be divided into identifiers and characterizers. Both can either positively or negatively affect clinical interactions.

Identifiers. Identifiers are isolated phonemes or combinations of phonemes that are not words. These include such sounds as "uh-uh," "ah," and "um." Sounds of these types are often used by stutterers as ways of initiating speech. An increased use of identifiers has also been found to be an indication of general discomfort (Vrugt, 1990).

Characterizers. Characterizers are sounds that can stand by themselves. These include laughing, crying, yawning, belching, swallowing, coughing, yelling, whispering, sneezing, snorting, and groaning. The appropriate use of characterizers facilitates the flow of conversations. "Uh-uhs" said in response to clients' discussions can indicate that clinicians are following clients' train of thought and encouraging them to continue. A moan or groan when clients are relating particularly painful experiences can convey to them that clinicians are empathetic. Laughter when clients are talking about a particularly humorous experience indicates that clinicians also can share the humor of the experience.

While all of the above are appropriate uses of characterizers, clinicians should be aware of when they are not using them appropriately. One of the biggest problem for some clinicians is the inappropriate use of laughter. Unfortunately, it is a common practice to use laughter as a way of hiding nervousness. It is inappropriate for clinicians to use laughter to hide their nervousness. It can convey to the client a cavalier attitude that may affect the relationship.

COMMUNICATING AT THE CLIENT'S OWN LEVEL

It is important that the words and linguistic constructions you use are appropriate for the linguistic level of your client. Studies have shown that matching the clinician's linguistics with the client's ability to understand the communication is correlated with both outstanding teaching (Meredith, 1985) and perceived effectiveness (Shaffer, Murillo, & Michael, 1978). Methods for effecting the matching appear in Table 5–5.

Communication Style

There are various communication styles clinicians can use with their clients. Usually the style that is used is similar to the one the clinician uses in nonclinical settings. The clinician who normally uses humor in interactions will probably rely on it in clinical settings. The clinician who interacts in a confrontative manner will probably bring that style into the clinic. Depending on the client, clinicians may need to restructure their nonclinical style of communication into one that is more appropriate for clinical interactions.

Professional Jargon. The use of professional terminology and jargon reduces the positive feelings of clients toward clinicians (Kratz & Marshall, 1988). Additionally, the choice of words used to express ideas and respond to clients' utterances will be important in conveying the clinician's therapeutic approach (Frosh, 1991). To effectively help our clients, we will need to clearly communicate instructions, provide feedback, and describe behaviors.

Profanity. A misguided approach taken by a very small number of clinicians is to use profanity to make the session more informal. Some believe that by using a few select terms, the distance between the client and the clinician can be minimized.

Nothing can be farther from the truth. The use of even mildly profane words by clinicians has been shown to negatively impact on therapy, both in terms of clinician evaluation and retention of information presented during the session (Sazar & Kassinove, 1991). Interestingly, the level of religiosity of the clients has no affect on the acceptability of profanity by clinicians. Clients think less of clinicians who use profanity, even if the words used are routinely contained in the speech of the client. Clinicians are not perceived as peers. The standards used by clients to evaluate them are higher. It makes little difference about how one thinks clients *should* evaluate clinicians. Of more importance is how they *do* evaluate them.

The use of profanity also reduces the ability of clients to recall the content of the session (Sazar & Kassinove, 1991). It appears that what clients focus on is the unexpected or unacceptable characteristics of the clinician's speech, rather than on the idea that is being conveyed.

Age Considerations. Adolescents were found to prefer a communication style that was friendly, attentive, and relaxed in comparison to ones that were dominant and contentious (Potter & Emanuel, 1990). Although there was no direct correlations between outcome and preferred style, there are other benefits for using a style preferred by the client. By choosing a style that adolescents find acceptable, a basis for establishing a more trusting and compliant relationship is developed. Adolescents are, by nature, not too enamored with adults. Adults represent for many teenagers that which they do not want to become. By using an acceptable style of communication, some of the barriers that are in place even before therapy begins are reduced.

Just as adolescents have difficulty understanding adults, so do adults have difficulty with the elderly. Whether it is a fear of what we will become, or an unfounded

TABLE 5–5
Self-analysis of Clinician Communication

Audiotape your therapy session for 30 minutes. Then analyze your speech in terms of the following eight characteristics. After you have described each characteristic, determine if it was inappropriate or appropriate for the client and the context in which it was used. If inappropriate, propose how you would revise it.

COMMUNICATION STYLE	DESCRIPTION	APPROPRIATE ✔	INAPPROPRIATE ✔	PROPOSED REVISION
Objective	1. _____ 2. _____ 3. _____	☐ ☐ ☐	☐ ☐ ☐	1. _____ 2. _____ 3. _____
Compassionate	1. _____ 2. _____ 3. _____	☐ ☐ ☐	☐ ☐ ☐	1. _____ 2. _____ 3. _____
Peer-like	1. _____ 2. _____ 3. _____	☐ ☐ ☐	☐ ☐ ☐	1. _____ 2. _____ 3. _____
Authoritative	1. _____ 2. _____ 3. _____	☐ ☐ ☐	☐ ☐ ☐	1. _____ 2. _____ 3. _____
Humorous	1. _____ 2. _____ 3. _____	☐ ☐ ☐	☐ ☐ ☐	1. _____ 2. _____ 3. _____
Use of Professional Jargon	1. _____ 2. _____ 3. _____	☐ ☐ ☐	☐ ☐ ☐	1. _____ 2. _____ 3. _____
Use of Profanity	1. _____ 2. _____ 3. _____	☐ ☐ ☐	☐ ☐ ☐	1. _____ 2. _____ 3. _____
Age Related Features	1. _____ 2. _____ 3. _____	☐ ☐ ☐	☐ ☐ ☐	1. _____ 2. _____ 3. _____

belief in their universal diminished capacity, the style of communication used with the elderly is often inappropriate. It has been suggested that communication with the elderly should emphasis six principles (Gross, 1990). The first is that the clinician should focus on topics of shared interest. The second is that communicative interactions should involve more dialogues than monologues or directive interactions. The third is that the values and feelings of elders should be accepted, rather than criticized. The fourth is that the client should perceive that treatment is personalized, not a set of standardized procedures which do not allow for individual differences. Fifth, clinicians should be perceived as being open, rather than restrictive. And sixth, discussions of issues should be focused on the here and now, rather than on the past or future.

Communicating for Client Comprehension

Much of what happens in therapy is the conveying of information from the clinician to the client. It is important that clinicians do not assume that what they have communicated is automatically understood. Often clients think that they understood what the clinician has said, but in fact, either through selective attention or misunderstanding, have constructed something that the clinician could not have even imagined. At other times, they may be too embarrassed to admit that they did not understand. It is important for clients to comprehend what is being said to them, whether it is a set of instructions or a description of a behavior or attitude. There are four ways of making sure that clients do in fact understand what is being communicated to them. Suggestions for accomplishing this appear in Table 5–6.

Often clinicians will find that they need to describe a behavior that they wish to be performed by clients. The principles used for describing behaviors are similar to those for "Communicating Instructions" in Table 5–6. Suggestions for how to describe behaviors to clients appear in Table 5-7. When communicating instructions, clients are asked to perform the behavior as a way for clinicians to determine if the instructions were understood. When describing behaviors, clinicians should now do the

same with their clients. That is, after clinicians have verbally described the behavior, they should perform it for their clients.

Preceding Statement. One of the simplest ways of enhancing comprehension is to precede instructions or descriptions with a statement asking clients to let you know if there is anything in what you said that they do not understand. Although one of the simplest of clinical techniques, it is often forgotten. An example of an effective preceding statement would be, "Mrs. Jones, I'm going to explain to you how I would like you to practice at home. If there is anything I say that you don't understand, please interrupt me. It's important that you understand exactly how to do it."

Asking Questions. There is a natural tendency on the part of clinicians to reduce the complexity of questions and narrow the parameters of responses for younger clients. Many questions require only simple yes/no responses or short answers. The rationale for reducing the demands of the question is that appropriate responses will be more likely. However, one study showed that there is no correlation between age and the ability to answer more complex questions (Wittmer & Honig, 1991). By asking more open-ended questions of all clients, clients are required to engage in remembering, comparing, reasoning, and organizing thoughts, all of which enhance the development of language.

Questions can also be characterized as having either a positive or negative overtone. An example of a positive question would be, "Can you tell me how you were able to do so well on that task?" A negative question would be, "Can you tell me why you always get up out of your chair and run around the room when you are supposed to be working?" Clinicians often try to structure their questions to facilitate changes in the clinic. For example, some clinicians astutely avoid the use of negative questions because they believe that it directs the ses-

TABLE 5–6
Communicating Instructions

SUGGESTION	METHOD	CULTURAL CONSIDERATIONS
Statement Preceding Instructions	"I'm going to explain to you now how I want you to do ____. If there's anything I'll be saying that you don't understand, let me know right away."	**Language.** Statement is particularly important with clients whose second language is English. **Ethnicity/Socioeconomic.** When using this statement with a client who is from a different ethnic or socioeconomic background from the clinician, care needs to be taken that the statement is not perceived as being ethnocentric or condescending. **Age.** The younger the client, the simpler the words and concepts used. **Disability.** The more cognitively impaired the client, the simpler the words and concepts used.
Short, Clear Statements Without Professional Terminology	"First I want you to ____." "Then you can _____." "At the very end I want you to do ____ 3 times."	**Ethnicity/Socioeconomic.** If clients are reluctant to indicate they did not understand, clear simple statements may prevent the problem from occurring. **Age.** See above. **Disability.** See above.
Graphic or Visual Representation	"Let me draw for you a little picture of how I want you to do this."	**Ethnicity.** Especially important when working with Native Americans. **Age.** The younger the client, the more important are graphic or visual representations. **Disability.** The more cognitively impaired the client, the more important are graphic or visual representations.
Confirming Behaviors and Client Summaries	"Ok, now that I have explained what I want you to do, please do it for me, just like I explained it." "I've suggested a number of things for you to think about. It will help me know that I explained them well if you could briefly summarize them for me."	No cultural considerations are necessary for this method.

TABLE 5–7
Describing Behaviors

SUGGESTION	METHOD	CULTURAL CONSIDERATIONS
Statement Preceding Instructions	"I'm going to describe for you what I'd like to see you do. If there's anything I'll be saying that you don't understand, let me know right away."	**Language.** Statement is particularly important with clients whose second language is English. **Ethnicity/Socioeconomic.** When using this statement with a client who is from a different ethnic or socioeconomic background from the clinician, care needs to be taken that the statement is not perceived as being ethnocentric or condescending. **Age.** The younger the client, the simpler the words and concepts used. **Disability.** The more cognitively impaired the client, the simpler the words and concepts used.
Short, Clear Statements Without Professional Terminology	There are __ things you need to think about when you do this behavior." "First is _____." "Second is _____." "And third is ____."	**Ethnicity/Socioeconomic.** If clients are reluctant to indicate they did not understand, clear simple statements may prevent the problem from occurring. **Age.** See above **Disability.** See above
Graphic or Visual Representation	"Let me draw for you a little picture of what it should look like." "Let me show you what it should look like."	**Ethnicity.** Especially important when working with Native Americans. **Age.** The younger the client, the more important are graphic or visual representations. **Disability.** The more cognitively impaired the client, the more important are graphic or visual representations.
Confirming Behaviors and Client Summaries	"Ok, now that I have explained what I want you to do, please do it for me, just like I explained it." "I've suggested a number of things for you to think about. It will help me know that I explained them well if you could briefly summarize them for me."	No cultural considerations are necessary for this method.

sion to aspects of the client's behavior that are to be minimized. Rather, the approach taken is to use only positive questions because it focuses therapy on desired behaviors. Other clinicians believe the opposite. That is, negative questions are necessary to make the client aware of unacceptable behaviors that are occurring. In actuality, neither type of question has much clinical relevance. In a study examining the effects positive and negative questions had on performance, it was found that the type of questions asked had no relationship to success or failure (Chang, 1994). Rather, the responses provided by the clinicians to clients were correlated with performance. Positive feedback resulted in greater gains than either neutral or negative feedback.

Simplification. A second way to enhance comprehension is to keep your statements short, clear, and without professional terminology. Not only will the elimination of terminology make statements simpler, but will also enhance the client's perception of the clinician (Frosh, 1991; Kratz & Marshall, 1988; Thompson, Hearn, & Collins, 1992). One way of simplifying statements is to limit each to one main idea, concept, or construction. If compound sentences are used, clients may lose part of the message. Although you should not simplify your speech so as to make it condescending, try to avoid terminology that would be unfamiliar to someone who is not in the field of speech-language pathology. Obviously the younger the client, the simpler the instructions should be.

Visual and Graphic Instructions. The third way to enhance comprehension is to provide some form of visual or graphic representation along with your verbal explanation. In the section on stimulus configurations, various suggestions for constructing graphic stimuli were presented. For example, if you are trying to com-

municate to a child who has some minor cognitive problems and the words you will be working on have two parts, a visual representation of two units would greatly facilitate the child understanding the instructions. This can be as simple as using two pieces of paper that are colored or shaped differently.

Confirming Understanding Through Demonstration. The fourth enhancing method involves asking clients to immediately demonstrate what you have asked them to do, or to summarize what you have just explained. This should be done with all clients for all instructions. This method is particularly effective for clients who have attending problems or whose second language is English. In many Asian cultures the "yes" responses or the affirmative head nods do not necessarily mean that what is said is either comprehended or accepted. These two affirmative behaviors may mean " Yes I am *listening* to what you are saying" (Dresser, 1996). In some cultures, it would be embarrassing to state that what was said was not understood. Requests for demonstration or summations are a form of retrieval that allows clinicians to assess clients' ability to understand instructions and descriptions.

RESPECT

Showing respect for the clients' beliefs, feelings, and attitudes results in positive changes and a willingness to engage in clinical activities (Hector & Fray, 1987). Respect can be shown in three areas: (1) culture, (2) personal needs, and (3) use of a caring interaction style.

Cultural Values

The cultural values of clients may differ from those of clinicians. With differences in values also come differences of what may or may not be acceptable in therapy.

These may involve both goals and clinical activities.

Acceptable and Unacceptable Clinical Activities.
Because cultural values form the basis of many types of behaviors, it is possible that behaviors clinicians ask clients to engage in violate one or more of their cultural values. For example, asking a Chinese American father to publicly display affection towards his son would be contrary to the father's cultural values, regardless of how much he loved his son. Although the clinician may believe that this behavior would enhance the development of the client's language, respect for the father's cultural values would rule out this possibility. The clinician should attempt to find alternative methods of accomplishing the same goal. By referring to the suggestions made in Chapter 3 regarding cultural sensitivity, appropriate clinical activities can be selected.

Goals.
Although the primary goal of therapy should be the remediation of the communication problem, goals are not created within a vacuum, nor do communication disorders occur in a sterile environment. The treatment of a communication disorder is always in relationship to the client's functioning in a nonclinical world. The goal of therapy, therefore, is not just the remediation of the disorder, but rather the enhancement of communication within the client's world. For example, when treating a retired Filipino American who spent a considerable amount of time prior to the stroke playing dominos and discussing politics at a community center, a goal of therapy should not be learning strategies for retrieving unrelated words. Rather, the strategies should be taught that will enable the client to retrieve the numbers on the dominos and words that related to the political issues that were of interest to him.

Personal Needs

In therapy we try to remain focused on the task at hand, and we expect our clients to do the same. Although our rigor may have rewards in achieving goals, it may be at the cost of our clients' feeling that we are respecting their needs. Regardless of the type of disorder or its severity, it is important that clinicians are aware of needs clients have that may not be related to the therapy task, and allow clients to express them (Smith, 1994).

Effects of the Disorder.
Take, for example, an aphasic client who just had a humiliating experience where a store clerk misinterpreted his difficulty in retrieving language as a sign of retardation. Instead of working on the language goal for the session, the clinician spent the entire session allowing the client to discuss how he felt as a result of the experience. This choice conveyed to the client a feeling that the clinician was not only interested in his ability to communicate, but also in him as a person. It is very important that clinicians do not view clients as their disorders. Communication is such a complex behavior that its disruption may affect all aspects of the person's life.

Acceptance of Clinical Activities.
The development of new communicative behaviors often requires activities that would appear comical, simplistic, or self-deprecating if done publicly. Children do not slide a finger down their arms in order to produce /s/. Adults do not use a pencil and paper to write the words they are about to utter. Adolescents do not prolong their speech in order for their words to be produced smoothly. Yet clients are routinely asked to engage in activities such as these and others that would be viewed by the general populace as abnormal. Clients cannot help but to view many of these as demeaning, though necessary. The level of acceptability increases significantly when they are

told why they are being asked to do it and the effects it will have on the development of more normal communication.

Caring Interaction Style

Clients and their families not only value competence on the part of their caregivers, but they also wish that the clinician's expertise is communicated in a manner that conveys compassion for their problems and respect for their feelings (Knafl, Breitmayer, Gallo, & Zoeller, 1992).

Conveying Painful Information. Often prognostic information has to be conveyed to clients and their families that may be painful. The wife of a university professor who had suffered a stroke with massive damage asked if he would ever be able to communicate normally again. The mother of a profoundly deaf child wanted to know if her daughter's speech would ever sound normal. The father of a young child with severe motor apraxia wanted to know the possibility of his child ever using oral speech. In all of these cases, the information that needed to be conveyed may be painful to articulate and painful to hear. The upsetting effects of the messages can be reduced by using a communication style that is compassionate. For example, a mother of a moderately retarded child asked the clinician if her daughter would ever be able to communicate normally. Based on an extensive diagnostic assessment, medical reports, and 2 years of therapy provided by an excellent clinician, the prognosis for the development of normal communication was very poor. Although the clinician could have merely presented the above facts to the mother, she phrased them in a manner that suggested that, although normal communication was not a possibility, the behaviors that her daughter already had and the potential to learn would allow her to lead a noninstitutionalized life, doing meaningful work under the guidance of a sheltered home environment.

Instead of feeling depressed about her daughter, the mother now felt at ease that after her death, her daughter would still be able to remain outside of an institution.

MAXIMIZING RESPONSE OPPORTUNITIES

The retrieval of information or behaviors is the only way clinicians can know if clients have learned specific behaviors. For some clients, although learning took place, the ability to retrieve the information may be enhanced or reduced by clinician behaviors. Two of the most significant considerations involve the amount of time given to respond and the use of retrieval cues.

Response Time

Clients who have closed-head injuries often require more processing time to respond than other clients (Wertz, LaPointe, & Rosenbek, 1991). Although information may have been learned, the amount of time required for these clients to retrieve it may be significantly different than for cognitively unimpaired individuals. Clinicians who do not provide adequate time for responding may incorrectly assume that the difficulties the client has in responding is related to conceptual problems rather than to retrieval.

Complexity, Age, and Practice. Various studies have shown that with age, subjects require more time to respond to complex stimuli (Rogers & Fisk, 1990). For clinicians, this translates into providing additional time for older clients to respond to complex stimuli or to produce behaviors that require retrieval of complex patterns. This relationship between complexity and age is not static. In one study, older subjects were allowed to practice responding to a complex stimulus (Rogers & Fisk, 1990). Researchers found that when the subjects were allowed to practice, the response time was dramatically reduced. For clinicians this finding should indicate that as clients become more adept at producing the desired behavior, it is appropriate to require a shorter processing time.

Interpretations. Clients respond with varying speeds. Regardless of the correctness or incorrectness of the response, important information can be derived regarding clients' response certitude by observing the time required to respond and the vocal pattern of the response. In a study conducted by Smith and Herbert (1993), response patterns of subjects were studied. Some of the conclusions of this study were that (1) the less conviction subjects had in their answers, the slower their response, and (2) answers with less conviction were correlated with rising intonation patterns, hedges (I guess), fillers (uh, um, etc.), and self-talk. The presence of these behaviors can provide clinicians with indicators of how well clients have comprehended something or believe in explanations or suggestions provided by clinicians. It is important to note that there is no one standard for all clients. Clinicians should become aware of each client's response repertoire and make conclusions based on a client's past performance and the presence or absence of the indicators previously listed.

Response Cuing

Although one way of allowing for additional processing time is to extend the amount of time provided to clients after a question or stimulus is presented, another method has been shown to provide better results. Deacon and Campbell (1991) found that when subjects with closed-head injuries were provided with response cues, responding time dramatically decreased. When the cues were phased out, the subjects still retained lower response times in similar tasks.

Types of Cues. Cues can be visual, auditory, or tactical. Regardless of the modality, the cuing system that is used should be one that was similar to one used in learning the behavior. For example, if when teaching the production of stops to children with phonological disorders a hand movement with an abrupt termination was used, clinicians may wish to use the same cue when asking the child to retrieve the placement of the articulators. If the target sound was /d/, the clinician may wish to demonstrate the hand movement as she says, "Now remember our sound. What's in this picture?"

Cue Fading. Although the use of cues is effective for retrieving behavior already learned, obviously it is not something that should be continually used. Eventually, clients should be expected to retrieve the information without any cues being present. In Chapter 8, suggestions are provided for how to fade out cues, going from most concrete to most abstract.

ATTENTIVENESS

One of the most common problems of new clinicians involves attentiveness (Sommers-Flanagan & Sommers-Flanagan, 1989). When clients believe the clinician is being attentive to them, their perception of the clinician is more positive (Meredith, 1985; Shaffer, Murillo, & Michael, 1978). Another description of attentiveness is *active listening*. There are two behavioral components to clinical active listening: conversational follow-through and asking relevant questions. Each contributes to the perception that the clinician is attentive, but in different ways. Suggestions for their use appear in Table 5–8.

Conversational Follow-through

The use of conversational follow-through is a fairly easy skill to use. It requires only

TABLE 5-8
Enhancing Attentiveness

Audiotape your session for 30 minutes. Identify at least five client communications. These can either be single or multiple utterances. Describe how you respond to each communication. Then identify the response type. The first three types enhance the perception of attentiveness, the last three reduce it.

CLIENT UTTERANCE	CLINICIAN RESPONSE	CLINICIAN RESPONSE TYPE	REVISED RESPONSE
1.		☐ Asked relevant question ☐ Reiteration response ☐ Expanded on response ☐ Unrelated question ☐ Change of topic ☐ No response	
2.		☐ Asked relevant question ☐ Reiteration response ☐ Expanded on response ☐ Unrelated question ☐ Change of topic ☐ No response	
3.		☐ Asked relevant question ☐ Reiteration response ☐ Expanded on response ☐ Unrelated question ☐ Change of topic ☐ No response	
4.		☐ Asked relevant question ☐ Reiteration response ☐ Expanded on response ☐ Unrelated question ☐ Change of topic ☐ No response	
5.		☐ Asked relevant question ☐ Reiteration response ☐ Expanded on response ☐ Unrelated question ☐ Change of topic ☐ No response	

that there is some form of "connective tissue" between what clients say and responses provided by clinicians. Essentially it is an example of topic maintenance.

Importance of Statements. Often in therapy, a client will begin discussing something that may not have any relevance to the clinician-set agenda. A usual response for clinicians is to politely listen and then redirect the focus of the interaction by saying something like, "That's very interesting, but now it's time to work on your speech." Although it may put the session back on track, it could result in a message to clients that may affect either the development of trust or the level of trust already established. A good starting point in understanding the relationship of conversational follow-through and trust is to assume that whatever clients are saying has importance to *them*. The key word here is importance.

Relevance. The fact that what a client is saying may not be directly relevant to therapy is unimportant. When someone shares information that they view as important with another person, they hope that the listener is at least being attentive to what is being said and hopefully placing as much importance on it as they are. The same situation is true in therapy. By assuming that everything clients are saying has importance to them, clinicians' automatic responses should be to provide verbal utterances and engage in nonverbal behaviors that indicate to the client that the clinicians were attending to the topic.

Asking Relevant Questions

The use of relevant questions adds an additional dimension to conversational follow-through. Topic maintenance requires a basic following of the conversation that adds little to the therapeutic processes other than the development of trust. The use of relevant questions, however, not only en-

hances trust, but also may provide clinicians with additional useful information.

Going Beyond Listening. When clinicians ask relevant questions of their clients, it indicates that they not only were following the clients' thoughts, but went beyond just listening and analyzed what was said. It takes a greater amount of concentration, and possibly interest, for someone to listen to what is being said, analyze and digest it, then produce a question about a specific aspect of the conversation.

Expanding Areas of Interest. Relevant questions result in the client responding in a manner that provides additional information for the therapeutic process. When a clinician asks a client how his day was and the client says, "Great except for English class," the client is inviting the clinician to ask about English class. If he did not wish this to be a topic of conversation, he would have just said, "Great." When given an invitation, clinicians should always accept. At a conscious or subconscious level, clients expect clinicians to follow-through with a question relevant to the topic or area clients highlight.

FLEXIBILITY

Most people like to believe that they are flexible and can "roll with the punches." Flexibility seems to be a trait that is highly valued in our society. In the clinic, the perception of flexibility results in positive evaluations of the clinician (Kivlighan, Mullison, Flohr, Proudman et al., 1992). In this section, specific areas of flexibility will be identified and methods for achieving it will be described.

Areas

There are two areas of clinical practice where flexibility on the part of the clinician can significantly impact therapy. The first occurs when the client and clinician have different cultural values and experiences. The second area involves age.

Cultural Differences. Although the ability to be flexible in a clinical setting is important in establishing rapport with all clients, it is especially important when the clinician and client are from different ethnic cultures (Darou, 1987; Lockhart, 1981). The distrust that is associated with ethnic nonmatches between clients and clinicians often is translated into clients believing that the clinicians' rigidity is related to an ethnocentric orientation, where clients needs are subverted for the sake of the clinicians' needs to function within the parameters of their own culture, without regard to the cultures of the clients. By being flexible, clinicians can minimize this misperception or prevent it from occurring.

Age. Being flexible seems to be more important in developing good perceptions of the clinician with younger than older clients (Morris, 1991). Flexibility is not defined here as a willingness to allow clients to engage in any activity or discussion of their choice. Rather, it means that clinicians are willing to modify the activity or discussion in order to meet clients' needs, within specific parameters. Although older clients may have a sense of when it is appropriate to initiate changes in an activity, younger children may not. For example, during a language activity, a clinician noticed that a child was not responding appropriately and would engage in a variety of delaying behaviors. In response to a question about what was happening in class, the child burst into tears and said she hated her teacher. The clinician immediately stopped the language activity and allowed the child to discuss the problem. If the clinician had attempted to stop the discussion and minimize the problem in order to continue with the language activity, a very negative message would have been conveyed to the child.

Components

There are two important components of flexibility that should be addressed by clinicians. These are the concept of freedom within established parameters and knowing how to shift the focus of therapy.

Freedom Within Parameters. Ford car dealers who sold Model As would jokingly tell potential customers that they could order the car in any color, as long as it was black. Parameters, whether they involve the selection of colors or clinical behaviors, are determined by the reality of the situation. In a few clinical situations, it is not possible to provide any choices. What you see is what you get! However, the majority of interactions between clients and clinicians can be structured to provide some degree of flexibility within well-defined parameters. Parameters should be considered as end points of acceptability. Anything occurring within the parameters is acceptable. Anything outside of the parameters is not. The parameters can be as wide as keeping a discussion on how family interaction patterns are affecting the recovery of communication skills of aphasic clients or as narrow as allowing children to change an activity, as long as the new activity still accomplishes a phonologically specific goal.

When working with children, the trick is to keep the parameters fairly narrow while giving the appearance of being flexible. By their very nature children will test parameters. They are not trying to be disobedient, defiant, uncooperative, or any of the other negative labels attached to children who test parameters. They are engaging in normal childlike activities of trying to understand the adult world in which they live. Unfortunately, many clinicians believe that flexibility means that parameter lines can be crossed. This tactic usually has an unwelcomed effect. For example, during a small group session a clinician wanted to create an impression that she was flexible.

When one child engaged in a minor disruptive behavior, she ignored it, hoping that her neutrality would show the children that she was flexible. The child interpreted her behavior very differently. For him, what he had just done was an acceptable behavior. Within 5 minutes, he engaged in another unacceptable behavior that was slightly more disruptive than the first. Again the clinician did not respond. She believed that now the child must surely view her as very flexible. And again her nonresponse was followed by an even more disruptive behavior. The sequence of events progressed until the child was out of control. Finally, totally exasperated with his behavior, the clinician spoke harshly to him, saying that if he did not immediately sit down and shut up, there would be no reward for coming to therapy. The child was utterly confused. Why was this behavior any different from the others that were accepted by her? By failing to initially establish the parameters of acceptable behavior, she was perceived as arbitrary and unpredictable, rather than flexible. Flexibility should always have limitations, clearly articulated before any activities begin.

Shifts in Clinical Focus. The course of a clinical session should shift with important events that occur within it. There may be times when the best planned intervention program should be placed on the shelf and the personal problems brought up by the client given center stage. When an intervention program is going nowhere, it makes little sense to persist with it. Usually, the shift should be made obvious to the client, especially children. To do otherwise could convey a message to clients that they are making the decision to shift the focus of therapy. For example, when working on an articulation exercise with an adolescent girl, the clinician could tell that the client was upset. During the past session they had talked about the upcoming school dance and that the girl still had not been asked. When she asked the girl about the dance, the client became visibly upset and said that she still did not have a date. The clinician said,

> I know that we were supposed to work on your lisp today, but it sounds like you are upset about the dance. Would you like to talk about it? We can work on articulation next session if you'd like to.

The clinician accomplished many things by her statements. First, she showed the client that she was concerned over her welfare. Second, that she was flexible enough to modify the therapy plan to meet the needs of the client. And third, that she respected the client enough to allow her to choose between alternatives.

CLIENT DECISION MAKING

Involving clients in determining the course of their therapy has been shown to positively affect the commitment to therapy, outcome, and development of trust. (Billings, 1994). When given the opportunity to select goals of importance, clients seem to learn more quickly, develop better strategies, and stay focused on acquisition activities (Butler, 1995). Few things enhance motivation as easily as allowing clients to be involved in the selection of goals (Archer, 1994). Clients with severe cognitive impairments obviously will not be able to participate in the decision process as much as clients with no cognitive impairments. For those clients, decisions should be allowed if the areas under discussion are ones where the clients' perspectives are realistic and compatible with those of the clinician (Goodwin & Bolton, 1991). These clients should be provided with simple choices that have been structured by the clinician. Decisions need not involve hard choices which result in including some areas and excluding others. They can be structured in terms of hierarchies of importance or immediacy (McCollum, 1994). Examples appear in Table 5–9.

TABLE 5–9
Client Involvement in Decisions

The areas for involving clients in decisions which appear below are only general guidelines. Adults with cognitive impairments may only be able to provide limited input. Children who are very attuned to their communicative disorder may be able to provide input in all decision areas.

AREA FOR DECISIONS	ADULTS	ADOLESCENTS	CHILDREN
Overall Goals (General)	✓		
Methodology for Learning Goals	✓		
Context for Applying Goals	✓	✓	
Assessment of Goal Attainment	✓	✓	✓
Reinforcement	✓	✓	✓

Models for Involvment

Although various ways for including clients in the decision-making process are possible, two basic ones are provided below. The first is very simple and requires little in the way of clinical sophistication. The second is more complex.

Simple. A model proposed for school professionals is adapted here for clients with communicative disorders of various ages (Jayanthi & Friend, 1992). It identifies three basic areas in which clients are asked to provide input to the clinician. The first area involves goals. Of all three, this is the most important one. The importance of involving clients in determining goals is addressed in a later section in this chapter. The second is to allow clients to be involved in the selection of methods and techniques, and the third is allowing clients to select their own reinforcers.

Sophisticated. A more elaborate model has been developed for treating adult drug and alcohol addicts (Chandler & Mason, 1995). Although developed for another population, it is applicable to individuals with communicative disorders. There are three phases in the use of this model. During the first phase of therapy, an atmosphere is created in which clients are empowered to direct their own treatment. Assumptions include the notion that change is possible and that clients have had successes in creating solutions. During the second phase of therapy, changes that the clients want are identified, clarification of how they will be beneficial occurs, and work on the behaviors begins. During the third phase of therapy, there is an identification of changes that have occurred and an elaboration of how they have made a difference in clients' lives.

Determining Goals

It is a normal response of clinicians to base the selection of goals on assessment results. After all, if the client has a specific disorder it is only reasonable that correcting the disorder should be the focus of therapy. The disorder, however, affects the client's life in many ways. Every attempt should be made to involve clients in decisions regarding both the goals and tactics that will be used in therapy. Involvement in decisions has been shown to minimize resistance and increase the likelihood that the goals will be accepted (Sagie et al., 1990). The degree of input varies with age. Children should have the least input, followed by adolescents, and finally adults should be given maximum input in the selection of goals. Also, by having clients determine the goals that will be addressed in therapy, they need to carefully examine how their communicative disorder is affecting their life and how the remediation of it will change their life. This process of self-reflection can be important for clients to understand the full dimensions of their problem.

Children. Although many children with communication disorders are aware of their problem, their understanding of what should be strived for as a goal is minimal. It makes little sense under the guise of being *client oriented* to give children the freedom of choosing therapy goals. Remember, when you give someone the ability to choose, along with it comes the capacity to accept their choice.

Adolescents. Although the period of adolescence is often identified as the time when poor choices abound, the independence so highly valued by this age group should not be disregarded. To do so invites rebellion, both blatant and subtle. In a therapeutic context, the rebellious adolescent may only go through the formal steps of therapy. You cannot force an individual to develop communication skills if they have no desire to do it. With adolescents, it is important to give them meaningful, yet limited input into the selection of goals for their therapy. The easiest way to do this is to allow them to choose between several acceptable goals *after* you have asked them to describe for you the incidents in their lives where their communicative problem causes them the most problems.

Adults. Unless adult clients have cognitive impairments, they can tell you in general what the goals of therapy should be. Most adult clients come to therapy because their communication problem is impacting at least one aspect of their life. An executive cannot get a promotion unless he speaks fluently, a singer is unable to audition at times because her voice turns gravelly after a performance, or a recent emigre is unable to make herself understood with colleagues because of her thick accent. There is a relatively easy way to determine the goals of adults. You ask them the following question, "Why did you decide to have therapy *at this time*?" The operative words here are "at this time." Unless the individual had recently suffered a stroke, their communicative disorder usually has been present for a long period of time. They may have had therapy in the past or never have attempted to change their communicative behavior with professional help. The answer to their timing of therapy is of crucial importance. It provides you with information regarding the most debilitating aspect of their problem from the clients' viewpoint, which some believe should be the only valid viewpoint of therapy (Baer, 1990).

When the above procedures still do not result in a level of specificity necessary for selecting the goals of therapy, a modified balance-sheet procedure used in some forms of clinical psychology can be used (Oz, 1995). A format for communicative disorders is provided in Table 5–10. On the left side of the sheet, a goal is described. To the right are two columns. In the first, all of the costs involved in

TABLE 5–10
Selecting Goals for Therapy

1. Choose up to four possible goals that you would like to work on in therapy.
2. List the costs involved in achieving each goal, then list its benefits. Costs and benefits can be emotional, psychological, physical, social, or monetary.
3. After you have listed the costs and benefits for each goal, rank order them in terms of when you would like to work on them, with 1 being the first and 4 being the last.

RANK ORDER	GOAL	COSTS	BENEFITS
☐			
☐			
☐			
☐			

achieving the goal are specified. In a column to its right are listed all of the benefits if the goal is achieved. After completing the procedure for each goal, clients are then asked to make a decision as to which goal will be addressed. This procedure has been found to be effective with clients who are either not sure of what goals to work on or have clearly delineated the goals for the clinician.

Selecting Methods and Techniques

Rarely is there only one way of accomplishing a goal, clinical or otherwise. Although the logic of sequencing the steps in goal attainment may be set, such as successive approximations, the way in which it can be accomplished may be infinitely variable (Culatta & Goldberg, 1995). The

1960s adage "different strokes for different folks" is true in all aspects of life, including therapy. However, the degree to which clients are allowed to select the strokes differs with their age. Allowing clients to have a significant input into the methods and techniques to be used for addressing their problems has many beneficial consequences. Besides allowing the clients to focus on what is most important and intrinsically reinforcing to them, it also conveys to them the idea that they are capable of exercising control over their own lives to affect positive change (Rudd & Comings, 1994).

Children. Children should always be allowed to choose the activity through which therapy will be provided. Their involvement in the decision process is thought to be a fundamental component of successful therapy (Ellinwood, 1989). This entails clinicians providing at least two activities for children from which to select. Regardless of what activity is selected, the same therapy objectives are used. The seemingly additional work for clinicians in developing at least two activities is more than compensated for by the benefits resulting from choice. First, children, by their behavior, are providing information to clinicians about what activity they find reinforcing. Children do not choose boring activities when interesting ones are available. However, clinicians often do. Second, it teaches the concept of contingencies if the selection of an activity is accompanied by a statement indicating that the child can choose whatever he or she wants, with the understanding that the activity has to be engaged in for a set amount of time or for a specific number of behaviors. This is a very important lesson for children to learn, both in and outside of the clinic. Children, just as adolescents and adults, need to become responsible for changes in their communicative behavior. Along with responsibility comes choice. They can choose to do cer-

tain things which will increase the likelihood that their communication will improve, or they can elect not to do these activities. By allowing them to choose activities and then complying with their consequences, self-responsibility is nurtured. Third, it provides clinicians with insights as to what types of objects and activities will be appropriate for the child in the future. Certain children gravitate toward activities containing one type of critical feature, such as movement, whereas others may prefer other types of critical features, such as construction.

Adolescents. Although most adolescents are grateful for the opportunity to act independently and respond responsibly, others may take delight either in the selection of shocking activities or ones that may not be socially acceptable. When you provide clients with an opportunity to select, there is an implicit assumption that you are willing to accept the selection and its consequences. Few things are as harmful to establishing a therapeutic relationship than is the disregard of a commitment. Therefore, care needs to be taken when providing adolescents with choices in how therapy will be implemented. For some adolescents, it may be fine to allow them to select from an open-ended list of activities. However, for most, a more appropriate method would be to provide an extensive, but controlled list of activities, all of which are acceptable.

Adults. Adults should be provided with a full range of choices in activities, as well as all other aspects of therapy, unless their cognitive abilities are so compromised as to limit their ability to understand the concepts of choice and responsibility. Involvement in the selection of activities and strategies for remediating the communication problem has an added benefit. By shifting emphasis from the negative effects of the problem to methods for remediating it, the affect of clients becomes more positive (Elliott, Sherwin, Harkins, & Marma-rosh, 1995). Positive affect associated with problem-solving approaches has been found to significantly enhance the attainment of goals (Wilkinson & Mynors-Wallis, 1994).

Selecting Extraneous Reinforcers

What is extraneously reinforcing to one client may not be to another. Some children would do anything for stickers, others find them boring. The "one size fits all" approach is totally inappropriate for the selection of extraneous reinforcers.

Children. Given children's vivid imagination and desires for almost everything, choices of what will constitute extraneous reinforcers should be limited. There are various ways of accomplishing this. If the extraneous reinforcer is an object or an activity, a token economy can be established in which children could exchange a specified number of tokens for various inexpensive items or specified number of minutes engaging in an activity. Items and activities could be arranged by their token cost, with more expensive and desirable toys and activities costing more tokens. By having more desirable toys and activities cost more tokens, long-term attentiveness toward engaging in therapeutic activities may be enhanced. Care should be taken so that the number of tokens necessary for purchasing a desirable object is not so large that reinforcement is delayed for a long period of time. Delayed gratification often can reduce the attentiveness of children towards an activity (Sloane & MacAulay, 1968). This problem can be easily overcome by instituting multiple extraneous reinforcement schedules, where one reinforcer can be acquired during a session, and the second requires multiple sessions. For example, if something like a balloon costs the child 5 tokens, when the tokens are exchanged for the balloon, a special token is also given. After accumulating 10 of these special tokens, a larger more desirable toy is then given. With a multiple reinforcement schedule of this type, the child has immediate gratification while waiting for the object that involves delayed gratification. Parents can be important in the selection of the long-term reinforcer. Have them identify an object or activity that they propose giving to the child when a significant goal is achieved. It is important that the selection is the parents', because cultural variables will be important, with the most significant one being socioeconomic.

NONVERBAL BEHAVIORS

It is only reasonable that the main focus of speech-language clinicians' attention is on the speech and language behaviors of their clients. After all, whose behaviors are targeted for change? However, an enormous amount of information about the clients' feelings toward the clinicians, the clinical process, and what they are discussing can be obtained through the skillful observation of their nonverbal behaviors.

Clients

When observing the nonverbal behaviors of clients, it is helpful to reduce the entire body to distinct units for observation. The easiest and more beneficial division is face, arms/hands, and legs/feet. Posture, which is another unit of analysis, incorporates all of the body. Tables 5–11 and 5–12 are provided for analysis.

Facial Behaviors. In most Western cultures, the area most often observed during interactions is the face. With hundreds of muscles, the face is capable of conveying a multitude of visual messages. These be-

TABLE 5–11
Behavioral Repertoire of Client Self-Directed Behaviors

Videotape an interaction between you and your client for a 15-minute period. Make sure that both of you are facing the camera with a clear view of both of your bodies. Analyze only one of the categories of behaviors at a time. Then proceed to the next one. For the four categories, you will need to view the videotape four times. Identify only those behaviors that are not intended to communicate.

FACE	ARMS/HANDS	FEET/LEGS	POSTURES
1. _____	1. _____	1. _____	1. _____
2. _____	2. _____	2. _____	2. _____
3. _____	3. _____	3. _____	3. _____
4. _____	4. _____	4. _____	4. _____
5. _____	5. _____	5. _____	5. _____
6. _____	6. _____	6. _____	6. _____
7. _____	7. _____	7. _____	7. _____
8. _____	8. _____	8. _____	8. _____
9. _____	9. _____	9. _____	9. _____
10. _____	10. _____	10. _____	10. _____

haviors may regulate the interaction or relate to the verbal message. Regulators are the behaviors that regulate the rate and flow of interactions between two or more people. In American cultures, they consist mainly of head nods and eye movements. In a clinical interaction, a client's head nod often indicates agreement with the clinician's verbalization with an implicit understanding to "keep talking."

The use of the face is more important in relation to verbal messages than in its use as a regulator. It is the part of the body most often used to convey a message intentionally. The speaker can easily control it since awareness results from kinesic feedback and listener reactions. Because the face is so visible and controllable, it becomes the principal nonverbal avenue for displaying both truthful and deceptive messages. The passive adolescent, who is dreading the thought of being pulled out of her class, may smile during the clinician's explanation of the therapy process. The stutterer who, when describing a particularly painful experience, smiles throughout her story in order to hide the humiliation she felt. Of all nonverbal behaviors, facial behaviors are the ones to which clinicians are most attuned. Since deceptive nonverbal messages are most likely to occur through the use of the client's face, clinicians should not routinely accept a pleasant smiling face as something that is necessarily positive.

Arms/Hands. Because the arms and hands are less visible than the face, they have less communicative ability (Bull, 1987). Since they are used less to convey messages, they become more available for self-directed behaviors. The arms and

TABLE 5–12
Behavioral Repetiore of Clinician Self-Directed Behaviors

Videotape an interaction between you and your client for a 15-minute period. Make sure that both of you are facing the camera with a clear view of both of your bodies. Analyze only one of the categories of behaviors at a time. Then proceed to the next one. For the four categories, you will need to view the videotape four times. Identify only those behaviors that are not intended to communicate.

FACE	ARMS/HANDS	FEET/LEGS	POSTURES
1. _____	1. _____	1. _____	1. _____
2. _____	2. _____	2. _____	2. _____
3. _____	3. _____	3. _____	3. _____
4. _____	4. _____	4. _____	4. _____
5. _____	5. _____	5. _____	5. _____
6. _____	6. _____	6. _____	6. _____
7. _____	7. _____	7. _____	7. _____
8. _____	8. _____	8. _____	8. _____
9. _____	9. _____	9. _____	9. _____
10. _____	10. _____	10. _____	10. _____

hands, therefore, differ from the face in that they display less communicative information but more self-directed behaviors. Intentional or other-directed behaviors can be divided into emblems and illustrators.

Emblems are behaviors that have been assigned an arbitrary meaning and function as pictures, sometimes conveying to listeners complex messages. For example, spinning the index finger around the side of one's head while looking at a person may indicate that the person is not making any sense or is acting in a crazy manner. The hitchhiker's extended thumb indicates that here is a person who needs a ride, does not have access to his own car, and possibly is without much money. The clinician giving the client a thumbs-up sign at the end of a session may be indicating that the ses-

sion went extremely well and she is proud of the client. Because emblems can be used instead of words, they may at times be substituted for words by clients who have certain types of communicative disorders. This is especially prevalent with clients who are aphasic or who stutter. Some aphasic clients have vast repertoires of emblems that allow them to convey information when words cannot be retrieved. Stutterers will also use emblems when a verbal response may involve words on which they believe they will stutter.

Illustrators are behaviors directly related to verbalizations and either emphasize what is being said, point to objects, or visually construct thoughts of objects (Feyereisen & de Lannoy, 1991). An example would be an aphasic client who, unable to remember the word comb, pantomimes the action of combing his hair and says, "Ya know, it's this, like this." Illustrators can also provide information about the intensity of a verbalization. Imagine a session between a parent and a clinician where the discussion involves a particularly disturbing interaction the parent observed between her child and the clinician. The child refused to listen to the clinician and physically accosted her when asked to sit down. The mother is now directing the clinician on how to prevent this episode from occurring again. Imagine that the clinician and parent are sitting comfortably on two couches at right angles to each other. Without any movement, the mother says, "I was very upset when I saw how he hit you. If he ever does that again, grab hold of his shoulders very tightly and tell him to sit down or you will come get me." Now imagine the same scenario with the following changes. The mother is leaning forward and when she says, "Grab hold of his shoulders very tightly," she held her two tightly clenched fists in front of her and shakes them violently. She had increased the intensity of the verbal message by adding illustrators.

Self-directed movements such as nail picking, scratching, hair preening, leg rubbing, and finger tapping are called adaptive, because they provide a means for individuals to adapt to stress or to emotional or environmental demands. *Self-directed behaviors* are usually beyond the awareness of the individual and therefore provide an opportunity for the observer to have insights into the nature of an interaction. The behaviors are habitual and routine, having been formed early in the person's developmental history. By carefully observing a client's self-directed behaviors, the clinician may be able to predict a client's receptivity to an activity or statement. For example, when faced with stressful tasks, some children may begin random hand movements as an attempt to calm themselves. When bored, other children may engage in finger tapping.

Specific self-directed behaviors do not mean the same thing for every client. There is a tremendous diversity in self-directed behaviors and their possible meanings. It is fallacious to assume that something like repetitive finger rubbing means *anxiety* for all people. The importance of self-directed behaviors is derived from their association with other nonverbal behaviors and verbal behaviors. For example, suppose that a 5-year-old child consistently begins swinging his arms 5 to 10 minutes prior to becoming uncooperative during language therapy. The behavior could have meant that he was bored, unable to focus, unable to comprehend the task, or just tired. Regardless of what it meant, the occurrence of the behavior was a prognostic indicator that, if the current activity persisted, the child would become uncooperative. Once the association was observed, the occurrence of arm swinging, regardless of what it meant, became a signal to switch activities. Looking for associations between specific self-directed behaviors and other aspects of the clinical session is more important than trying to determine what the true meaning of a nonverbal behavior may be. General feelings of uncomfortableness have been correlated with symmetrical arm positions (Vrugt, 1990).

Legs/Feet. The feet and legs are the parts of the body that have the least amount of visibility, the least amount of communicative ability, and the greatest percentage of self-directed behaviors. The range of behaviors is limited when compared with the face and the arms/hands area. There are three major types of behaviors associated with the feet/legs area. The first is repetitive movements, such as a rapid up and down movement of a leg. The second involves the degree of muscular tension observed in the upper and lower portions of the leg. The third involves a leg-crossing position that actually could be considered a posture behavior.

Posture. Postural configurations are reliable indicators of three aspects of communication (Scheflen, 1967).

1. *Interaction components*. They demarcate components of individual behavior that a person contributes to group activities.
2. *Relates contributions*. They indicate how individual contributions are related to each other.
3. *Interaction steps*. They define the steps and order in a interaction.

Postures cannot be viewed by themselves as distinct, meaningful units of behavior. They must be related to the overall interaction. In an early study that examined postures in 480 cultures, Hewes (1957) found that the human body could assume approximately 1,000 steady postures, some of which are universal. It appears that posture is a complex entity that is determined by many factors, serves numerous functions, and can be analyzed in terms of its component parts. Research into postures has shown that there is a relationship between some emotions and postural positions (Rossberg-Bempton & Poole, 1993). It appears that clients who assume a more closed posture are experiencing more unpleasant emotions than clients who assume a more open posture.

Clinician Self-Monitoring of Behaviors

Clinicians should not only observe the nonverbal behaviors of their clients, but also their own. This involves monitoring facial expressions, arms/hands behaviors, legs/feet position, and behaviors and posture. The behaviors that are most important to monitor are those that are self-directed and not intended to communicate. It is these behaviors that may convey messages to clients that can interfere with therapy. Table 5–12 is a form that can be used for analyzing one's own nonverbal behaviors. It is best that at least a 10-minute segment of therapy is videotaped. Analysis has shown that each individual tends to have a particular behavioral repertoire that is repeated throughout the session. During even a 10-minute segment, many of these behaviors will become evident.

Facial Expressions. Facial expressions can be modified easily, are quite visible, and are intended to communicate. Therefore, few self-directed behaviors occur in the facial area. The most studied behavior cited in the literature is the smile (Ekman & Friesen, 1971; Scheflen, 1967). One study of clinical importance dealt with the effects of smiling on perceived masculinity. It was found that smiling decreased ratings of masculinity, but not expertness or trustworthiness (Kratz & Marshall, 1988).

Arms/Hands Behaviors. Some commonly observed self-directed behaviors of clinicians are finger tapping, finger rubbing, clenched fists, and crossed arms. If a table is between the client and clinician, most of these are not visible. When they are observed, clients may perceive finger tapping as a sign of boredom, finger rubbing as a sign of nervousness, and clenched fists and crossed arms as a defensive or negative reaction to what is being said (Ekman & Friesen, 1968). Although there may be a great variability in clients' interpretation of these behaviors, none are positive. The presence of each can either shift the focus from what is being said, or distract from it. For example, while a client was explaining to the clinician how it felt to have her voice break while speaking publicly, the clinician was unconsciously tapping his fingers on the table. Observing this, the client assumed that what she was saying was trivial or unimportant to the clinician. Al-though very interested in what the client was saying, the clinician was also thinking about a boring meeting he would be attending after the session ended. Although the finger tapping was related to the meeting, the client perceived it as being a comment on her statements.

Feet/Legs Behaviors. Unless there is nothing between the client and clinician, the feet/leg behaviors of the clinician generally are not visible. Behaviors that are perceived as negative by clients involve repetitive foot movements, tapping, and legs tightly crossed. The first two are generally perceived by clients as indicative of boredom. The last can be perceived as indicating defensiveness or being distant. A neutral position is one where both feet are either firmly on the floor, or legs are crossed, but with an open position facing the client (Rossberg-Bempton & Poole, 1993).

Posture. Posture tends to be related to the overall nature of the interaction (Siegel, Friedlander, & Heatherington, 1992). For example, individuals leaning forward tend to be exerting control or trying to assert control over the interaction. Sitting upright is a neutral position. Leaning backwards is related to a more passive role in interactions. Clinicians can use this information in controlling aspects of the session. For example, clinicians may wish to lean toward clients when they wish to gain or regain control of the session. Conversely, if they wish clients to take a more active role in a discussion, they may wish to lean backward. Obviously, by merely changing body position the global characteristics of the session may not be changed. Postural changes should be used to compliment the verbal aspects of the interaction.

Functions

The claim is often made that an analysis of nonverbal behavior contributes little to the understanding of clinical interactions that cannot be supplied by an analysis of the linguistic portion of the interaction. Such an assertion is made without fully understanding the functions of nonverbal behaviors. Their functional importance can be appreciated by examining how they affect the verbal behaviors of clients and clinicians in four different ways: (1) amplifying, (2) contradicting, (3) qualifying, or (4) sending an unrelated message.

Amplification. A verbal message can be amplified or strengthened by nonverbal behaviors. The use of illustrators or facial expressions can emphasize how strongly people feel about what they are saying. The client who explains in a monotone that she understood the point the clinician was making is conveying a different message than the client who says the same thing but emphasizes each word in a slow precise manner.

Contradiction. Nonverbal behaviors can negate what is being said. For example, a client may be commenting on how relaxed and good he is feeling at the same time he is clenching his fists and holding his body in a stiff position. Since many clients resist examining their feelings honestly, an apparent contradiction between a verbal and a nonverbal behavior can become the vehicle for discussing emotions. Frederick Perls (1965) in a classic filmed interview noted that even though the client said she was afraid of him, she laughed. He commented that "frightened people don't laugh." This observation and comment became the starting point for examining the woman's use of a manipulative role that was negatively affecting her life.

Qualification. Often when someone is expressing a verbal message that involves feelings, desires, or commitments, the connotative aspects of the message may be less intense than its denotative aspects. An example would be a farewell scene in which a person says, "I really will miss you a lot" but barely touches the other person during a hug. In therapy, clients who have been led logically to an important conclusion by the clinician may say that they realize its importance without fully understanding it. This lack of understanding may become evident by the use of an emotionless speech pattern while saying, "Yes, you are right. I can see how that is the core of my speaking problem."

Unrelated Message. Nonverbal behaviors are not always related to the verbal message. At times, a person can engage in an interaction while thinking about something else at the same time. The parent, for example, who is explaining how she is using the generalization procedures at home, may be exhibiting self-directed behaviors not because of any concern with the procedures, but rather because she is worried about the health of another child.

SECTION III

TRANSITIONAL SKILLS

CHAPTER
6

Transitional
Technical Skills

*T*ransitional skills fall between those that are foundational and those that are complex. There are four categories of transitional technical skills that will be presented in this chapter: (1) control of the session, (2) response differentiation, (3) parental involvement, and (4) process of learning. Within these four categories, there are 44 techniques and behaviors. The listing can be found in Table 1–2.

CONTROL OF THE SESSION

At the ends of a continuum of control are client-driven and clinician-driven sessions. Client- driven sessions tend to allow clients to be more involved in setting the sessions' agenda. The reverse is true for clinician-driven sessions. While each serves as end points on a continuum of control, rarely are any sessions completely client or clinician driven. Sessions tend to combine elements of both. Usually, some form of control will need to be exerted by the clinician. This can be accomplished through verbal interac-

tions, contingencies, and the structure of materials and activities.

Verbal Interactions

The structure of verbal interactions with children, adolescents, and adults should be different both in terms of style and context.

Children. Of all three age groups, children are the least likely to be offended by direct controlling statements, probably because they are most used to it. A vast amount of children's interaction with adults involves adults telling them what to do, where to go, and when to do things. Although children expect adults to converse in this way, it may not be the most beneficial form of communication in a therapeutic context. By constantly using verbalizations to control the session, children may not feel that they are involved in the sessions' structure and in the outcome of therapy. In other words, while it is necessary to exercise control in therapy, the use of verbalizations with children may prevent them from assuming a more active and responsible role in the remediation of their communication problem. During those times when no other alternative is possible, the statements need to be clear, unambiguous, and make reference to conditions or rules that were initially discussed before the session began. By referencing them to conditions that were discussed and agreed upon prior to the beginning of the session, clinicians will not appear arbitrary in their exertion of control. Examples of appropriate controlling statements for children appear in Table 6–1.

Adolescents. Many adolescents resist direct control by adults. Some parents would maintain that it is as natural to them as is breathing. Although the same admonitions apply here, regarding the use of controlling statements, as was given for children, an additional problem exists with this age group. Whereas with most children, the relative strength position of clinicians increases with more and more direct controlling statements, the reverse occurs with adolescents. The more controlling the adult, the more resistive the adolescent will become. With adolescents, the key is to have them believe that the controlling statements you are using are no more than affirmations of what they had earlier agreed to do. "Should" statements are to be avoided at all costs. Adolescents quickly tire of hearing from adults what they should be doing. Statements should be phrased in a way that allows the adolescent to choose a course of action that they believe they initiated and is completely acceptable to the clinician. Examples of these types of statements appear in Table 6–1.

Adults. Controlling statements with adults can be even more problematic than with adolescents, but in different ways. When adults decide to enter therapy, they do so because they believe that they are not in control of their problem. If they felt otherwise, they would not be there. An important goal of therapy is to give them a feel-

ing of control: that they have the ability to do certain things that will remediate or control the problem. Everything done by clinicians should reinforce this concept, including the use of controlling statements. Obviously, the situations requiring the use of controlling statements will be different for adults than for either children or adolescents. Adults will not have a behavior problem. However, they may resist controlling statements if they believe that the clinician is exerting a culturally embedded style of therapy that is not acceptable to them, or is exerting an authoritarian style of therapy that is unacceptable, regardless of the acceptability of the clinicians' cultural values or sensitivity. Control through verbalizations will most likely have to be exercised when clients stray off-task, discussing things that are not related to the task at hand. Usually this occurs either because the topics are of importance to clients, or the focus of therapy is not sufficiently clear to them. In the first case, clinicians should note the topic, but suggest that this be discussed at a later time. In the second case, clients should be gently reminded of the goal of the activity. Suggestions for how to construct controlling statements for adults appear in Table 6–1.

Material and Activity Design

One of the best and simplest ways of exercising control over a session is through careful attention to the design of materials and activities. Suggestions appear in Table 6–2. The activity for which the material is designed should appear in the upper left hand side of the form. Each step of the activity should be listed under "Number of Steps." There are no specific number of steps an activity should have. Below the "Number of Steps," indicate the purpose of the activity. Then indicate the consequences for correct responses, incorrect responses, and maladaptive responses. For each critical feature of the material, the appropriate box on the right hand side of the form should be checked. Below that, in-

TABLE 6–1
Verbal Control
Examples

	CHILDREN	ADOLESCENTS	ADULTS
Purpose of the Session/Activity	Today, we will be doing _____. We do this so that you can _____.	Today, we will be doing _____. The reason is so that you can _____.	Today, we will be doing _____. The purpose for this activity is that you will be able to _____.
Consequences for Correct Responses	**1:1 Reinforcement Schedule** Now, every time you say _____, I will give you _____. **Fixed Ratio Reinforcement Schedule** When you have _____ pieces, then you can get a _____.	See Children for younger adolescents.	None
Consequences for Incorrect Responses	Now, when you don't say _____ just right, you won't get _____.	See Children for younger adolescents	None
Consequences for Maladaptive Behaviors	**(use only when maladaptive be-haviors are antici-pated)** It's really hard for you to say _____ when you are running around the room. Whenever you leave your seat, I will take away one of your tokens.	See Children for younger adolescents	None
Redirecting While Acknowledging	That's very interesting. I would like to hear more about that later. Now you remind me and we will talk about it after we finish this.	I can tell that what you just said is important to you. I would like to hear more about it. But right now, let's finish this activity, then we can talk about it.	That obviously had a big impact upon you. I think that it's important that we discuss it further. But right now I would like to continue working on this activity. When we are done, let's talk about it.

dicate the type of reinforcement involved with the material. Finally, in the boxes at the bottom of the page, indicate how each step will be explained to the client.

Some activities and materials exert minimal control in the session. Clay, for example, is malleable into an infinite number of things, has no logical structure to it, defies

TABLE 6–2
Material Design

Activity _____

Number of Steps _____
    Step 1_____
    Step 2_____
    Step 3_____
    Step 4_____
    Step 5_____

Purpose _____
_____

Critical Features
❏ Mobility   ❏ Flexibility
❏ Construction   ❏ Surprise
❏ Destruction   ❏ Competition
❏ Movement   ❏ Completion

Reinforcement
❏ Intrinsic_____
❏ Extrinsic_____
❏ Extraneous_____

Consequences

Correct Responses _____
Incorrect Responses _____
Maladaptive Behaviors _____

	Step 1	Step 2	Step 3	Step 4	Step 5
Instructions					

any sort of sequencing, and resists closure due to its always not being completed. At the other end of continuum would be games that have a specific number of steps, that are sequentially ordered, and whose structure sets the rules for the activity.

Sequentially Ordered Activities. An activity is sequentially ordered if it has a progression of steps. With the completion of one step, the next is engaged. By understanding what each step in the activity entails, clients are able to structure their behaviors to conform with the requirements of the activity. If the activity has intrinsic,

extrinsic, or extraneous reinforcing elements, the need for clinician control will be minimized. An example would involve an activity designed to teach children with pragmatic problems how to place telephone calls. The activity would be sequentially ordered from dialing the number through completing the call and hanging up.

Structured Activities. Although sequential ordering can impose control over an activity, a certain degree of chaos may occur if the expectations within each step are indeterminate. This can be avoided if rules are provided for how each step is to be completed. Let us use the above example of pragmatically disordered children. They were informed that to make a telephone call, they would need to: (1) dial the number, (2) introduce themselves, (3) engage in a conversation, and (4) finally say good-bye and hang up the phone. If no further instructions were provided, they may correctly go through the sequence, but the activities may not bear any resemblance to what a normal telephone interaction should include. What is additionally required for each step in the sequence are the pragmatic rules for interacting with the person at the other end of the telephone line. When activities contain both a sequencing and logical structure, clinicians can take less responsibility for controlling the session and allow the materials and activities to do it for them.

Contingencies

Contingencies can offer clinicians the element of control through the logic of their structure and the desirability of the consequence. Additionally, it reinforces the notion for clients that they are responsible for their actions, both those that are beneficial and those that are not.

Consequences for Actions. Throughout this book, it has been emphasized that clinicians cannot change client behaviors. At best, they can provide clients with the methodologies, strategies, and conditions necessary for clients to change their own behaviors. Clients must make a decision to do those things that facilitate change. Conversely, deciding not to do facilitating behaviors is in fact making a decision not to change. All clients have this freedom, whether or not clinicians want them to. Unfortunately, many clients of all ages do not see the relationship. Often, both failure and success are attributable to the efforts of clinicians rather than to their decision to engage or not engage in certain behaviors. By emphasizing consequences for actions

the direct relationship between choice and success is highlighted. For children, the use of extraneous reinforcers such as toys, food, or activities are often necessary. For adolescents and adults, the relationship is more direct. Focus should be on how engaging in specific behaviors will have a direct consequence on minimizing or remediating the problem in those areas of their lives that they indicated are causing them the most problems.

Representing Contingencies. Contingencies are merely the consequences for actions. If x occurs, then y will follow. If an activity is engaged in, then a token will be received. If a given number of correct responses are produced, then a desired game can be played for 5 minutes. If you want to be able to communicate with your friends, you will need to practice retrieval exercises every day. Although each of these consequences differ, they are all identical in that there is a logical relationship exerting control rather than the clinician. If you want x to happen, then y must occur. With children and some younger adolescents, the structure is clear. However, for very young children and clients with severe cognitive or emotional problems, a graphic representation may be necessary. For example, if an autistic client is on a 5:1 fixed ratio schedule of reinforcement, the concept of having to wait for five correct responses to be reinforced may not be understandable through the use of words. However, it can be easily displayed graphically using something similar to what appears below.

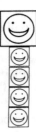

Whenever a correct response is given, a token is placed on the lowest square. With each new correct response, additional tokens are placed on the squares until the final, or fifth correct response is given. At that point, a reinforcer is provided. Visually, it becomes very apparent to even severely impaired individuals that not only are there positive consequences for desired behaviors, but after a specific number of responses the reinforcer will be given.

If there is something an individual is truly interested in accomplishing, the desirability of that event, object, or behavior may be sufficient for guaranteeing cooperation in clinical activities, regardless of how onerous or difficult they may be. This is the advantage of having something being either intrinsically or extrinsically reinforcing. For many stutterers, the ability to speak without a disfluency is so intrinsically reinforcing that they are willing to try almost any form of therapy, regardless of how little sense it intuitively makes to them. For children with language disorders, the ability to have an adult respond to their needs and desires, through the use of linguistic utterances, is sufficiently extrinsically reinforcing that they will use a strategy in a variety of situations without being asked to do so. A great deal of attention should be paid by clinicians on the selection of appropriate consequences for therapeutic activities. Obviously, if nothing intrinsically or extrinsically reinforcing can be found, then extraneous reinforcers will be required. In previous chapters, suggestions were provided for how to determine what may be extraneously reinforcing.

When jointly deciding with the client what will be intrinsically or extrinsically reinforcing, the activity or behavior should not be one that is so difficult or complicated that it will only be achievable with great effort. If it is, not only will opportunities to receive reinforcement be reduced, but the likelihood of failure will be increased. To minimize this, a procedure called response differentiation should be used.

RESPONSE DIFFERENTIATION

Most clients enter therapy with a history of failures: failure at determining how to correct a communication problem and failures in attempting to use normal communication. The self-images that disabled communicators have can be all encompassing and result in a set of values, beliefs, and behaviors that may be self-effacing or even humiliating. If not structured correctly, therapy may reinforce these negative views. Take, for example, a client who continues to fail at a specific task without substantial improvement on subsequent trials, or improves only slightly but does not approach an acceptable criteria level. The clinician may repeatedly ask the client to engage in the same activity, hoping that eventually the task will be learned. In many instances, after a number of failed efforts it will be mastered, but at the cost of reinforcing client's views that the development of normal communication is difficult and its path strewn with punishing failures. When self-doubt develops clients can be become immobilized, refusing to further participate in therapy (Harlow & Cantor, 1994).

Some have argued that the process of failure is not negative, since it develops determination and a strength of character that helps in the development of the individual. This, however, seems to be contradicted by studies that have shown that errorless learning produces significantly better results than learning that is characterized by errors (Wilson, Baddeley, Evans, & Shiel, 1994). The development of communicative competency need not be associated with failure. One proven clinical method of reducing failures is response differentiation. This is a term that refers to the gradual development of a goal. Usually two different types of response differentiation can be made. One involves a structure where a number of goals are specified. This is known as *successive approximations*. The second type involves cues or aids that the client can use to achieve success. With both procedures, the task size of the client's performance is reduced. Reductions of these types has been shown to substantially increase performance both in terms of accuracy and time (Dunlap & Plienis, 1991).

Successive Approximations

With the inability to solve problems, individuals begin developing doubt in their ability to meet the challenges involved in changing any aspect of their behavior (Harlow & Cantor, 1994). With doubt, various psychopathogical conditions can develop which may interfere with clients' abilities to use new or difficult modes of functioning (Brackney & Karabenick, 1995). One of the most important ones is the lack of "self-efficacy" (Zimmerman, 1990). This is a term used to identify a condition where individuals do not believe they possess the ability to change fundamental aspects of their functioning. Given these problems, it becomes important for the clinician to utilize techniques that can change clients' self-image. Although counseling can be used to reverse these negative attitudes, a more efficient and effective method is demonstrating the ability to change. Nothing reverses the feeling of failure as much as success that is easy and rapid. An effective way of accomplishing this is through a process known as successive approximation.

Successive approximations involve the identification and teaching of sequentially ordered behaviors, whose completion will lead to the mastery of a target behavior. One complex behavior is reduced into several simple ones. An example appears in Table 6–3. The completion of one behavior serves as the basis for learning the next behavior. You can use this method for most behaviors that can be divided into units. For example, it may be difficult to go from never having jogged to 30 continuous minutes of running as a first goal for an individual who is not in good physical condition. Although the person may eventually achieve the goal, an enormous amount of failures probably would occur along the way, each event creating doubt in the mind of the runner that the goal can ever be achieved. However, if the goal for the first week was 5 minutes each day, the likelihood of success would be greatly enhanced. Each successive goal could be an additional minute. By structuring goals in this way, the probability of success is maximized and failure minimized (Fabiani, Buckley, Gratton, Coles et al., 1989; Frederiksen & White, 1989). When deciding to use successive approximations, first select the end behavior. Then specify individual steps. And finally, design the components of each step.

Selecting End Behaviors. When deciding on what should be an appropriate end behavior, two basic considerations need to be made. The first is determining if the goal can be reached in measurable steps. These steps should each be an approximation of the final goal. There are three types of approximations that can occur. The first is magnitude. In our jogging example, each step could involve an additional 5 minutes. If there were six steps to the program, our individual still is doing the same thing at step six that she did at step one, but just for a greater amount of time. Many types of communicative behaviors fit into this category. For example, increasing the amount of time stutterers are expected to produce fluent speech, increasing the amount of time someone with spastic dysphonia speaks without vocal breaks, and expanding of the length of time aphasic clients or children with auditory difficulties are required to attend to auditory stimuli.

The second type of behavior that can be modified with successive approximations is anything whose proficiency is gradually improved. Although many clinicians use successive approximations in this way, it can be problematic. Take, for example, the child with a lateral lisp who distorts the production of /l/. The clinician may wish to initially accept a distortion of the /l/ as ac-

TABLE 6–3
Successive Approximations

Target Behavior	Controlled normal fluency
Starting Behavior	Disfluency with periods of uncontrolled fluency
Steps in Program	5

Critical Features

❐ Mobility ❐ Flexibility
❐ Construction ❐ Surprise
❐ Destruction ❐ Competition
❐ Movement ❐ Completion

Reinforcement

❐ Intrinsic Fluency & control
❐ Extrinsic Fluent completion of utterance
❐ Extraneous _____

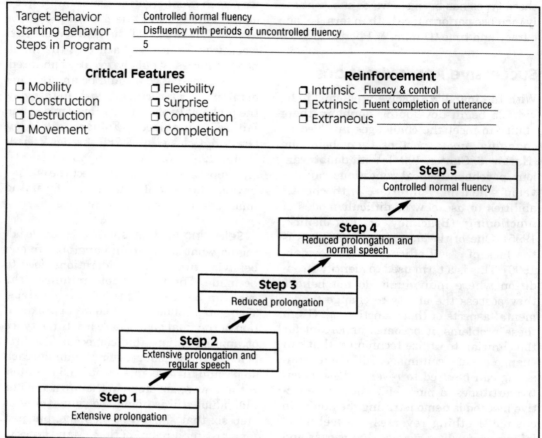

Step 5
Controlled normal fluency

Step 4
Reduced prolongation and normal speech

Step 3
Reduced prolongation

Step 2
Extensive prolongation and regular speech

Step 1
Extensive prolongation

ceptable if it contains less distortion than was present before an intervention program began. Although both the clinician and the client may hear the difference, it may be difficult to identify why the change occurred other than to just state that less air escapes laterally. The use of successive approximations in this case will probably be framed in terms of quality. One production of /l/ is better than another production. The problem with using quality as a measure of improvement is that it may not provide clients with the specificity of feedback necessary for changing behaviors.

The third way of using successive approximations is to identify a specific be-

havior that has individual components, all of which are sequentially related. This form of successive approximations is frequently used to teach cognitively impaired individuals pragmatic language skills and work skills (Hunt, Goetz, Alwell, & Sailor, 1986). For example, there are certain verbal and nonverbal rules of greeting, all of which must be performed sequentially. The first is to walk close to the person who is to be greeted, look them in the face, extend your hand, utter a greeting (Hi, my name is _____), shake their hand for a limited amount of time, then release it. This greeting ritual can be divided into each of the steps listed. The individual would first practice walking toward the person being greeted. With this behavior mastered, the additional component of looking them in the face would be added. With each new mastery of a component, the chain is increased and practiced. Finally, the whole sequence is performed.

Approximation Steps. As a society, we wish for everything to happen rapidly in giant steps. Change is something that we desire to occur in units that are substantial (Harre, 1988). Nobody wants to improve only a little. We want big changes to occur in our lives. A salary increase of only $5 a week is considered insulting. A weight loss of only 1/4 pound a week is disappointing. An increase in a grade point average from 3.0 to 3.1 is discouraging. Yet, in therapy it is the small changes that should be strived for, not the massive ones. With a history of failure, clients have a psychological need to be successful. There are two rules that should never be forgotten when selecting steps in an intervention program.

1. The smaller the steps in changing behaviors, the more likely success will be achieved.
2. The greater the steps, the more likely failure will result.

The number of steps in any successive approximation program should be determined by logic and the features of the end goal. Logically, a program should have a minimum of three steps and maximally not so many that the achievement of the goal takes so long that the client loses sight of it. The number of steps will be governed by the type of successive approximation approach clinicians use. For example, if clients are currently producing only single word utterances, and clinicians wish to increase the length to two words, a program might involve three steps: (1) production of action words, (2) production of object words, and (3) production of action + object constructions.

Step Components. After having decided the steps that will be used in achieving the goal, the components of each step will need to be specified. Basically this involves three parts. The first is having an understanding of what may be involved in the mastery of the task. The second is deciding what materials to use, and the final part is setting a criterion for feeling reasonably sure that the client is ready to progress to the next step. This procedure has been incorporated into a method that is called a Competency Based Format for Clinical Intervention (Goldberg, 1993). Examples for using this format are provided in Tables 6–4 to 6–7. Table 6-4 shows a completed articulation program with each of the four levels completely delineated. Tables 6–5 to 6–7 illustrate partial programs for the treatment of other disorders, with only the first level under the first competency described. The examples in Tables 6–5 through 6–7 are provided to show the structure of competency-based instruction. They are not suggested intervention programs.

The *terminal competency* is an end product, the specific behavior the clinician would like the client to achieve. It can be as small as the identification of car toys, or as large as the correct usage of grammatical rules in all contexts. As a matter of practicality though, the smaller the terminal competency, the easier it will be for the clinician to construct a manageable intervention program. It is clinically a more viable approach to have a series of small interrelated intervention programs rather than one very complex and cumbersome one. The designation of a behavior as a terminal competency is more a matter of ease than rigid guidelines. For example, *normal language usage* as the terminal competency for a nonverbal child would prove to be too complex a goal to develop, given the number of behaviors that would have to be traversed to achieve it. In Table 6–4 the terminal competency that is used as an example is "production of /r/ in all contexts." This constitutes a unit of behavior that has

TABLE 6–4
Competency-Based Format
Complete Articulation Program

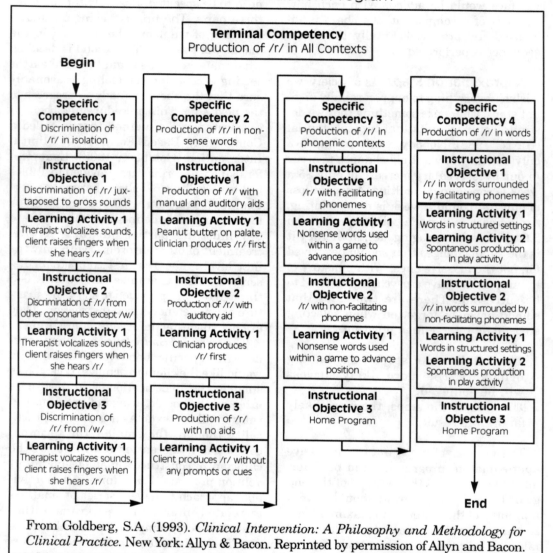

From Goldberg, S.A. (1993). *Clinical Intervention: A Philosophy and Methodology for Clinical Practice*. New York: Allyn & Bacon. Reprinted by permission of Allyn and Bacon.

well-defined limits and lends itself to being divided easily into basic component parts. Each component is designated as a specific competency.

Each terminal competency has two or more *specific competencies*. The specific competencies should be viewed as the major components of a terminal competency.

The number of specific competencies that should be included under a terminal competency is determined by the scope of the terminal competency and the preferred method of acquiring it. The question of scope is illustrated in the following example. If driving a car is a terminal competency for a 16-year-old new driver, the spe-

TABLE 6–5
Competency-Based Format
Asphasia Example

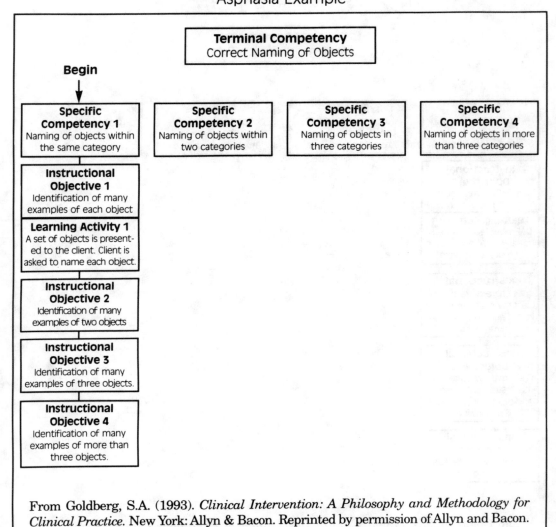

From Goldberg, S.A. (1993). *Clinical Intervention: A Philosophy and Methodology for Clinical Practice.* New York: Allyn & Bacon. Reprinted by permission of Allyn and Bacon.

cific competencies might be (1) knowing basic car controls, (2) understanding the rules of the road, and (3) being able to maneuver in traffic. The terminal competency for a new NASCAR racing driver might be (1) knowing controlled sliding techniques, (2) knowing the rules of slipstreaming cars, and (3) being able to pass at very high speeds. In the area of speech-language pathology, similar differences exist. The specific competencies necessary for attaining the appropriate use of modifiers would look very different for a language-impaired child than for an adult aphasic who was a college professor before her stroke occurred. Differences in methods of acquiring the terminal competency may be reflected in the choice of specific competencies. For

TABLE 6–6
Competency-Based Format
Stuttering Example

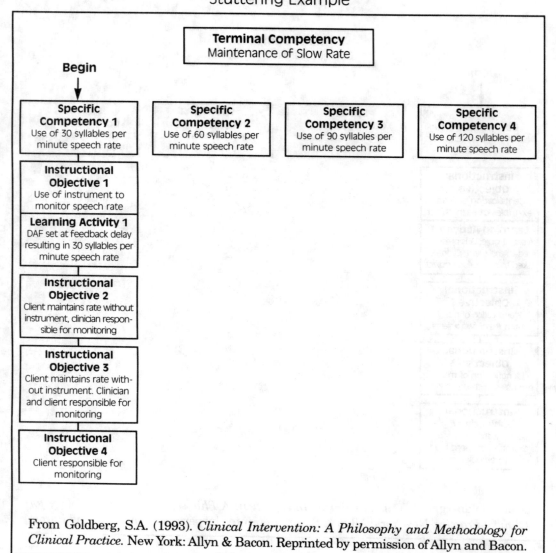

From Goldberg, S.A. (1993). *Clinical Intervention: A Philosophy and Methodology for Clinical Practice.* New York: Allyn & Bacon. Reprinted by permission of Allyn and Bacon.

example, a traditional method for training race car drivers involves the early placement of a driver in a low-powered car on a track. A more technologically based approach may use computerized simulations before actual track experience. In speech-language pathology, one's theoretical position is often reflected in the choice of specific competencies. For example, in stuttering therapy, someone who espoused a two-factor learning theory of stuttering may include the elimination of secondary behaviors in the terminal competency of increased fluency (Brutten & Shoemaker, 1967). For someone who views stuttering as purely an operant behavior (Shames & Florance, 1980), the

TABLE 6–7
Competency-Based Format
Voice

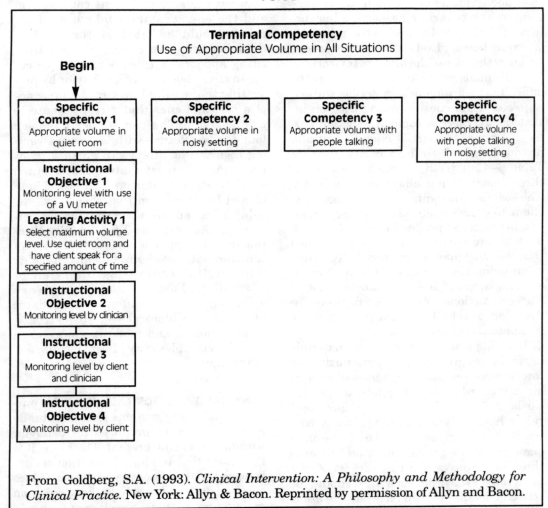

From Goldberg, S.A. (1993). *Clinical Intervention: A Philosophy and Methodology for Clinical Practice.* New York: Allyn & Bacon. Reprinted by permission of Allyn and Bacon.

elimination of secondary behaviors would not be a separate, specific competency. Table 6–4 lists four specific competencies. These involve discrimination, production of /r/ in isolation, production of /r/ within various phonemic contexts, and the production of /r/ in words. The selection of these four specific competencies reflects three theoretical positions. The first is that target sounds should be discriminated from error sounds before production begins (Winitz, 1969). The second

position is that the easiest way to break the automaticity of error productions is the use of unfamiliar contexts in which the target sound is produced (Holland, 1967). And the third is that the production of words should not be separated from their normal use within sentences (Elbert, 1989). Obviously, if one did not believe that these theories were relevant for the remediation of phonological disorders, a different set of specific competencies might be used.

Instructional objectives are the means by which specific competencies are acquired. Often, the instructional objectives for more than one competency are identical or very similar. The criteria for selecting instructional objects usually involve the principles of acquisition and retention. For example, we know that one of the problems of learning for individuals with cognitive deficits is the difficulty of learning new materials without concrete visual cues. Knowing this, an instructional objective could specify that easily discriminable visual cues be initially provided when learning any new task. In Table 6–4, under Specific Competency 1, three instructional objectives are listed. The goal for this competency is to teach the client to discriminate between the correct and his incorrect production of /r/. From educational research it has been determined that the most appropriate way to teach discrimination tasks is to do it with ever-increasing levels of fineness (Bandura, 1969). The instructional objectives are therefore designed to take the client from gross to fine phonetic discriminations.

Learning activities refer to the materials or actual progression of events during an intervention program. Examples of materials are board games, puppets, or picture cards. An example of an event is "client raises hand before beginning fluency contract." It is a common mistake of new clinicians to focus more attention on this area than on the preceding three levels of construction. Learning activities should be constructed that (1) will facilitate the use of instructional objectives, (2) will hold the client's interest, (3) are safe and inexpensive, and (4) facilitate the generalization of the behavior being developed. The primary purpose of learning activities is to facilitate the completion of an instructional objective.

Multiple Cuing

When using a successive approximation program, clients may have difficulty in mastering a particular task. When this occurs, clinicians should attempt to determine if a step is missing. In other words, the jump from one step to another is greater than the client can handle. If no other steps can logically be placed between the step the client can perform and the one constantly failed, multiple cuing should be tried at the level of the failed step. An example of multiple cuing appears in Table 6–8. Multiple cuing involves learning of a behavior by presenting the required task in the presence of a series of cues that directly relate to the behavior. The use of cues has been found to be effective with learners of varying cognitive abilities, with greatest gains occurring when cues are supplemented with strategies (Bernard, 1990). There should be no concern that clients will develop a dependency upon the cues for performing the behavior. By gradually eliminating the cues clients not only can function without them, but also have no difficulty in generalizing the behavior (Foxx, Kyle, Faw, & Bittle, 1989). When selecting cues, consideration needs to be given to a hierarchy of abstractness, form, number, and modality, since each of these variables may affect the outcome of therapy.

Hierarchy of Abstractness. The purpose of all cuing systems is to eventually enable clients to produce the behavior without cues being present. Therefore, it is important that the initial selection of cues be based on their eventual phase out. Since cues are designed to help in the acquisition of behaviors, their phasing out should progress from most concrete to most abstract. For example, if a client is attempting to learn the rule that articles precede nouns in sentences, the clinician may construct some form of visual representation were *the* is highlighted by a big blue square with the word *the* printed in the middle of it, similar to what appears below.

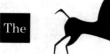

TABLE 6-8
Multiple Cuing

Target Behavior _____

Number of Cues _____

Cue Hierarchy (most abstract to most concrete)	**Modality**		
_____	❏ Visual	❏ Auditory	❏ Tactile
_____	❏ Visual	❏ Auditory	❏ Tactile
_____	❏ Visual	❏ Auditory	❏ Tactile

No Cues

↗

One Cue

↗

Two Cues

↗

Three Cues

As the clinician points to each visual representation of a word, the client would produce the correct one. When the client is able to consistently produce the article when highlighted by the blue square, she may wish to eliminate the color, leaving only a thick border around the word.

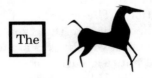

And then use only the word *the* and eliminate the square.

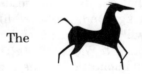

Types of Cues. Cues that are provided to clients can take many forms, some of which are more helpful than others. There is evidence to indicate that color coded cues result in faster response time than cues which rely only on shape (Jubis, 1990). This does not mean that only color should be used in designing cues. They can be combined with shapes and interlocking pieces to emphasize differences and specific behaviors on which to focus. In the example for teaching articles above, both color and shape were combined in order for the client to focus on the production of articles. Color should be faded out first, followed by shapes.

Number of Cues. It is a common practice to provide clients with multiple cues in order to facilitate correct responses (Goldberg, 1993). Although it seems logical that a greater number of cues will result in quicker acquisition of the correct behavior than a fewer number of cues, a recent study suggests the opposite. In a study conducted by Jubis (1990), subjects with normal cognitive abilities responded more quickly when provided with one visual cue rather than with two visual cues. These findings need to be qualified in issues of clinical design. In the Jubis study, the two-visual cue condition involved two cues that were not related. In the design of clinical cues, all cues used during a specific acquisition activity should be related. In the above example of teaching the article *the,* the word, shape, and color were all presented as an integrated unit. This allowed the clinician to gradually fade out portions of the cue. There is evidence to suggest that the greater the distinctions that can be made between what clients should focus on and what is background, the more likely the behavior will be acquired and retained (Gagne, Briggs, & Wager, 1988). Therefore, the practical implications of the Jubis study are that when more than one cue is used in teaching a behavior, they all should be related and perceived as an integrated unit.

Modality of Cues. Cues that are provided to clients can be tactile, visual, and oral. There is evidence to suggest that visual and oral cues provide different degrees of help to the client, depending upon what the desired task is. Ward (1994) found the following: (1) visual cues positively affected response time for both nonverbal and auditory behaviors,

(2) auditory cues were effective only for auditory responses, (3) when both visual and auditory cues were presented together, attention toward the cue was dependent on the task. Tasks requiring auditory behaviors resulted in attention being directed toward auditory cues, and tasks requiring nonverbal behaviors resulted in attention being directed toward visual cues. Many clinical implications can be drawn from this study. The first is that, if clinicians are asking clients to either produce an auditory response or to nonverbally identify something through a behavior, visual cues are appropriate. The concreteness of visual cues provides an easy method for most clients to focus on, and may be critically important for clients with cognitive impairments. Second, if clients are being asked to produce a nonverbal response, visual cues tend to be more effective than auditory ones. This is most evident with the modeling process, where clinicians demonstrate to clients exactly what they want them to do rather than by explaining it. Third, if the task clients are being asked to perform is nonverbal, it is more likely that their attention will be directed more toward visual cues than auditory cues.

Combining Successive Approximations with Multiple Cuing

A very effective way of structuring and designing therapy programs is to use successive approximations with multiple cuing when required. The basic format of teaching behaviors should be successive approximations. The majority of behaviors lend themselves to this type of format. Communicative behaviors are usually complicated entities, easily broken down into specific units. Although a successive approximation format may be the basis of an intervention program, it often is not sufficient. At times, even with the best designed program, clients may fail to progress. If clinicians are sure that a step is not missing, they have two options. One is to persist with the activity, hoping that the client will eventually be successful. As was previously discussed, learning through failures has undesired consequences. A better approach would be to institute multiple cuing at that step in order to achieve successful productions. For some clients, the use of multiple cuing may be necessary for only one step. For other clients with more severe cognitive impairments, the multiple cuing may be needed at each step. In Table 6–9 a schematic for combining successive approximations and multiple cuing is presented.

PARENTAL INVOLVEMENT

Just as with clients who are communicatively disabled, parents come to the clinic with a history of failures. In spite of their best efforts they have been unable to substantially improve the communicative ability of their children. If they are to become an integral part of the therapy process, their self-image as failures must also be changed. This can be done through a systematic process or recruiting parents into the therapy process with the same type of thought that goes into the construction of intervention protocols for their children.

In this section parent counseling will not be covered. Although many of the techniques and behaviors presented in this text can be used to counsel parents, a comprehensive approach to parent counseling goes beyond the scope of this book. There are many appropriate books and articles available on this subject (Andrews & Andrews, 1990; Crais, 1991; Donahue-Kilburg, 1992; Shipley, 1992).

TABLE 6–9
Combining Successive Approximations and Multiple Cuing

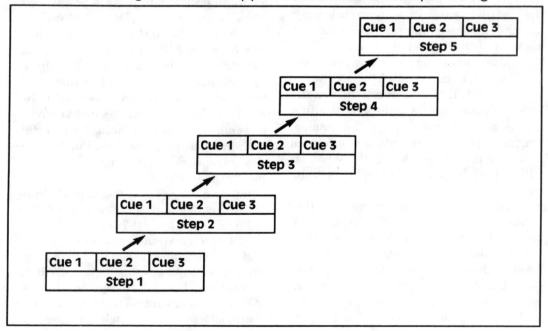

Initial Contact and Recruitment

It is important for parents to become involved in the therapy of their children. If this is to occur, they need to be brought into the process systematically, slowly, and carefully. Table 6–10 is a summary of suggestions that can be provided to parents. It contains five general suggestions for *what* they can do in the clinic and home, *why* it should be done, and *how* to do it. A copy of this form should not be given to the parents without an oral explanation. If possible, at least 30 minutes of a session should be allocated for a discussion of the material contained in the form.

Although in some public school districts the involvement of parents is an important goal, in others, involvement is limited to being informed at the Individualized Therapy Plan meeting (IEP) about the intervention plan that is being proposed for their child. After spending a considerable amount of time developing the proposal, everyone hopes that the parent will approve it without many changes. Although theoretically the plan is to be developed at the meeting, it is a rare occurrence when speech-language clinicians do not already know what they would like to do.

Involvement of parents in private practice, hospital, and rehabilitation sites is somewhat different. There will usually be weekly discussions with parents either at the beginning or end of the session. During this time, parents are informed about the progress of their child. When facilities permit, observation of the session may be possible.

What is common to all settings, whether public or private, is the lack of meaningful consultation *prior* to the development of an intervention plan. Parents are a valuable asset to therapy and should always be included in discussion prior to the development of the intervention plan. Christenson and Cleary (1990) presented a six-part consultation program for parents whose children are being treated in the public schools. Although designed for public school counselors, the program is applicable to the area of speech-language pathology and can be used in various clinical settings.

Step 1: Increasing Parent-Clinician Interactions. The amount of school-home interaction between parents and clinicians tends to be minimal. Rarely is it due to parents not caring. It is incumbent upon the clinician to find ways of circumventing the multitude of problems that make this difficult, such as parent work schedules and large case loads. Monthly group meetings and telephone conferences are just two ways of increasing contact with parents. Many parents feel that they are unwanted in the clinical process. Clinicians tend to be surprised how much interaction is possible when parents are welcomed into the process.

Although interactions with parents in private facilities are not as problematic as in the schools, important ones exist. Therapy provided in private practice settings is generally expensive. Many parents believe that if they are paying someone between $45 and $90 an hour, that individual needs to assume all of the responsibility for behavioral changes. And many clinicians would agree with this. Additionally, the attitudes and behaviors of some parents may actually interfere with the therapeutic process. Finally, there are parents who are in the process of mourning the loss of normality in their child, and may find it too overwhelming to be involved in the therapy of their child (Kubler-Ross, 1979).

The role relationship of *pure* provider and *pure* consumer is one that may glorify professional images, but is usually detrimental to effective change in children. When possible, parents need to become co-therapists, providing insights, suggestions,

TABLE 6–10
Suggestions for Parents

WHAT	WHY	HOW
Involvement: Become involved in your child's therapy.	Therapists see your child for only a limited amount of time each week. Unless you become involved, little progress can be made.	Ask the following: 1. anything you do not understand 2. how you can help in therapy 3. what you can do at home
Consistency: Be consistent in how you treat your child.	Children expect parents to behave the same way they did the last time they did something. When they don't, children become confused.	First, decide how you want to react to what your child is doing. Write it down in a notebook. Then at the end of each day, see how well you did.
Reward: Reward (reinforce) your child for doing something you want him or her to do.	Everybody, including children, learns best and does better if what they are doing is rewarding.	There are 3 types of rewards you can use with your child: 1. choose an **activity** that is rewarding. 2. have the **completion** of the activity be rewarding. 3. provide something to the child that is reinforcing that **may not have anything to do** with the activity. Your activity should use at least 1 of these rewards.
Make Change Easy: Whatever you want your child to do differently, make it easy to achieve.	Change is hard for everybody. The easier it is to achieve, the more likely your child will be successful.	There are two ways to make change easy: 1. **Small steps** take the behavior you would like your child to learn and break it into small steps. 2. **Cues:** provide hints or cues to your child.
Memory: Do things to help your child remember better.	Many times when children can't do certain things, it isn't because they don't want to. Rather, they forgot how to do them.	There are many things that can be done to improve your child's memory: 1. **Interesting.** Make materials and activities interesting. 2. **Use in Many Areas.** Whatever you are trying to teach your child should be usable in many areas. 3. **Organize Your Child's Thinking.** Before beginning any activity tell your child what he or she will be doing, how he or she will do it, and why it will be done. 4. **Emphasize the Activity.** Whatever the activity is, make it stand out from everything else.

and a questioning attitude if the best and most efficient therapy is to be provided to their children. By not involving parents in therapy, the amount of time necessary to change behaviors increases dramatically.

Step 2: Problem Identification and Monitoring. Parents should be involved in the initial identification of the problem and then the monitoring of their child's progress. The identification should occur during the initial diagnostic assessment. Some authors believe that some of the most important information about the child is provided by parents during the diagnostic assessment by asking open-ended questions (Culatta & Goldberg, 1995). Once therapy begins, it is important that the child's progress is monitored at home. Although verbal reports are better than nothing, reliance on memory has been shown to be both selective and faulty (Frensch & Miner, 1994; Frank and Keene, 1993; Starnes & Loeb, 1993). Monitoring should involve a written format that can be easily used. An example of a form used to monitor the child's behaviors outside of the clinic will appear in the section on parental training.

Step 3: Sharing Relevant Information. Since the purpose of therapy is to develop behaviors which clients can use in nonclinical settings, it is critical that clinicians share both the content and progress of therapy with individuals who have contact with the children. This involves both teachers in the school and parents. The openness displayed by the clinician often results in a reciprocity of information giving that has only been waiting for an invitation. Each individual only sees a small slice of the child's behaviors. Often what occurs in one setting is not present in another. In therapy, children may not have much of an opportunity to demonstrate spontaneous speech. Yet it is abundant in the home. The classroom teacher may only be able to assess the child's behavior in terms of the chaos which may be occurring

in the presence of an additional 30 children. Information provided to her by the clinician regarding how the child functions individually or within a small group can be immensely important for interpreting classroom behavior. Parents who only know the effects of their interaction style upon their children could benefit from knowing the effects of other interaction styles.

Step 4: Understanding Behaviors. Clinicians may be in the best position for understanding how the behaviors of clients are affected by their communicative disorder. The reticent child who refuses to speak may be embarrassed by her articulation problem. The child who appears to always speak in a loud voice may be using a compensatory strategy for his hearing impairment. The child who is a bully on the playground may be acting aggressively to prevent others from laughing at his stuttering problem. The child who never appears to be able to listen may not be purposely inattentive, but unable to focus on the teacher's instructions because of an auditory processing problem. In all of these cases, and countless others, individuals who do not understand the impact of the communicative disorder may inappropriately infer explanations for the child's behavior that are inaccurate. By providing an understanding of the behavior to parents and teachers, many of the punishing consequences associated with the communicative disorder can be minimized.

Step 5: Supporting Parents. It is difficult to be a parent of a disabled child. The guilt associated with a child who is not normal can be overwhelming: guilt about having a child who is not normal and guilt about wishing that the child was normal. Disabilities affect not only the individual, but the whole family. Family constellations are reconstructed to meet the needs of the disabled child, often by sacrificing the needs of other family members. Even the best, most efficient parents require support from the clinician. It can be as minimal as providing verbal reinforcement for their involvement and concern about their child. Or the clinician's support can be as aggressive as becoming an advocate for needed services. By offering support to parents, problems that are interfering with their involvement in therapy are minimized. An example was a mother of a 5-year-old child who was prematurely exposed to a variety of drugs and alcohol. The child was nonverbal, had bizarre behavioral patterns, and needed constant supervision, both at school and at home. During all of his waking hours at home, the parent was involved in making sure that her child did not injure himself or destroy the apartment. When he slept, she slept. When he woke, she woke. When he went to school, she began her job. For this single mother, there never was any respite. Her life was tragically focused around meeting the needs of her disabled child for whom she knew she was responsible. To ask this mother to become involved in the therapy process, given what she faced daily, would be fruitless and possibly unconscionable. What the mother needed was some respite care, not additional work. The clinician was able to find a social service agency that would send someone to her house for a few hours a week, so that the mother could relax. The effects of this care were dramatic. Not only was the mother's mental health rescued, but the minimal help she experienced allowed her to feel that her involvement in therapy would not be an burden.

Step 6: Examining Overlapping Roles.
Speech-language clinicians, parents, and teachers have overlapping roles. Each cajoles, instructs, disciplines, admonishes, reinforces, and nurtures the child. There is always the possibility that the role behaviors of these adults will conflict. The conflicts can be minor or can have serious impact upon therapeutic progress. It is best that clinicians not only clarify the roles of each of the relevant adults who interact with the child, but also their own role behaviors.

General Considerations

When training parents, there are two general considerations that should be made. The first is that there should be a focus on training parents to use intervention strategies, rather than on how to correct specific behaviors. The second is that intervention strategies should be comprehensive. That is, they should not only deal with the communicative problem. Rather, they should address the relationship between the disorder and the child's functioning.

Use of Strategies. Most parents want to teach their children to do new behaviors, think more maturely, and achieve goals. The problem encountered is that, although motivation is high, parents tend to focus on specific behaviors and goals, rather than on the strategies for achieving them. The problem is even more acute with parents who have children with disabilities (Lyytinen, Rasku-Puttonen, Poikkeus, & Laakso, 1994). When training parents to be involved with teaching or generalizing new behaviors, clinicians should focus on the strategy that is being used and how the strategy can be incorporated into other learning situations. Take, for example, the use of a visual aid to signal a phonologically impaired child that a word has three parts. In teaching the parent how to use the aid, a discussion should occur in which the clinician explains how the use of this device is also applicable to other words in which her child leaves off the final consonant.

Comprehensiveness. Rarely is a child's communicative disorder an isolated event that has no or little effect on the child's socialization and the family's functioning. Communication is such an intertwining event that it affects everything. When designing training programs for families, it is important for their clinicians to stretch the areas of treatment. For example, not only does a child's phonological disorder affect her communication, but may also result in behavioral problems related to difficulties in being understood. By addressing those areas tangential to the basic problem, but significantly affecting the life of the family, commitment to therapy, positive feelings toward the clinician, and more involvement are substantially increased (Pfiffner, Jouriles, Brown, Etscheidt et al., 1990).

Rigor

When one thinks about parent training, what usually comes to mind is teaching parents how to implement or generalize a specific behavior already taught to the child in the clinic. An explanation is provided to the parent, usually orally, and possibly the parent can observe how to engage in the desired behavior. Observation alone, however, does not result in the development of those competencies necessary for parents to effect changes in their children (Wilkinson, Parrish, & Wilson, 1994). Parent training should have the same amount of rigor and thought given by the clinician in designing the intervention program for the child or adolescent. Just as we teach clients how to use specific behaviors and develop problem-solving skills, so we should do the same with parents. There are few differences between teaching children new behaviors, training parents to become co-therapists, and involving classroom teachers in the clinical process.

Procedures

Although generalizing a specific behavior is important for the child, showing the parent how to change their interaction patterns with their child is even more significant (Pfiffner, Jouriles, Brown, Etscheidt et al., 1990; Webster-Stratton & Herbert, 1993). Both can be accomplished by training parents through a systematic process which involves goal selection, written directions, observation, joint therapy, solo therapy, and home therapy.

Goal Selection. The first step in designing a successful experience for parents is in the initial selection of goals. Of prime importance is that you structure the activity so that the probability of succeeding is maximized and the possibility of failing is minimized for parents. This can be done by selecting a goal that the child can already perform. There are certain characteristics that the goal behavior should have. Namely, it should already be in the child's behavioral repertoire, be simple, requiring a minimal amount of time to produce, quantitatively scorable, and generalizable in the home. A format for goal selection is provided in Table 6–11.

The behavior should be in the child's *behavioral repertoire* and one that can be consistently produced. It need not be a behavior that is fully developed through a successive approximation approach. It can be an intermediary goal. Do not choose a behavior that the child has just mastered, since it may not be consistent. Remember, the initial purpose of selecting the goal is to provide the parents with a successful experience. This can be enhanced by choosing a behavior that the client is more likely to produce at home. A benchmark number would be consistent productions over a two-session period.

Do not choose a behavior that has many parts. It is best that at this early stage of parent training, the behavior is one that is *simple* and easily produced. The simpler a behavior is, the easier it will be to produce it correctly. Additionally, simple behaviors are easier for parents to assess than those that are more complex. For example, it takes a very little amount of sophistication for parents to determine if their child used articles during a home therapy session. It would take a greater degree of sophistication for parents to determine if the distortion created by a lateralization this week

TABLE 6–11

Preparation for Selecting and Rank Ordering
Behaviors to be Trained by Parents

Behaviors Recently Trained in Clinic (rank ordered from simple to complex)	Time Required To Complete	Method for Quantitative Scoring		
1. _____	_____	❒ Presence	❒ Correct	❒ Other
2. _____	_____	❒ Presence	❒ Correct	❒ Other
3. _____	_____	❒ Presence	❒ Correct	❒ Other
4. _____	_____	❒ Presence	❒ Correct	❒ Other

List generalization activities that can be done by the parent for each behavior in the home, while traveling (e.g., in the car), and in other settings. Try to identify at least three activities in each setting (e.g., eating, playing, and going to bed in the home)

BEHAVIORS	Home	Travel	Other
1.	1. _____ 2. _____ 3. _____	1. _____ 2. _____ 3. _____	1. _____ 2. _____ 3. _____
2.	1. _____ 2. _____ 3. _____	1. _____ 2. _____ 3. _____	1. _____ 2. _____ 3. _____
3.	1. _____ 2. _____ 3. _____	1. _____ 2. _____ 3. _____	1. _____ 2. _____ 3. _____
4.	1. _____ 2. _____ 3. _____	1. _____ 2. _____ 3. _____	1. _____ 2. _____ 3. _____

was less than what occurred last week.

Because the activity will most likely be done in the home, it should require a *minimal amount of time* to produce. Of importance is that the activity should blend in as much as possible with the parents' normal activities. The more special time required to set up doing the activity and completing it, the more likely its interference value will impede further parental involvement. Even having one normal child takes a great deal of time for parents. Children with disabilities will require additional time. It is very easy to blend in the activities even with very busy families. The key

is to incorporate therapy into activities that parents are already doing on a daily basis. For example, if everyone gathers around the table to have dinner together, it would make sense to incorporate the speech or language task within the activities required for making meals and eating them. If the child is given a bath every evening during which the parent is required to monitor, incorporate an activity into bath taking.

An important feature of any program that involves parents is that their involvement should lead to very clear indicators of how they are helping their child. This can be best done by selecting behaviors parents can *score* either to their correctness or number of times they occur. With data such as these, it becomes possible to unequivocally show parents how their involvement is helping their child. Scoring methods should be extremely simple, using nothing more than a ✔ for correct responses and an ✗ for incorrect responses.

The purpose of teaching any behavior in the clinic is so that it can be used in nonclinical settings. Not only should the behavior be *generalizable,* it should be something meaningful that can occur in the home. There are two advantages to this. The first is that it is easy for the parent to do and therefore will occur more likely than if it can only be done in a non-home setting. The second reason is that its occurrence can be easily reinforced. And we know that the more a behavior is reinforced, the more likely it will be strengthened and integrated into the child's behavioral repertoire.

Written Instructions. Before observing the clinician elicit the behavior from the child, parents should be provided with a single page of typewritten instructions clearly describing what they will be observing and the steps in which the clinician will engage. The clinician should not be attempting to impress parents with vocabulary. The words selected should be simple, descriptive, and nonprofessional. By adopting this approach when interacting with parents, a more collaborative relationship is developed (Fine & Gardner, 1994). Two good rules to use when selecting words are: (1) Would someone totally unfamiliar with the field of speech-language pathology understand what the word means? (2) Is there a synonym for the word that is simpler? It seems that sentence structures grow and get more complex as the number of years in education expands. Where simple and concise sentences would suffice, more obtuse and complicated ones are substituted. The re-

verse should be true. It takes more effort and knowledge to simplify a thought and have it be clear than it does to make it complicated. Sentences should be short with the thoughts appearing in them ordered sequentially. In other words, if parents are first to provide their child with a model for producing an utterance and then reinforce its presence, that is the order it should appear in the instructions, not the reverse. Again, simplicity is the key here. Parents will be asked to engage in new and structured activities in ways that may be unfamiliar to them. Since there will probably be anywhere from two to five very specific things the clinician will want them to do, one sentence should be used and numbered for each thing the parent is to do.

When the instructions are presented to the parent, they should be oriented to their purpose. Essentially, they are being provided with the material so that they can follow what they will be observing and then asked to do with the clinician and finally do on their own at home. When provided with the material, the clinician should go through everything on the page with them, reading each line verbatim and if necessary, orally and or visually, describing what each thing will look or sound like. Then they should be asked if there was anything that they did not understand or would like to go over again.

Wording. There is a natural tendency to improvise in therapy as the need arises. In the case of parent training, the opposite must occur. The clinician is providing a model that will be emulated by the parent. The replication will at best be only as good as the model, and usually contain some differences. If the model provided is from the start different from what the parent is to do, what the clinician will get back may be significantly different from what it was hoped the parent would do. As clinicians, you will be responsible for training up to four different classes of individuals: (1)

clients, (2) guardians and family members, (3) professionals, and (4) aides. Although the specific procedures will differ for each group, the basic methodology is identical.

Steps

Four steps are involved in training parents to become co-therapists. They involve: (1) observation of the activity, (2) performing joint therapy with the clinician, (3) doing solo therapy, and (4) engaging in home therapy. A sample written format for these steps appears in Table 6–12.

Observation. Ideally, the observation should occur through a one-way glass or on a video monitor so that parents can devote their full attention to observing rather than be distracted by their child. Even if this is not possible, observation within the clinic room will work. The most important thing about the observation is that the parent is able to follow therapy along with its written description. Therefore, there are a few things that should be done to insure that this will happen: (1) use the words and behaviors in the description, (2) call off the

TABLE 6-12
Sample Format for Parent Training

Behavior to be Trained _____

There are four training steps that you will be doing. Each is described below. Please read through everything before you begin observing. If there is anything you do not understand, please ask me when you come into the therapy room.

STEP 1: OBSERVATION
1. You will see me doing the activity I would like you to do with your child.
2. I will do it exactly as I want you to do it.
3. I will do it __ times in order for you to see how it is done.
4. After I have finished the activity, I will call you into the room.
5. Please bring this sheet with you.

STEP 2: JOINT THERAPY
1. When you are in the room we will do the activity together.
2. I will tell you what to do.
3. As soon as you complete it, I will tell you if it was correct or what needs to be done differently.
4. We will repeat the activity until you feel comfortable doing it. If you need more time please tell me.

STEP 3: SOLO THERAPY
1. I will ask you to do the whole activity by yourself.
2. If I see any problems while you are doing the activity I will tell you.
3. If you are not sure about something, please ask me if you are doing it correctly.
4. I will ask you to repeat the activity until you feel comfortable doing it. If you need more time please let me know.

STEP 4: HOME THERAPY
1. On the following page you will see a form that you will be using at home.
2. The form contains a description of what you did with your child, and places and times to practice the behavior.
3. We will complete the form together at the end of the session.

numbers for each of the prescribed parent and child behaviors, and (3) verbally note any exceptions or important features that will enhance the parent's understanding of what is occurring.

Joint Therapy. In joint therapy, parts of an activity can be assigned to the parent or, after the clinician models the behavior, the parent can engage in it. It is best to start with a modeling procedure and then advance to a shared responsibility approach. As parents become more proficient and consistent, their responsibilities can be increased. It is important not to rush the learning process. Parental confidence, competency, and consistency should be the primary goals, regardless how long these goals take to achieve.

Solo Therapy. Once parents have demonstrated the ability to perform an activity with the help of the clinician, they should be asked to perform the entire sequence by themselves. During this process, clinicians should provide immediate feedback regarding the appropriateness of parents' behaviors. If verbal feedback is not sufficient, modeling should again be performed. This should be followed by a second attempt at solo therapy. The process should be repeated until there is little or no difference between the parents' and clinicians' delivery of the activity.

Home Therapy. If the goal chosen for the first home therapy project was simple and the training in the clinic was complete, there should be few problems carrying out the activity in the home. However, it is not sufficient to merely ask parents to go home and do the activity with their children. Structure has to be provided. In Table 6–13 a sample format is provided. As you can see, *everything* that needs to be done is provided in writing for parents. This is critical. It is too easy to forget something 2 or 3 days after it occurs. Also, parents may

inappropriately believe that modifications can be made in the program. The activity is not only described in detail, but provisions for easily scoring children's responses are included. It is also a good idea to have the parents call clinicians after their first attempt to discuss the outcome. It makes little sense for the parent to work inappropriately on a behavior for a week before being given feedback.

THE PROCESS OF LEARNING

To understand the cognitive processes that clients use to learn new behaviors, two areas of learning must be addressed: stages and levels. A schematic for understanding the relationship is provided in Table 6–14.

Stages

There are four stages of learning that are sequentially ordered. Problems in lower stages of learning usually result in problems in subsequent stages.

Apprehending. Apprehending refers to an individual's ability to be aware of a particular stimulus configuration. For example, when teaching a child to discriminate between a correct and an incorrect production of /r/, the child must apprehend differences before he can acquire an understanding of the differences. Without apprehending, learning may be difficult or impossible. To establish attending behavior, use stimuli configurations that focus attention on whatever is to be learned. In Chapter 4, very specific suggestions were provided for constructing stimulus configurations that would facilitate apprehending.

Acquisition. Acquisition refers to the process by which the components of a new behavior or idea are recognized. In the preceding example, the child may now under-

TABLE 6-13
Home Therapy example

Behavior: Describing things that move

1. Here is a list of words we want your son to use.

Action	Objects
push	ball
throw	car
hide	doll

2. They can be used in any combination as long as an action word is first and an object word is second.

3. Place the strategy card in front of your son and hold up an object.

4. Say, "Charlie, what should I do?"

5. A correct response would be one of the following:
   1. He touches the cards and says the two words (i.e., "push car").
   2. He says the two words without touching the cards.

6. In the far left hand column under "Situation," list the situations in which you did the activity. Place a ✔ or an ✘ for each attempt your son made. Place these marks in the columns listing the days of the week. Try to do at least ___ activities each day.

7. Please call during the week if you have any questions.

8. Bring this sheet with you next week for therapy.
   ✔ = correct   ✘ = wrong

Situation	Sunday	Monday	Tuesday	Wednesday	Thursday	Friday	Saturday
Home 1. ___ 2. ___ 3. ___							
Driving 1. ___ 2. ___ 3. ___							
Other 1. ___ 2. ___ 3. ___							

stand the distinctive features of /r/ and therefore be able to apply this knowledge to differentiate between correct and incorrect productions of /r/. Acquisition can be facilitated by having components that "stand out" or have figure-ground differences. Take for example the three different auditory discrimination tasks that appear below:

/w/ from /r/
/w/ from /p/, /d/, /c/
/w from "gross sound"

In the first line, discrimination between /w/ and /r/ is difficult because the two phonemes are different in only one distinctive feature. If this was the first step in acquiring and understanding of the distinctions, numerous errors would probably result. Contrast this with the second activity in which /w/ is differentiated from /p/, /d/, and /c/. Because the distinctive features of these three sounds differ from /w/ more than /r/ does from /w/, it is more likely that the discrimination will be acquired. Now contrast both activities with the final one, which has the clinician contrasting /w/ with gross sounds such as belching, groaning, and chirping. Obviously, with contrasts such as these, the client would probably be able to identify the /r/ phoneme 100% of the time. Acquisition is enhanced if the critical elements of what is being acquired stand out.

Retention. Retention refers to the memory processes that result in information being stored in a manner that allows for retrieval at a later time. It is hypothesized that retention involves two memory processes: short-term and long-term (Frensch & Miner, 1994). When the child learned the distinctive features of the /r/ phoneme, the initial knowledge involved short-term memory. After being processed in short-term memory, the information was transferred into long-term memory, where storage involved electrochemical processes. Retention is facilitated by creating multiple associations. Methods for doing this were discussed in Chapter 4. The only way clinicians know if clients have retained information is through the retrieval process.

Retrieval. Retrieval is the ability to recall information that will allow an individual to produce a previously learned behavior. Retrieval is the best method available for determining whether the information was learned. Until the child is asked to differentiate between correct and incorrect productions of /r/, it can never be known whether she learned the discrimination. During any testing procedure, retrieval is being used. It is often mistaken for intervention. For example, when pictures are shown to clients and they are asked to do activities such as identification, use the word in a sentence, and say the word using correct articulation, it is a retrieval activity unless they are using a strategy. Contrast the following two situations below:

Retrieval (Assessment):	A series of objects are placed in front of an aphasic client and she is asked to name each one.
Acquisition (Intervention):	A series of objects are placed in front of an aphasic client and she is asked to name each one.

On each picture there is a colored dot. The colored dots correspond to larger categories such as "transportation," "tools," and "money." On the table a card has a picture of each category, which are colored to correspond to the dots on the pictures.

Before trying to say the word, the client has been instructed to first match the colored dot with the larger category, think of other objects in the same category, then try to retrieve the word.

TABLE 6-14
Stages and Levels of Learning

1. Identify a behavior that you wish your client to learn.

2. In the appropriate boxes indicate the activities that will occur in order for your client to learn a behavior.

Stages of Learning	LEVELS OF LEARNING					
	Stimulus Response	Chaining	Discrimination	Concept	Rule Governed	Problem Solving
Apprehending						
Acquisition						
Retrieval						

Repetition of questions or demands may result in learning taking place. When this occurs, clients are internally generating instructional methodologies. There is no clinician guidance, and as a result, this is a very inefficient method of learning. A good rule of thumb is that, if clients have not been provided with a strategy to produce a behavior or utterance, the activity is more than likely a retrieval or assessment activity, rather than an acquistion or intervention activity. One defining feature of the therapy of master clinicians is that most of the time spent interacting with clients involves acquisition activities. The time spent on retrieval activities is minimal. In Chapter 8, specific strategies will be presented.

Levels

Gagne and his associates (1970, 1988) maintained that learning occurs at eight hierarchical levels, each one being dependent on the one that preceded it. His model of learning provides clinicians with a framework for understanding some of the cognitive problems clients have. The acquisition of a behavior that requires a higher level of learning assumes that the individual is able to use all of the lower, sequentially ordered levels of learning. Understanding Gagne's levels of learning can help the clinician not only to identify a client's cognitive deficits, but also to construct intervention protocols.

Type 1: Signal Learning. Another term for signal learning is reflexive conditioning. The most well-known example of how it occurs is the salivation condition Pavlov achieved in his dog experiments. Three steps are involved in signal learning: (1) eliciting an unconditioned response, (2) pairing a neutral stimulus with an unconditioned stimulus; and (3) transforming the neutral stimulus into a conditioned stimulus. Pavlov's classic experiment illustrates how the process occurs.

In step 1 food powder is placed in a dog's mouth, and he salivates. This would be an unconditioned response.

Food Powder → Salivation
(unconditioned (unconditioned
stimulus) response)

In step 2 a few seconds before the food power is placed in the dog's mouth, a bell rings. The dog will eventually associate the bell with food. Until that happens, the bell is called a neutral stimulus

Bell + Food → Salivation
(neutral (unconditioned (unconditioned
stimulus) stimulus) response)

In step 3 if the dog has associated the bell with the presentation of food powder, we should be able to ring the bell without any food powder present, and create the salivating response. If this occurs, then the bell is now called a conditioned stimulus and the salivation a conditioned response.

Bell → Salivation
(conditioned (conditioned
stimulus) response)

The preceding example is one that illustrates the process involved in conditioning an involuntary behavior. This type of learning does not occur when the behaviors are voluntary, such as learning to write or speak specific sounds.

Type 2: Stimulus-Response Learning.

Stimulus-response learning differs from signal learning in that it involves precise voluntary responses. A person or animal produces a behavior, with or without help, and is then reinforced. The behavior is produced as a consequence of being reinforced. An animal example would be teaching a dog to shake hands. A human example would be teaching a child to produce a combination of phonemes. Four conditions are usually associated with stimulus-response learning.

First, the act is learned *gradually*. Initially the person does not perform it perfectly, and repetitions of the presentation and reinforcement are necessary. For example, children who have a lateral lisp will not immediately produce /s/ correctly on their first attempt when provided with an appropriate model. Most likely, it may sound like a distorted /s/ with less lateralized sounds than was produced prior to instruction. There may not be any firm lines between the lateralization and subsequent distortion.

Second, there is an *increasing proficiency* of the act. The behavior that is performed becomes more refined with practice. The behavior is *shaped* by aiding the person with various types of cues. Gradually, the cues are reduced. This process is known as response differentiation. In our example the child may have been instructed with the use of a mirror in which she observed herself and the model. The clinician may also have used her fingers to reduce the child's lateralization.

Third, there is an *increasing strength of the controlling stimulus*. Initially, the response may have occurred not only in the presence of the controlling stimulus, but of others as well. With increased presentations, the response is elicited only in the presence of the controlling stimulus.

And fourth, the clients will be *reinforced* when a correct response is emitted. They will not be reinforced when an incorrect response is emitted. This type of learning, originally explored by B.F. Skinner, is commonly referred to as operant conditioning. Skinner (1957) contended that this type of learning can account for all of linguistic acquisition, a position strongly disputed by many linguists (Chomsky, 1972; Huxley & Ingram, 1971; Kausler, 1974; Naremore, 1984). Although operant conditioning may not be able to account for language learning, it is an important technique for the acquisition of new behaviors.

Type 3: Chain Learning: Chaining occurs when two or more previously learned stimulus-response events are sequenced together. An example of this would be some of the very early naming activities of children. At some time in the past, a child has learned that a doll is used for hugging, kissing, and cuddling. Whenever the child's parents give him the doll, the above activities occur. This is the first part of the chain. Also in the past, the child has been reinforced for imitating the mother's production of the word *doll*. This is the second part of the chain. The child is now laying in his crib, which he associates with *doll* playing. The doll is seen outside of the crib. He points to the doll, looks at his mother, and says the word doll. The child has just exhibited an example of type 3 learning. Three conditions are necessary for chaining to occur: First, *each link of the chain must have been previously learned.* Second, there must be a *continuity of links.* Each new link of the chain must follow the preceding link. And third, there must be an *immediate acquisition of the behavior.* If the two previous conditions are met, the acquisition of a chain is not a gradual process, but rather occurs on a single occasion.

Type 4: Verbal Association Learning: Learning: Verbal association is a subvariety of chaining that involves associating one word with another, for example, learning the French word for *match*. Four conditions must be present for verbal association to occur. First, *each link of the chain must have been previously learned.* In our example, the person must know what a match is and know the English word for it. Second, there must be a *production of the verbal associate.* The person must be able to correctly pronounce the French word for match. Third, there must be an *available coding connection.* The English and the French words for the object must be connected by a code that would be visual. And finally, fourth, there must be a *continuity of links.*

Each new link of the chain must follow the preceding link.

Type 5: Discrimination Learning. In discrimination learning, two or more previously learned chains are juxtaposed. The individual is now expected to identify each type of chain correctly when in the presence of other previously learned chains. Two conditions are necessary for learning discriminations. The first is that each of the chains with their identifying responses must have been previously learned. If the responses have been learned, it is assumed that the stimulus that elicited them can also be readily identified. The second is that interference must be reduced. If the stimuli of two or more chains or the responses of two or more chains are similar, it will become more difficult to differentiate between the chains. This is known as interference. Specific procedures need to be undertaken that will reduce interference.

Type 6: Concept Learning. Concept learning depends on the neural processes of representation and involves classifying stimulus situations in terms of abstracted properties, such as color, shape position, number, and others. In concept learning, the individual learns to classify objects or events according to specific discriminative stimuli or critical attributes. For example, if a child uses the word *table* to refer only to one specific piece of furniture in his house, even when other tables are present, he is using the word in the context of type 3 learning: chaining. However, if he appropriately used the word table to correctly identify various types of tables, he is operating at the level of concept learning, since he is able to use one word to label items that are similar, yet have dissimilarities. Three necessary conditions must be present for concept learning to occur.

First, there must have been a *prior learning of a stimulus.* The stimulus portion of the chain must have been previously learned, as must the response. Second, there must be a *variety of stimulus situations*. The concept that is to be learned must be presented in various ways. By doing this, the learner can identify the critical attributes of the concept when it appears in objects or events that have differences but are still occurrences of the concept. Third, *learning is gradual*. The concept may be learned gradually over a period of time.

Type 7: Rule Learning. A rule is a chain of two or more concepts. In its simplest form, a rule would have the structure of "If A, then B." Rule learning is more than just the memorization of verbal facts. Otherwise, rule learning would be identical to stimulus-response chains. In rule learning, the individual is expected to apply the rule to a variety of situations. For example, a simple early linguistic rule that children use in describing objects and people is "color + object." A child who understands this rule can apply it in a multitude of ways, such as "red ball," "black doggie," and "blue car." Three conditions must be present for rule learning to occur.

First, *concepts had to have been previously learned*. The concepts that are linked in the rule must have been previously learned. Second the *rule needs to be applied*. Understanding the rule results in its application to a variety of situations involving previously learned concepts. Third, there is *immediate learning*. The learning of a rule takes place on a single occasion.

Type 8: Problem Solving. It has been proposed that problem solving may be accomplished in three ways: (1) trial and error, (2) linear step, and (3) intuition (Brammer, 1990). In trial-and-error learning, the person repeatedly tries to solve a problem, eliminating solutions that do not fit. In linear step learning, problems are solved through a logical progression of decisions and insights. Intuition, the most difficult problem solving technique to describe,

involves an inductive reasoning process where the individual refers back to various experiences and sets of knowledge acquired in the past. Regardless of the process used, the individual combines two or more previously learned rules to address a problem not previously solved. For example, let us assume that a child has learned two basic linguistic rules that are appropriate for describing objects. Rule 1 is *color + object*. Rule 2 is *size + object*. In the past, the child has said "blue ball" and "big ball." As he is sitting in the living room, he notices a very large blue ball that is out of his reach. He would like his father to give it to him and is about to formulate the verbal request. Since there are other balls of various shapes and colors next to the big blue ball, the application of either the previously learned rules would not assure him of receiving the big blue ball. He now combines the two rules into a new one having the formula *size + color + object*, and he says *"big blue ball."* The child has solved a problem by chaining and synthesizing two previously learned rules. In one study, the ability to use problem-solving strategies appeared to be influenced by the emotional state of the client (Rueter and Conger, 1995). Subjects whose interaction styles were identified as hostile showed poor problem-solving skills Four conditions are essential for problem solving to occur. First, there needs to be an *identification of essential features*. The person must identify the essential features of the response before he produces it. In other words, he must know what the activity's goal is. Second, there must be a *recall of past rules*. All past rules that will be relevant to solving the problem must be recalled. Third, the *recalled rules must be combined*. The rules that have been recalled are combined to formulate a new rule. And fourth, there must be a *sudden solution*. The processes involved in combining rules may be lengthy and complex, but the solution appears suddenly. Repetition plays no part in problem solving.

C H A P T E R

7

Transitional
Process Skills

The therapy setting is not a sterile environment in which only speech and language disorders are addressed. It is as messy as life is, compounded by client fears, joy, anger, pain, and disappointments. Clients enter into this relationship with an expectation that everything they bring into it, including very private emotional issues, is appropriate for discussion. Within this milieu, clinicians should be prepared to use some basic counseling skills that will satisfy client needs, yet protect standards of professional ethics. In this chapter, six categories of skills containing 34 techniques and behaviors are presented.

ACKNOWLEDGMENT

Clients often want to discuss issues of an emotional nature with their clinicians that they may not feel comfortable discussing with anyone else. Many clinicians, however, are reluctant to allow, no less encourage, clients to bring up emotional issues. This may be due to a professional convic-

tion that speech-language clinicians should not be engaging in counseling activities or a personal discomfort they experience in examining clients' feelings and emotions. There are various viewpoints concerning the extent to which clinicians should do counseling. At one end of the continuum are those who believe that without extensive psychological training, exploration of clients' feelings and emotions should be kept to an absolute minimum (Barbara, 1954; Sheehan, 1978). At the other end are clinical educators who maintain that the feelings and emotions of clients cannot be separated from their communicative disorders, and therefore extensive counseling, possibly to the exclusion or minimization of direct speech or language therapy is appropriate (Rollin, 1987). In the middle are those who maintain that counseling is an appropriate activity if it focuses on an exploration of feelings and emotions that are directly related to the disorder (Donahue-Kilburg, 1992; Culatta & Goldberg, 1995). Clients are impervious to the niceties of academic discussions on counseling. When an aphasic client, whose wife has sexually rejected him because of his condition, comes to therapy, his mind is not on the retrieval of common nouns. When parents have just compared the behaviors of their language-delayed child with a normal child of an identical age, they need to grapple with the feelings they have of disappointment and fear. When a young stutterer has just had a group of children laugh at her speech, her thoughts will not be on a fluency exercise. Who is better suited to share these feelings with than the speech-language clinician? Nobody. At the very least, clinicians need to acknowledge what the client is saying. To do otherwise can have a significant negative impact on the clinical relationship and eventually on the progress of therapy (Ozechowski, 1994). There are very specific verbal and nonverbal methods that can be used to acknowledge the emotionally loaded topics that clinicians inevitably want to discuss.

Verbal

There are various ways of verbally acknowledging clients' expression of feelings and experiences. They can range from the simplicity of using some of the previously discussed techniques, such as conversational follow-through and asking relevant questions, to the sophistication of nondirective therapy. A summary appears in Table 7–1. This form can be used to analyze the methods used to acknowledge clients' communications. Regardless of how one shows attentiveness, it has been shown to correlate positively with positive perceptions of the clinician and therefore contributes to the development of trust (Meredith, 1985; Shaffer, Murillo, & Michael, 1978).

Conversational Follow-through. Conversational follow-through is probably the easiest method to use to acknowledge client emotions. The guiding principle is topic maintenance. Essentially, whenever

a client ends his or her verbalizations, whatever is said by the clinician should directly relate to what was said by the client. Take, for example, the following sequence:

> *Parent:* Yesterday was horrible. I was in the supermarket and Henrietta was out of control. No matter what I said to her, she just wailed and acted like a little beast. It was so embarrassing.
>
> *Clinician:* I shop in that store also. I know how easy it is for children to reach those shelves.

In this example, the clinician maintained the topic of conversation. By doing this, she not only indicates that the parent's conversation is being followed, but there is an implicit assumption that, although this was not necessarily the thrust of the session, it is all right to continue. Contrast this with a very different kind of response from the clinician. Assume that the parent's statement remains the same, but this time the clinician says, "I shop at the store also. Now let's talk about the home program I asked you to do last week." At the very least, the parent may feel that her introduction of the topic was inappropriate. At the very worst, she may feel hurt that the clinician does not feel that an extremely embarrassing event is worthy of discussion. Regardless of the parent's reaction, damage has been done to the clinical relationship.

Asking Relevant Questions. An excellent and easy way of acknowledging clients' statements is through the use of relevant questions. A relevant question is one that directly pertains to what the client has just said. It results in answers that elaborate on the topic. Using the

TABLE 7–1
Analyzing Verbal Aknowledgment

Describe five communications your client made and your response to them. Analyze each response in terms of the type of verbal acknowledgment you used. Then offer a revision of your acknowledgment if necessary.

CLIENT COMMUNICATION	CLINICIAN RESPONSE	TYPE OF VERBAL ACKNOWLEDGMENT	REVISION OF VERBAL ACKNOWLEDGMENT
1.		❑ Conversational Follow-through ❑ Asking Relevant Questions ❑ Simple Rephrasing ❑ Client-centered Techniques ❑ None	
2.		❑ Conversational Follow-through ❑ Asking Relevant Questions ❑ Simple Rephrasing ❑ Client-centered Techniques ❑ None	
3.		❑ Conversational Follow-through ❑ Asking Relevant Questions ❑ Simple Rephrasing ❑ Client-centered Techniques ❑ None	
4.		❑ Conversational Follow-through ❑ Asking Relevant Questions ❑ Simple Rephrasing ❑ Client-centered Techniques ❑ None	
5.		❑ Conversational Follow-through ❑ Asking Relevant Questions ❑ Simple Rephrasing ❑ Client-centered Techniques ❑ None	

above example, a relevant question would take the following form:

| Parent: | Yesterday was horrible. I was in the supermarket and Henrietta was out of control. No matter what I said to her, she just wailed and acted like a little beast. It was so embarrassing. |
| Clinician: | What did she do that was so embarrassing? |

In this example, asking a question indicates two things to the parent. First, that the topic is worthy of discussion. And second, it is important enough that the clinician would like additional information.

Paraphrasing/Simple Rephrasing.

Paraphrasing, or simple rephrasing, is the process where clinicians slightly modify what clients say. Take for example the following interaction:

| Client: | I was so frustrated when a couldn't remember her name. She's my best friend! |
| Clincian: | I can see how that would make you frustrated. After all, she's your best friend. |

Although the clinician added nothing to the client's statement, the act of repeating what the client said is a form of acknowledgment. After all, in order to repeat something, it has to be attended to. Although this technique does acknowledge the feelings of clients, its overuse can trivialize it. During one session in which a client was presenting the clinician with many personal problems that the clinician felt unable to competently handle, virtually every statement by the client was followed by a sim-

ple rephrasing, similar to the above example. Instead of leaving the session believing that the clinician was acknowledging what he was feeling, the client now viewed the clinician as an "air head," because, "all he kept doing was saying what I said. He never even offered his opinion or gave me anything I could use." Paraphrasing and simple rephrasing is appropriate if it is not overused. Often, people mistake this simple technique for a more advanced one found in client-centered therapy, in which new insights are provided to clients through restructuring of their utterances.

Client-centered Therapy Techniques.

One of the most effective and commonly used methods for acknowledging the feelings of clients is client-centered therapy (Rogers, 1965). The basic tenet of client-centered therapy is that clients bring to the therapeutic relationship the ability to heal their emotional problems. The role of the clinician is to structure the therapy session in a manner that will facilitate the development of solutions from the client's perspective. The individual, not the problem, is the focus of therapy. The goal of therapy is not to identify nor solve clients' problems, but rather to help them gain insight into their behaviors so that they may cope better with them in an integrated manner. Because clients' perceptions of their problems influence their behavior, the approach concentrates on helping clients fully understand these perceptions. Because perceptions are personal, it is inappropriate for clinicians to impose their own frame of reference to explain the perceptions of clients. By providing a guided opportunity for clients to fully explore their own feelings, they are able to understand them, individually, and in relation to their communicative disorder. The approach is less intimidating to both clinician and client, as there is no highly structured and theoretically rigid framework with which verbalizations are made.

Vocal

In Chapter 5, vocal behaviors were divided into two categories, prosody (intonation) and paralanguage. Prosody, or intonation, includes the qualities of intensity, pitch, register, tempo, duration, and tension. Paralanguage consists of sounds that are not words. In Table 7–2 a form is provided for analyzing how clinicians vocally acknowledge the feelings of clients.

Prosody or Intonation. It is rare that anyone's speech is so monotone that no inferences can be made regarding its emotional overtones. Even in the driest of lectures, the instructor's intonation patterns can convey a level of commitment to the content. Listeners will often focus on the intonation patterns of a speaker to determine their feeling levels. This can be very useful in therapy. Although everyone could probably simulate what it sounds like to be *compassionate, empathetic, angry, bored,* or *interested*, when asked to behaviorally describe it, they might be at a loss. Unfortunately, very few studies have attempted to find the discriminative features of these feeling states. However, just like pornography, listeners can identify it when they hear it. Therefore, when responding to clients' emotional concerns, clinicians should attempt to use intonation patterns that *they* associate with *compassion, empathy, concern,* or similar feelings. Regardless of how clients interpret them, all are positive, and indicate to clients that their topic of conversation is acceptable and of interest to the clinician.

Paralanguage. Paralanguage can be divided into identifiers and characterizers. *Identifiers* are isolated phonemes or combinations of phonemes that are not words. These would include such sounds as "uh-uh," "ah," and "um." The interjection of these sounds by the listener often serves as verbal lubricants for the speaker. It is as if the listener is saying, "Yes I understand, continue on with your story." It is an easy way to acknowledge what clients are saying. *Characterizers* are sounds that can stand by themselves, such as yawning, belching, swallowing, coughing, yelling, whispering, sneezing, snorting, and groaning. Although more difficult to use clinically, they can be as effective as identifiers. For example, a client who had a laryngectomy was explaining to the clinician the intense pain he was experiencing following an operation to increase the size of his stoma. At the end of the description the clinician groaned, then said "God, that must have been so painful for you." By groaning, the message was amplified. It was very clear to the client that the clinician not only acknowledged his feelings but was empathetic to them.

Nonverbal

Clinicians engaged in therapeutic interactions tend to consciously rely heavily on verbal communication as the primary method of conveying information to clients. Unfortunately, the body is similar to a giant billboard which continually thrusts messages in front of all who can see it. Some of these messages can be easily controlled by clinicians while others cannot. A summary of nonverbal behaviors appears in Table 7–3.

Intentional Messages. The area of the body that is most often used to convey intentional messages is the face. In clinical interactions, a clinician's head nod often indicates agreement with the client's verbalization and is also interpreted as the message, "Continue talking. This is information I think is important." The clinician can easily control it since awareness results from kinesic feedback and listener reactions. This is also the area of the body clients feel most comfortable observing during interactions. Facial configurations of listeners can also be used to mirror the emotions expressed by speakers. If clients

TABLE 7-2
Analyzing Vocal Acknowledgment

Use the five communications listed in Table 7-1. Analyze each response in terms of the type of vocal acknowledgment you used. Then offer a revision of your acknowledgment if necessary.

CLIENT COMMUNICATION	CLINICIAN RESPONSE	TYPE OF VERBAL ACKNOWLEDGMENT	REVISION OF VERBAL ACKNOWLEDGMENT
1.		❑ Intonation Pattern ❑ Amplitude ❑ Intensity ❑ Identifiers ❑ Characterizers ❑ None	
2.		❑ Intonation Pattern ❑ Amplitude ❑ Intensity ❑ Identifiers ❑ Characterizers ❑ None	
3.		❑ Intonation Pattern ❑ Amplitude ❑ Intensity ❑ Identifiers ❑ Characterizers ❑ None	
4.		❑ Intonation Pattern ❑ Amplitude ❑ Intensity ❑ Identifiers ❑ Characterizers ❑ None	
5.		❑ Intonation Pattern ❑ Amplitude ❑ Intensity ❑ Identifiers ❑ Characterizers ❑ None	

are expressing especially painful experiences, a painful expression displayed by the clinician indicates that the topic is acknowledged as something that is causing emotional distress.

Because the arms and hands are less visible than the face, they have less communicative ability (Bull, 1987). If they are used to intentionally communicate, two forms of behavior are possible: emblems

TABLE 7-3
Analyzing Nonverbal Acknowledgment and Unintentional Messages

Use the five communications listed in Table 7-1. Analyze each response in terms of the type of nonverbal acknowledgment you used. Then offer a revision of your acknowledgment if necessary.

CLIENT COMMUNICATION	CLINICIAN RESPONSE	TYPE OF VERBAL ACKNOWLEDGMENT	REVISION OF VERBAL ACKNOWLEDGMENT
1.		❏ Facial Expression ❏ Arms/Hands ❏ Feet/Legs ❏ Posture ❏ None	
2.		❏ Facial Expression ❏ Arms/Hands ❏ Feet/Legs ❏ Posture ❏ None	
3.		❏ Facial Expression ❏ Arms/Hands ❏ Feet/Legs ❏ Posture ❏ None	
4.		❏ Facial Expression ❏ Arms/Hands ❏ Feet/Legs ❏ Posture ❏ None	
5.		❏ Facial Expression ❏ Arms/Hands ❏ Feet/Legs ❏ Posture ❏ None	

and illustrators. *Emblems* are behaviors that have been assigned an arbitrary meaning and function as pictures, sometimes conveying complex messages to listeners. They have limited use in acknowledging the feelings of clients. *Illustrators* are behaviors directly related to verbalizations and either emphasize what is being said, point to objects, or visually construct thoughts or objects (Feyereisen & de Lannoy, 1991). They may be useful when the clinician is responding to the clients' statements.

Unintentional Messages. Unintentional messages are self-directed movements such as nail-picking, scratching, hair preening, leg rubbing, and finger tapping that are related to current feeling states of the person using them. Self-directed behaviors are usually beyond the awareness of clinicians and therefore provide an opportunity for observant clients to assess the impact of what they are saying. The behaviors are habitual and routinized, having been formed early in the person's developmental history. Specific self-directed behaviors do not mean the same thing for every clinician. There is a tremendous diversity in self-directed behaviors and their possible meanings. However, most self-directed behaviors convey negative connotations to the listener. It makes little difference what the true meaning is of repetitive leg movements, finger tapping, muscle tension, or hair twirling. All of these, and similar behaviors, indicate to clients that clinicians are either not fully involved in what they are saying, or may not necessarily want to hear it. Self-directed, unintentional behaviors should be kept to a minimum. Their unconscious use can affect the therapeutic relationship.

ACCEPTANCE

Acceptance of a client's values does not necessarily mean that the clinician agrees with them. Rather, it refers to the legitimacy of those values or feelings. Legitimacy means that for that client, their feelings are genuine and understandable, given their value system and world-view. Acceptance of the client can be indicated in two ways. The first involves withholding judgments. The second restricts judgments to the behavior of the client.

Withholding Judgments

One of the important qualities of master clinicians involves timing, knowing when to say or do something and when not to. This is especially true for the use of judgmental statements. Although it is important to provide clients with feedback regarding inappropriate beliefs and behav-

iors, there are times when this type of feedback should be withheld due to the effect of prior judgments and not enough time to establish a trusting relationship.

Effects of Prior Judgments. When clients come into the clinical setting they usually tote along a history of value judgments made about them or their children. Although many of these judgments have been made by family, friends, and professionals, a significant amount may be self-induced. Until a strong interpersonal relationship is established, it is best not to be judgmental about any aspect of the client's behavior. A judgmental approach prior to establishing trust usually leads to defensive reactions, which tend to limit the amount of information clients are willing to accept or even hear.

Developing Trust. Clients and their families come to the clinic, not because they are successful communicators or parents, but rather because they were unable to develop a communicative skill in themselves or their children. Failures at achieving goals have been shown to lead to guilt, which can be debilitating (Williams & Bybee, 1994). By initially withholding judgment, an important component of trust is developed: acceptance.

Providing Judgments

It is difficult for some clinicians to criticize anything about clients who have a disability, especially those who have placed their trust in them. A similar uncomfortableness occurs with parents of disabled children. The assumption is that, if clinicians are judgmental, clients will not feel accepted. Although the assumption is true prior to the establishment of trust, it is not after trust has been established. Unfortunately, the compassion we feel towards the *current* situation of our clients and their families may adversely affect the development of positive *future* behaviors and attitudes.

Judgments can be made about the behaviors and attitudes of clients and their families that do not indicate a rejection of their cultural values or personhood.

Behaviors. As clinicians, one important role is that of an evaluator. We are responsible for evaluating the performance of clients until they can fulfill that role themselves. It is impossible to fulfill that role without being judgmental. However, it is important that judgments of behaviors are phrased in a way that do not imply anything negative about the individuals or their values. Take for example, a client who continually neglects to do vocal generalization exercises outside of the clinic. The purpose of the following interaction is to enable the client to begin consistently practicing the exercises. In the first dialogue, instead of concentrating on the behavior, the clinician impugns the personality of the client.

Client: Last week was very difficult. You see I had all of these social commitments to keep. What with the two parties and four meetings I just did not have time to practice.

Clinician: Are you telling me that you didn't have at least 5 minutes each day to practice? How can you delude yourself in that way? You'll never be able to develop good vocal quality unless you do your exercises.

The dialogue results in the client's perception that the clinician views him as foolish and a failure. It makes no difference if the clinician actually believes this. The clinician's statements will have the opposite effect of what she wanted to achieve. Instead of motivating the client to begin doing the

exercises, the client now feels guilty about not doing the exercises and views himself as a failure. Compare the above dialogue with the following one.

Client: Last week was very difficult. You see I had all of these social commitments to keep. What with the two parties and four meetings I just did not have time to practice.

Clinician: How much time did we agree on that you would practice each day?

Client: I believe it was 5 minutes.

Clinician: That's right, it was 5 minutes. How much time each day did the social functions take?

Client: It varied. Some days a few hours, other days many hours.

Clinician: What was the maximum amount of time on any day?

Client: I think it was about 4 hours.

Clinician: If you add these 4 hours to your normal 8 hour working day plus 8 hours for sleep that comes to 20 hours. What was occurring during the remaining 4 hours that made it impossible for you to find 5 minutes for the exercise?

Client: I can see where you are going. There was nothing that important that I couldn't find at least 5 minutes for the exercise.

Clinician: We had discussed that without doing the exercises on a daily basis, the probability that you would improve your vocal quality was very small. Have you made a decision about therapy that we need to discuss?

In the above dialogue, the clinician required a significantly longer amount of time to accomplish her objective. At no time was a negative judgment made of the client's personality. The focus was only on his behaviors.

Attitudes and Interaction Patterns.

The attitudes and interaction patterns of clients and their families can adversely affect intervention plans. Regardless of how supportive clinicians are in therapy, a parent who minimizes a child's progress can do more damage in one day than the good a clinician can do in a month. Obviously, there will be times when the attitudes of clients and their families will need to be changed. Head-on, direct negative judgments are rarely effective because they can impugn both cultural values and personality. The example below will illustrate this point. The clinician wishes to change the parent's attitude about the way he responds to his daughter's speech. She is now beginning to replace her stuttered speech with a controlled form of fluency. Although not completely normal sounding, it is significantly better than her stuttered speech. Unfortunately, the father still finds it unacceptable. The clinician wishes to have the father reinforce its presence whenever she uses it.

Clinician: Your daughter is using a controlled form of fluency at home that we have been working on for the past two weeks. She tells me that whenever she speaks that way, you criticize her.

Father: That's right. It sounds terrible. She can't talk that way in front of people.

Clinician: Of course not. But I want her to practice it at home. After she has practiced it for a while, we will change it to sound normal. What I would like you to do is tell her how much better it sounds than stuttered speech.

Father: I can't do that.

Clinician: Why not?

Father: It goes against everything in my value system. You don't tell someone that they are doing fine when they aren't. I wasn't raised that way and I don't raise my children that way.

Clinician: Well, I think you need to change the way you think. You should reinforce the way she is speaking even if you don't like it.

The interaction is a direct assault on the father's value system. With the clinician's last statements, the focus of the discussion shifted from the child's behaviors to the parent's cultural values. This is an unproductive and threatening approach. The focus should always be on the effect the attitude has on the behavior. Let's modify the clinician's last statements in the above dialogue and then examine its effects.

Clinician: I can see your point. You really don't want to tell someone that they are doing something perfectly when they are not. I can appreciate your viewpoint. But let's talk about how we can improve your daughter's speech so that it will sound perfectly normal. What I have noticed in therapy is that when I encourage her when she speaks smoothly, her speech gets even better. I say things like, "That sounds so good" or "That really was smooth. You are really working hard today. That's great!"

Father: You mean to say that just by saying those kinds of things her speech gets better?

Clinician: Yes.

Father: Well, I guess I could do that. It's not as if I'm telling her that her speech is perfect or anything.

Clinician: Exactly. And I think you will see that by reinforcing this intermediate step in the development of fluency, her speech will continue to improve.

With the above modifications, no judgments of the parent's values are made. Rather, the focus has shifted back to what can be done to help improve his daughter's speech.

SELF-DISCLOSURE

Self-disclosure is the clinical procedure where clinicians, after hearing or discussing a problem of the client's, offers a similar problem of their own. The use of this technique can facilitate the development of trust with some clients, especially if the client perceives the clinician as either cold or distant. The vulnerability displayed by clinicians when they reveal something about themselves can be critical in developing trust. However, the technique should not be applied equally to clients of all cultures.

Cultural Considerations

Caucasians. There is no data regarding the use of the self-disclosure technique with Caucasian clients. Clinically, the effectiveness of this technique with Caucasians will vary, as the reasons it is effective are based on variables other than ethnicity. The use of self-disclosure with Caucasians should be based on individual client characteristics, because there is nothing in the macroculture of the United States that would counter-indicate the use of this technique.

African Americans and Hispanics. With African American and Hispanic clients, it was found that self-disclosure by clinicians resulted in increased self-disclosure by clients (Berg & Wright-Buckley, 1988). For these two ethnic cultures, the reason the technique is useful is that it can reduce the effects of long-term discrimination. The values, beliefs, and behaviors of both cultures historically have been the subject of derision or criticism by members of the macroculture. It is only reasonable that African American and Hispanic clients would tend to feel some trepidation in revealing anything that makes them appear vulnerable. As a defense mechanism, African American and Hispanic clients may find it difficult to either volunteer sensitive information or provide it when requested, if the clinician is from another culture. When clinicians reveal an aspect about themselves that is vulnerable, the effect is disarming, often leading to clients freely discussing very personal issues.

Native Americans. Self-disclosure on the part of the clinician is not appropriate with clients who have a strong identification with the cultural values of Native

Americans. In Native American culture, the open expression of personal feelings is not something that is socially acceptable (Lockhart, 1981). The focus is on the larger social unit, the family or the tribe. It is more acceptable to convey personal feelings as an extension of family or tribal problems. The clinician's use of self-disclosure not only is unacceptable to Native Americans, but may also indicate an insensitivity toward their values. Regardless of its interpretation, it does not have the desired effect: it will not lead to self-disclosure by Native American clients.

Asian Americans/Pacific Islanders.

It is not the general practice of Asian Americans or Pacific Islanders to use self-disclosure, either in or out of clinical situations (Baptiste, 1990). To do so risks public humiliation. Personal problems are not things that are dealt with publicly. They are very private and often must be handled by the individual alone. That is why there is more reluctance on the part of Asian American/Pacific Islanders than most other ethnic groups to seek professional help (Gim, Atkinson, & Whiteley, 1990). When clinicians use self-disclosure, clients may react to them in a way similar to how someone in their culture would react to them if they said the same thing. It is embarrassing not only for the speaker, but also for the listener to publicly talk about private problems. Clinicians who have been held in esteem may now be viewed differently, having embarrassed themselves in the eyes of the client. As with Native Americans, the use of self-disclosure by clinicians does not result in self-disclosure by clients.

PREPARING FOR TERMINATION

The termination of therapy involves a considerable amount of preparation on the part of both clinician and client. To deter-mine if the client is ready to be terminated from therapy, some clinicians have maintained that specific criteria be used (Fortune, Pearling, & Rochelle, 1991); others rely on clients to make the decision (Goldberg, 1981). In the area of communicative disorders, it is best to use a combination of both. Procedures for termination are listed in Table 7–4.

Clinician

In each type of communicative disorder, unique criteria for termination have been developed. These criteria, which can be found in texts on the disorders, are based on the presence of specific behaviors. In addition to these criteria, there are others that are generic and crossover all disorders. They are: (1) prognosis, (2) utilization of strategies, and (3) generalization of the behaviors.

Prognosis. If clients plateau in their ability to learn or produce certain behaviors, should they be continued in therapy? The answer to this question involves how clinicians view their role as therapists. If the role of speech-language clinicians is merely to maximize the speech and linguistic abilities of clients, then clients who have plateaued should be dismissed. This role, however, is very limited and does not reflect what clinicians as professionals actually do. Their role is not to maximize specific speech or language behaviors, but rather to maximize the individual's ability to **communicate**. Just because a client is no longer achieving additional successes with specific behaviors does not necessarily mean that his or her ability to communicate is also maximized. Communication is dependent on many things including attitude, familiarity with content, and the ability to use strategies. A prognosis for the development of specific speech and language behaviors is not necessarily the same as a prognosis for communicative ability. When speech and language behav-

TABLE 7–4
Termination Plan

WEEK	CLINICIAN RESPONSIBILITY	CLIENT RESPONSIBILITY	SUPERVISOR RESPONSIBILITY
1	❏ Formulate prognosis ❏ Evaluate client's ability to use strategies ❏ Evaluate client's generalization of behavior ❏ Tell client that next week termination plan will be discussed		❏ Discuss plan with supervisor ❏ Receive approval from supervisor
2	❏ Ask client to perform self-analysis ❏ Ask client to think about when therapy should end. Discussion will occur next week	❏ Client performs self-analysis	
3	❏ Ask client to provide termination plan ❏ Discuss termination options	❏ Client provides termination plan	❏ Discuss plan with supervisor ❏ Receive approval from supervisor
4	❏ Begin termination plan		

iors have plateaued, the role of the speech-language pathologist is to provide the client with strategies, experiences, and emotions that will allow the client to maximize what he or she is capable of doing. With communicatively impaired individuals, rarely would a prognosis for communicative ability be so negative as to call for termination.

Utilization of Strategies. Is it necessary to keep clients in therapy if they have mastered and can use the strategies that lead to the maximization of communicative normalcy? The answer to this is a qualified no. In Goldberg's Behavioral Cognitive Stuttering Therapy (1991), clients are taught various strategies that they can use to produce fluent speech. The strategies are augmented with specific daily activities in everyday normal activities, without requiring the presence of the clinician. In this form of therapy, clients are rarely seen for more than 16 weeks. Termination takes the form of eliminating regularly scheduled clinician contact and substituting it with clinician-planned activities and occasional follow-up contact. Using this criteria to terminate is appropriate because there is still some form of clinician directed intervention.

Generalization of Behaviors. The ultimate goal of therapy with all communicatively disordered clients is the generalization of client-developed behaviors. If clients can generalize behaviors, they no longer need therapy. This is probably the easiest and most unequivocal criteria that clinicians can use in deciding when to terminate therapy.

Client

Clients need to be carefully prepared for termination. Preparation should include discussions of responsibility, on-going analysis of behaviors and goals, and phasing out of direct contact.

Responsibility for Change. Throughout the therapy process, clients should be continually told that they are responsible for changing their own behavior and that the role of the clinician is that of facilitator. One of the reasons this should have been emphasized is to prepare clients for the time when therapy is terminated. If this attitude was carefully nurtured by the clinician and reinforced, it should have been internalized when discussions about termination begin. If clients believe that the changes they experienced were due to their own involvement and commitment to change, the thought of not seeing the clinician is not traumatic. However, if clients still believe that change is attributable to the presence and intervention of the clinician, termination becomes an event that will be met with great anxiety. The relationship between clinician and client becomes symbiotic, establishing a dependency that is difficult to break.

Ongoing Analysis of Behaviors and Goals. Throughout therapy, clients and their families have been involved in setting the goals and accessing progress. The more

objective both of these activities are, the easier it will be for clients to accept the ending of an important relationship. Nobody wants to end a relationship that is positive and has significantly affected one's life, especially a facilitative one. However, if the goals on which the relationship is based have been accomplished, the relationship's reason for being ends. Clients can understand this. And as difficult as it may be for them to let go, it can be done with the understanding that they have accomplished what they set out to achieve. Termination becomes just another logical step in the clinical process.

Phasing Out of Direct Contact. If therapy is conducted weekly, a discussion of termination should begin at least 1 month prior to the beginning of the process. Clients need time to adjust and assess their willingness and ability to continue on their own. By gradually introducing the topic, there is an appropriate period of acclimation. The discussions after the initial introduction of the topic should focus on lines for termination with developing a schedule for gradually phasing out direct contact. If clients are seen once a week, it may be appropriate to begin termination by seeing them once every other week for a month, then once a month for a few months. During the phase-out period, clients should have a regular time during which they call the clinician to report progress and discuss problems. While therapy is phased out, clients should be provided with very specific written activities that they are to engage in between sessions. In some ways, the structured activities take the place of the clinician. Even when all regularly scheduled direct contact ends, clients should be assured that they can contact the clinician at any time in the future if new problems occur, or old behaviors recur.

EFFECTIVE USE OF TIME

Time is a precious commodity. Clients who are paying for a service have a right to expect that its use will reflect the money being paid for it. Public schools who are paying for the services of speech-language clinicians have the right to expect them to dispense the best possible, most efficient service under existing conditions. Methods for maximizing time appear in Table 7–5. The greatest proportion of time spent in therapy should be on the direct acquisition of new behaviors.

Minimizing Extraneous Activities

The reason people come to therapy is to have therapy. This may sound simplistic, but often clinicians lose sight of this self-evident statement. The way it is manifested with children, adolescent, and adults differs.

Children and Adolescents. It is a common practice to extend nontherapy time with children and adolescents more than adults. There is a strange concept espoused by some that 5 or 10 minutes at the beginning of each session should be used for "warm-up," which is defined as the time necessary for children to get ready for therapy. If children do not know why they are seeing the speech-language clinician, then the clinician was remiss in providing the explanation at the very first session. If a warm-up period is necessary to begin therapy, then they are warming up to an activity where there probably is something wrong. If activities are correctly structured and explained, children do not need any extra time to prepare for them. Given the limited amount of time available for speech-language therapy in the public schools, it is unconscionable to waste a third or half of it with activities that have absolutely nothing to do with the goals of the session.

Adults. Adults do not come to therapy to discuss the weather, talk about parking, or engage in activities or discussions that have nothing to do with their problem. This is not say that normal pleasantries should be ignored. However, after a few minutes, they are no longer pleasantries, but an inefficient and ineffective use of time. When clients persist in this practice, it can be an indication of reluctance to begin therapy. When this occurs, the problem should be directly confronted or subtly manipulated by the clinician with statements such as, "That was very interesting. I'm sorry we don't have more time to talk about it, but there are a number of things we need to do today. Possibly we can work that idea into our activities."

Maximizing Responses

It is a good rule of thumb to start with the assumption that the more responses that can be generated by the client, the more likely and quickly behaviors will be learned. Obviously not all behaviors should have the same response rate. For example, if working on a specific phonological or articulation problem, it is reasonable to expect the client to produce in excess of 200 responses during a 50-minute period. However, the same criterion would not be appropriate for eliciting spontaneous utterances from a language-disordered child. There are two very easy ways in which clinicians can maximize the number of responses clients are producing during a session: (1) reducing the amount of time spent on nonresponse activities and (2) requiring the client to produce multiple responses.

Efficient Structuring of Activities. A useful exercise for clinicians is to analyze the time spent on each component of therapy. For most interactions this would in-

TABLE 7–5
Effective Use of Time

Use this form to analyze one type of repetitive activity. Use a separate copy of this form to analyze each other type of activity performed during a session.

Activity_____   Total Minutes
_____   for Analyzed activities_____

RESPONSES	APPROXIMATE TIME SPENT ON EACH RESPONSE	APPROXIMATE TIME SPENT ON PRESENTING STIMULI/ ENGAGING IN RELATED ACTIVITY FOR EACH RESPONSE	APPROXIMATE TIME SPENT ON REINFORCING EACH RESPONSE
1			
2			
3			
4			
5			
6			
7			
8			
9			
10			

AVERAGE TIME SPENT ON EACH ACTIVITY			
PERCENTAGE OF TOTAL TIME SPENT ON EACH ACTIVITY			

volve (1) explanation of the activity, (2) presentation of the eliciting stimulus, (3) client response, and (4) reinforcement. Usually, these four components repeat themselves throughout the session. Of the four components, client responses are clearly the most important. Therefore, more time should be spent on them than on the other components. However, this rarely occurs. Clinical activities are notoriously inefficient in terms of the time required to complete them, in relationship to the amount of time clients spend on producing behaviors. This is especially true with children. Elaborate games are constructed which require rolling of dice, spinning spinners, moving pieces, pulling objects out of boxes, coloring squares, or a variety of other things that rapidly eat up the bulk of a 50-minute session. This is not to say that activities need to be stark and lifeless to be efficient. There are many justifications for using elaborate and time-consuming activities, such as intrinsic motivation and the use of stimulus configurations that facilitate memory and generalization. However, clinicians need to be aware of the time these activities consume and be prepared to justify their inefficiency.

An exquisitely efficient clinical activity is one in which the entire activity is the response. For example, when working with an adult aphasic client, the goal of the session was to improve the communicative ability of the client. To do this, the entire session consisted of a conversation between the client and clinician. Throughout the session, as problems occurred, they were addressed. When progress was made, the client was provided feedback. There was no way to be more efficient for this session. The client was responding for the entire 50 minutes.

Requiring Multiple Responses. At times there may be compelling reasons why an inefficient activity should be used. When clinicians are convinced that the activity warrants the amount of time spent

on engaging in it, a slight modification can substantially increase its efficiency. Very simply, they could double, triple, or quadruple the number of responses the client is required to produce. For example, if an elaborate play activity is used to elicit the production of a linguistic structure from a child, require two related utterances with the same structure before continuing. For instance, instead of a child having to say "push car here" (action + object + location), she might have to give directions for two objects "push car here; push boy there."

MATCHING ACTIVITIES TO LEARNING STYLES

It may be difficult for clinicians to match their approaches to therapy with the learning styles of clients. As difficult as it may be, appropriate matching has been shown to significantly affect the outcome of therapy in terms of the time required to acquire certain behaviors (Katz, 1990).

Individual Cognitive Styles

The two main individual styles of learning have been identified as reflective and active (Katz, 1990). Although preferences may differ among clients, one is significantly better than the other for the development and generalization of new behaviors.

Reflective Learning Style. A reflective learning style is one in which learning is passive. The person dispensing information or knowledge dispenses and the learner receives. It appears that one variable associated with a reflective learning style is a lack of knowledge on the subject being learned (O'Brien & Albrecht, 1991; Smith, 1993). It makes sense that, if individuals believe they know little or nothing about a subject being learned, they also will believe that they have little to add to the learning process. Although this may be a preferred style of learning for some individuals, it is not as conducive for therapy as a more active learning style.

Active Learning Style. An active learning style is one in which the learner engages in activities designed to demonstrate the knowledge that hopefully will be gained. Active learners appear to believe that they have something to contribute to the learning process (Sagie, Elizur, & Koslowsky, 1990). With active learning styles, clients become more involved in therapy and generally have better results. One key to transforming reflective learners into active learners is to provide them with information about the entire therapy process. This can be accomplished in two ways. The first is to explain the activity in terms of what, why, and how statements, discussed in earlier chapters. The second is to ask for continuous feedback from the client. By combining these two aspects of therapy, active learning may be facilitated.

Cultural Learning Styles

Much of the writing on cultural learning styles is tangential or anecdotal. The suggestions that have been provided in the literature tend to be based on personal experiences or gross generalizations. The problems associated with identifying particular learning styles with cultural values is that the amount of acculturation that occurs in individuals varies immensely and the effects of the learning paradigms used in the children's schools and homes may dominate the influence of the culture (Dunn & Griggs, 1990). This was very apparent in a study conducted in India in which learning styles of children from modern and traditional schools were compared (Mishra, 1988). Although all children had similar cultural values, the ways in which each group organized information differed. What appears below, therefore, should be viewed as very general guidelines for understanding how learning styles may be affected by culture.

Ethnic Learning Styles. It is a widely held belief that Asian Americans/Pacific Islanders tend to use deductive learning/response styles with narrow parameters (Kember & Gow, 1990). Drill and repetition activities are not only acceptable methods of learning, but ones that are desired. In a study of adolescents from Hong Kong and Malaysia, most of these accepted beliefs are questioned (Watkins & Ismail, 1994). The researchers found that both groups reported much less extrinsic motivation and fear of failure, and less use of superficial learning strategies, such as syllabus-boundness and verbatim reproduction, without understanding. Both Asian groups were also more likely to report using learning strategies designed to maximize understanding, including reading widely debating issues and reflecting on what they were learning. It has been asserted that cooperative learning styles are more appropriate for Asian Americans/Pacific Islanders than competitive ones. However, in a study comparing cooperative with competitive learning styles, no significant differences in performance were found in Maori, Samoan, and Pakeha children (Rzoska & Ward, 1991).

Most of the writings on learning styles of African Americans maintain that a cooperative learning style should be used. This belief is based on the cultural heritage, family background, and socialization of African Americans. Some studies seem to corroborate the use of a cooperative learning approach with African Americans (Haynes & Gebreyesus, 1992).

It has been hypothesized that Hispanics tend to prefer inductive learning/response styles with larger parameters. Unfortunately, much of what has been written has not been empirically validated. In a study of Puerto Rican children, it was found that when Puerto Rican clinicians modeled appropriate cultural values, some target behaviors were achieved, but others were not (Malgady, Rogler, & Costantino, 1990). The researchers concluded that it is too simplistic to attribute significant positive gains in therapy to cultural matching of client and clinician or to cultural sensitivity. They believe that any assertions relating to the positive effects of cultural sensitivity on outcome need to be empirically validated.

Most of the nonresearch articles on Native American learning styles emphasize the use of a holistic approach to learning, with cognitive connections that are loose, and extensive use of allegories and analogies. If these conceptions of Native American learning styles are accurate, therapy should be constructed which is holistic with reduced analytical thinking. Recent research on the acceptability of inductive/analytical reasoning classroom approaches with Navajo students has cast doubt on some of the basic assumptions of culturally sensitive approaches for Native Americans (McCarty, Wallace, Lynch, & Benally, 1991). Not only was the more western-technological approach accepted by the children, but the approach was positively assessed by both children and adolescents.

Religious Learning Styles. Virtually nothing has been written on the direct relationship between religions and learning styles. Most discussions are based on inferences from cultural values. For example, individuals who strongly identify with eastern religions tend to use holistic approaches to learning, accept the conditions of present circumstances, have an understanding of the interconnectiveness of events, and concentrate on the present more so than either the past or future (Suzuki, 1955). It has been asserted that individuals who strongly adhere to fundamentalist religions rely on literal interpretations and use linear thinking (Presley, 1992; Georgia, 1994).

Geographic/Regional Learning Styles. There is no data on learning styles associated with different regions of the country. Although differences may exist between individuals who live in rural, urban, and suburban areas, there are no experimental studies showing the relationship.

Socioeconomic Learning Styles. The socioeconomic status of clients has an indirect relationship on the learning styles of their members. In general, the lower the status, the more likely it is that the client's past and present educational experiences and resources will be inferior. Schools in more affluent settings have not only the finances, but also personnel who are committed to institutionalizing teaching methodologies that are conducive to learning (Sinatra, 1990; Valle, 1990). Less in-depth learning styles are not an inherent characteristic of lower socioeconomic status, but rather an economic by-product of it. Poor children rarely eat as nutritiously as children whose parents are not poor. Inadequate nutrition of mothers and children creates learning disabilities that are lifelong (Sigman, Neuman, Jansen, & Bwido, 1989). These clients are both medically and environmentally at risk.

Disability. The clearest effect of a disability on an individual's learning style involves disabilities that have a cognitive basis. The child with Down syndrome will rely more on concrete visual stimuli for learning than will a child without Down syndrome. A client with aphasia may use a variety of categorical retrieval strategies. The child with autism will learn and think in terms of pictures rather than words. These and other examples present fairly obvious parameters within which clinicians can design and implement intervention strategies. A more difficult-to-assess effect of disability on learning styles involves the psychological aspects of the disability. We are a product of our experiences. Clients who have experienced years of failure in achieving communicative normalcy may have few expectations for success and, therefore, may not take a very active role in learning or therapy. Clients who have continued to struggle, without losing hope, may wish to be actively involved in therapy. Relation-ships such as these should be considered when determining the effect of the disability on a client's learning style.

Age. Age has a direct relationship to learning styles, because learning styles are related to cognitive ability. With age comes the increased ability to use abstractions, complex relationships, and understand hidden meanings. Also, because learning styles are related to experiences, the more experiences an individual has, the more likely his or her learning style will be affected.

Section IV

COMPLEX SKILLS

CHAPTER

8

Complex Technical Skills

Although complex technical skills may be acquired early in the training of clinicians, they tend to be consistently applied only after extensive experience. There are seven categories of complex technical skills containing 62 techniques and behaviors. A list of these skills appears in Table 1–3 in Chapter 1.

CHANGING ATTITUDES

There are times in therapy when it is more important to focus on changing clients' attitudes than their behaviors. A voice client may believe that he will never be able to generate enough air volume to be heard in anything but a very quite room. An aphasic client maintains that she will never be able to comprehend anything spoken to her other than very simple linguistic constructions. A parent is convinced that his Down syndrome child will never be able to use utterances consisting of more than two connected words. For these clients, it may be more productive to address the attitude than work on

a behavior. There are two methods that can be used to change client attitudes: discussion and demonstration.

Discussions

If a discussion mode is to be used, two specific approaches can be taken: client-centered and logical structuring. Each is based on the assumption that clients can be *convinced* that an attitude they have is false.

Client-Centered. In a previous chapter, the basic tenets of client-centered therapy were discussed. In this approach clinicians enable clients to solve their own problems through rephrasing and restructuring what the client is saying, all from within the clients' frames of reference. The advantage of using this approach is that, when clients have insights into their attitudes and behaviors, it is through self-examination, an intellectual process resulting in deeper convictions. The disadvantage of this approach is that it is very time-consuming (Culatta & Goldberg,

1995). Clients often have a great deal of difficulty attacking their problems head-on. As the core of a problem is approached, clients will often feel discomfort or anxiety and veer tangentially in another unrelated direction.

Logical Structuring. A clinical approach that uses logical structuring is clinician-directed. Clinicians have a fairly precise idea of what they would like the client to believe. They know what the client currently believes. And thus, they structure a set of steps that will take the client from a belief system that is inappropriate to one that will facilitate forward movement in therapy. The best example of this approach in general counseling is rational emotive therapy (Ellis, 1962). A good example in the area of speech-language pathology is the cognitive stuttering therapy approach developed by Culatta and Rubin (1973). In both programs the client is led through a series of steps from one position to another. If the programs are applied properly, clients arrive at the desired attitude though a rational approach that leaves little room for irrational thought. The advantage of this approach is that it is fairly rapid. Instead of taking many weeks for the client to develop the desired attitude, if a client-centered approach is used, it may occur within one session. The disadvantage of this approach is that, although the client's head has been forced to accept the logic of the clinician's position, his or her gut may still reject it. Saying that something is, does not necessarily make it so. After spending 20 minutes leading a client through a series of logical steps and decisions, the clinician asked the client if he now realized that he was capable of doing a behavior. The client responded "yes, I guess." The "yes" came from his head, while the "I guess" came from his heart. Unfortunately, therapy is not a game of chess, in which one participant can overwhelm an opponent by the shrewdness of logical and tactical moves. In therapy, clients

have to willingly acquiesce, not be dragged, screaming to a more acceptable position.

Demonstration

The problems associated with changing attitudes through either a client-centered or logical structuring approach can be avoided if demonstration is used instead. Attitudes can be changed more quickly and more objectively by directing clients to engage in something and having them succeed. This method has been shown to be effective in counseling (Safran, 1989). The clinician could spend endless hours trying to convince a stutterer that he has the ability to speak completely fluently on demand without succeeding. However, if the clinician asks the client to engage in a simple behavior that produces fluency (albeit an exaggerated form), the effect is immediate and fundamental. Clients believe they can be fluent because they have just demonstrated it to themselves.

MONITORING

Monitoring involves providing auditory, visual, or physical cues which allow clients to focus on a specific task. These cues can be supplied by the client or the clinician. A summary of monitoring techniques and their application sequence appears in Table 8–1. This form can be used to identify the step in the monitoring process, the description of the method, the modality used, and the person responsible for performing it.

Effects

When clients are provided with a method for monitoring the production of a new behavior, their performance for the specific behavior improves (Kinnunen & Vauras, 1995) and also for other similar behaviors (Bielaczyc, Pirolli, & Brown, 1995). Interestingly, even when they are not accurate

TABLE 8–1
Monitoring Sequence and Analysis

Activity _____

STEPS	DESCRIPTION OF MONITORING METHOD	MODALITY	CLINICIAN MONITORING TYPE	CLINICIAN/CLIENT MONITORING TYPE	CLIENT MONITORING TYPE
1 Clinician Monitoring		❏ Auditory ❏ Visual ❏ Tactile ❏ Mental	❏ Interval Contingent ❏ Signal Contingent ❏ Event Contingent		
2 Client-Clinician Monitoring		❏ Auditory ❏ Visual ❏ Tactile ❏ Mental		❏ Interval Contingent ❏ Signa Contingent ❏ Event Contingent	
3 Client Monitoring		❏ Auditory ❏ Visual ❏ Tactile ❏ Mental			❏ Interval Contingent ❏ Signal Contingent ❏ Event Contingent

in monitoring a specific behavior, the process of self-monitoring appears to positively affect other behaviors (Whitney & Goldstein, 1989). When working with a child who had suffered seizures causing the complete loss of language usage, the clinician taught her to use a strategy which also served as a monitoring device. When asked to identify a picture of an object, the child would say, "Look all around," while she moved her finger in a circular motion. If she responded before her finger made a complete circle, she knew that her response was premature. The strategy was effective in reducing an immediate identi-

fication attempt when asked to point to a specific picture. The strategy, which was only taught for the picture identification task, was used by the child in other contexts to provide herself with additional time to process information.

Form

It is important to monitor new behaviors in a very simple manner, rather than behaviors which are to be replaced. In some forms of articulation therapy, a great deal of time is spent on auditory training, where children are taught how to differentiate between their current incorrect production of a sound and the correct production. The assumption is that by auditory bombardment of both incorrect and correct productions, their ability to monitor both types of productions in their own speech will increase. This is at best only an intuitively plausible position. Monitoring should be a fairly simple procedure, requiring concentration on only one behavior. For example, in the Behavioral Cognitive Stuttering Therapy Program, clients keep their hands raised while using fluency enhancing behaviors (Goldberg, 1981). Not only is the method of monitoring simple, but very effective.

Types

There are basically 3 different types of monitoring that clinicians and clients can do: (1) interval contingent, (2) signal contingent, and (3) event contingent (Wheeler & Reis, 1991).

Interval Contingent. In interval-contingent monitoring, clinicians or clients report on the clients' behaviors at regular intervals. *Interval* refers to a unit of time. The clinician or client is not necessarily monitoring individual behaviors, but rather more global features of the behavior. An example would be clinicians producing come sort of a monitoring gesture every 2 minutes in order that clients could refocus on the behaviors needed to produce a new vocal quality.

Signal Contingent. The second is signal-contingent monitoring. In this form of monitoring, the clinician uses a monitoring gesture after a specific event occurs. In our example, the client may be producing the appropriate vocal quality for 10 minutes. During this period of time, no monitoring gestures were used by the clinician. Then during an explanation of a painful experience, the client's voice breaks, and reverts back to a pretherapy vocal quality. The clinician immediately signals the client

with a monitoring gesture that indicates the behaviors are not being used.

Event Contingent. The third is called event contingent. Monitoring cues are provided whenever a defined event occurs. In our example, the clinician may have decided that a monitoring cue is necessary whenever the client begins speaking. At the onset of speech, a signal is provided that hopefully will focus the client's attention, during the entire utterance, on producing behaviors that will result in normal vocalization. Of the three, this last form of monitoring appears to be the most easily structured for self-monitoring, because it does not rely on the clinician.

Clinician Monitoring

Initially the clinician should assume responsibility for monitoring the client's speech. The monitoring can be either visual or auditory. Regardless of what modality is chosen, the responsibility for modeling should eventually be gradually shifted onto the client. If clients are to change behaviors, it is important that they are aware of what they are currently doing and what they should be doing. Feedback can take many forms from visual or verbal acknowledgment by the clinician to internal physiological sensations. Feedback can be fleeting, as with a smile, or lasting, as with cue cards. When clinicians are responsible for monitoring behaviors, attention should be paid to the modality used and the method for shifting responsibility for monitoring onto the client.

Modality. In the research cited earlier in this text, it was noted that, if a behavior the client is to produce is auditory, then either a visual or auditory stimulus configuration is appropriate. If the behavior is nonverbal, it is better to use a visual stimulus configuration. Further, if the client has any cognitive problems, both should be used. The same principles should be applied to clinician monitoring, but with some qualifications. If the behaviors clinicians want clients to produce are auditory, the use of an auditory monitoring signal may interrupt the flow of speech, resulting in a situation that is highly unnatural. For example, if a young client is producing a series of words with the target phoneme /s/ at the beginning of each, the clinician may wish to provide the client with a monitoring device that says, "Here it comes, here's the /s/ sound." If the monitoring device is the production of a 2-second hissing sound, the child will be provided with an appropriate monitoring device, but one that may interfere with the activity. For most clinician monitoring, it is appropriate to use visual cues, as they are applicable to both auditory and nonverbal behaviors and result in the least interference in the production of client behaviors. For the child in the above example, a downward sliding movement of the clinician's fingers on his arm would be just as effective as the hissing sound, and less disruptive.

Shifting From Clinician to Client Monitoring. There is no special number of responses for determining when monitoring should be shifted from the clinician to the client. However, there is a procedure that can be used to effect the transfer. Clinicians should view the movement from clinician monitoring to client monitoring as constituting three distinct stages. The first stage is clinician monitoring. How to do this was presented in the previous section. The second stage is shared responsibility, and the final stage is client responsibility. In this section, methods for using a shared responsibility approach will be provided. After clinicians are reasonably sure that clients are using the clinician monitoring cues to consistently produce the desired behaviors, they should introduce a means for sharing that responsibility. In the example in the previous section, the clinician used a downward finger movement on her arm to

help the child monitor when he would need to concentrate on using his new behaviors to produce /s/ phonemes. In this transition phase of monitoring, she could instruct the child that they will both do it together. Initially, the clinician should begin the monitoring cue with the same speed she demonstrated in the first phase of monitoring. When she noticed that there was a minimal delay between the time she initiated her cue and when the child initiated his cue, she would hesitate in cuing, so that the child could respond first.

Client Monitoring

There are various ways clients can assume the responsibility for monitoring behaviors. The initial monitoring should be simple and focus on a limited number of behaviors. Monitoring signals can be either nonverbal or verbal.

Nonverbal Signal. The initial nonverbal signal clients should use should be dramatic and visual. A raised hand works well, as does movement of an object to a particular place on a table. The advantage of using something like a raised hand is that it is amenable to shaping. Eventually, client monitoring should be phased out. Initially, clients can raise their hands to signal a monitoring activity. This movement can then be reduced to raising a finger, then placing two fingers together, and finally just thinking about what is to be monitored. Although equally effective initially, moving objects on the table does not lend itself to a fade-out procedure.

Verbal Signal. A very simple verbal monitoring technique that can be taught to clients is known as "private speech." This is the speech individuals use to talk to themselves while engaging in an activity. For example, while children are constructing a complex toy, they may be describing what parts should be selected in the construction and how each should be used. It was found that in children, when private speech is used, it tends to be correlated with better task performance (Bivens & Berk, 1990). Similar results were found with high school students (Watson & Lawson, 1995), college undergraduates (Cantor & Engle, 1989; Simpson, Olejnik, Tam, & Supattathum, 1994), and adults with severe cognitive disabilities (Belfiore & Browder, 1992). This technique can be used with clients of all ages. As they are to perform a task, the clinician can ask them to either silently tell themselves how each component of the task is to be produced or to just mouth the set of self-instructions. Although this form of monitoring is effective, clinicians may wish to supplement it by using a more permanent method of self-recording, such as a check-mark system for behaviors that lend themselves to it. Self-recording methods have been shown to significantly increase attending behavior and performance in individuals with and without cognitive problems (Lloyd, Bateman, Landrum, & Hallahan, 1989). For example, whenever the client can tell that she is using the strategy for retrieving words that the clinician taught her, she would make a mark on a sheet of paper.

STRATEGIES

Learning is a continual process for individuals of all ages and cognitive abilities. As we interact with the world around us, we are constantly encountering new situations and required to meet new demands. Even when something has been mastered, there always seems to be situational modifications that require us to alter previously learned behaviors or attitudes to meet the new conditions. It seems that few things recur exactly as they were originally encountered. What a text says should happen with an individual who has a specific communicative disorder, rarely is seen in the clinic exactly as was printed. We modify

our academic knowledge to accommodate the clinical reality of the disorder. When encountering a second individual with the disorder, the clinician again modifies his or her understanding, because the second client presents slightly different characteristics. Throughout the process of learning, clinicians are developing various learning strategies that allow them to understand the new situations, not by looking at each situation as if it was an isolated instance, but rather by using a strategy that allows clinicians to see their connectedness. *A strategy is an abstract relationship, concretely displayed, which allows clients to solve a variety of problems or engage in a variety of activities that, although similar in construction, have significant differences.* This appears to be one of the most crucial features for generalization. A significant amount of excellent clinicians' therapy time involves either the development or use of strategies to elicit responses. The use of strategies is one major variable that distinguishes successful from unsuccessful learners (Fenton & Levine, 1989; Loranger, 1994; Meltzer, Solomon, Reynolds, Shepard, Lapan, Kreek et al., 1990). Just as we use strategies to accommodate the continual uniqueness of our clinical experiences, so should strategies be taught to our clients if they are to be able to become successful problem solvers.

General Considerations

The ability to use strategies for learning is not only a natural process outside of the clinic, but should be our basic approach in the clinic. If strategies are correctly taught to clients and internalized by them, they become self-help tools. With these tools, clients attain a certain degree of independence, not having to rely on clinicians for improvement (Heather, Kissoon, Singh, & Fenton, 1990). When strategies are not present, learning suffers. Five reasons for the absence of strategies in learning situations have been postulated (Garner, 1990): (1) poor cognitive monitoring, (2) primitive learning routines that only focus on a specific outcome, (3) a meager knowledge base, (4) a setting that does not encourage the use of strategies, or (5) activities requiring minimal transfer.

Criteria for Selecting Strategies. In the sections that follow, you will be introduced to a number of different strategies that can be used for a variety of purposes. No one set of strategies is appropriate for all clients. No one set of strategies may even be appropriate for the same client on two different days! Although there are no studies in the literature that directly deal with selection criteria, a study which examined how children select their own learning strategies may provide an initial step in developing them. When examining the strategies children used in solving mathematical problems, Lemaire and Siegler (1995) found that children were drawn to the most efficient strategies. Therefore, when deciding between two or more strategies, clinicians should select the one which is most efficient. This usually will be the one that has the smallest number of steps and is simplest. By using the criteria of smallest number of steps and simplicity, it is more likely that the strategy will be acceptable to the client. Although the above study was done with children, it seems reasonable that the results would also apply to adolescents and adults.

Behavior vs. Strategy. It is very easy in therapy to be so consumed by trying a remediate communicative disorder that the focus is on changing the outward manifestations of the behavior, rather than teaching the client to use a strategy to correct the problem. Usually shortcutting the procedure does result in faster learning. However, a specific communicative problem is rarely an isolated disorder. The inability to use one type of syntactical structure most likely is related to other types of

syntactical problems. And even if it is an isolated problem, it will occur in many contexts other than in the clinic. If, for reasons of immediate expediency, the approach is taken to work on the behavior rather than teaching a strategy, the ability of clients to generalize the new learning will be severely limited (Balajthy & Weisberg, 1990). For example, if a client has difficulty asking questions, a shortcut approach involving appropriate question-asking utterances may be modeled and reinforced. Although the behavior might be acquired more quickly than if a strategy was used, the procedure would probably have to be repeated for each missing question form. A more difficult but better approach for the clinician is to first determine why the client is having difficulty in utilizing question rules, then devise a strategy that the client can use for understanding the nature of all question forms. The initial additional amount of time needed to devise a strategic approach is more than offset by the improved efficiency derived throughout the later learning and generalization activities.

Strategies and Intelligence. It seems reasonable to conclude that intelligence must be a factor in the selection and use of strategies. It is, if you are comparing individuals with normal intelligence and those with severe cognitive impairments. However, it is not a factor if comparisons are made only among individuals who have at least normal intelligence (Alexander & Schwanenflugel, 1994). Even when matched for intelligence individuals have different preferences. Although attempts to determine if specific cognitive attributes correlate with the selection of specific strategies, efforts are still equivocal, resulting in conclusions that are cloaked in qualifications.

Source of Strategies. Given the number of strategies cited in this section, it would seem reasonable that clinicians should select those they believe would be most beneficial to the client. This should be the last step in the selection of strategies. The first would be to ask the client to describe how he or she solves problems. The reason for this is that it has been found that learner-generated strategies produce better results, both in terms of initial performance (King, 1994; Wood, Willoughby, Kasper, & Idle, 1994) and retention of information (Wood, Miller, Symons, Canough et al., 1993), than those provided to them. Simply put, if clinicians allow clients to tell them how they learn best, the clients' selection of strategies will probably be at least as good as those selected by clinicians, and in all likelihood, better. With some clients, either because of cognitive problems or minimal insight, self-generated coping strategies may not be possible. For these clients, clinicians should match clients' abilities for choosing and understanding with their cognitive capacities. For example, you would not provide a choice of strategies for a severely language-impaired child. For a client of this type, clinicians should rely on the literature and complement the data with observations of how the client attempts to solve problems. The use of puzzle pieces or toys requiring construction may provide insights. For a client whose cognitive and linguistic abilities are more intact, selections could be made between two or three different types of strategies. A good approach would be to provide two different problems and instruct the client to use each of the alternative strategies to solve the problem. This procedure would allow the clinician and client to experimentally determine the most efficient and effective strategy to use.

Internal vs. External. Strategies can be internal or external. Internal strategies take the form of elaboration or rehearsal. An example for an aphasic client would be counting to him- or herself, starting from 1, when difficulties in retrieval occur. An external strategy would be the use of lists or notes designed to help solve problems.

Clients who are having difficulty remembering to do certain behaviors at specific times could set their watches to chime at the designated times. Both types of strategies work. And each has advantages and disadvantages. Internal strategies are less obvious because they do not rely on anything visible. Clients who may be embarrassed by needing to use a strategy may feel more comfortable with internal rather than external strategies. A second advantage is that, intuitively, internal strategies seem closer to the establishment of a more automatic form of behavior than external strategies. However, the main problem with internal strategies is their fragile nature. Reliance on internal mechanisms for producing new behaviors is notoriously unreliable. It is just too easy to forget. In a study done with elders, it was found that external strategies were not only preferred, but they also produced significantly better responses than did internal strategies (McDougall, 1995). The clinical application of these findings is that, although internal strategies should be a desired goal, they should be preceded by external strategies, which can slowly be shaped into internal strategies.

Training Requirements for Strategy Effectiveness. For clients who do not know how to use a particular type of strategy, training is required. There are various ways in which clients can be taught to use strategies including modeling, active participation, and guided demonstrations. Regardless of the method of training, before allowing clients to independently use the strategy, it is important to confirm that clients know how to use it. Two types of confirmation should be sought in training, both of which are thought to be critical for the independent use of the strategy (Melot & Corroyer, 1992). The first is that clients understand how the strategy can be generalized to other behaviors or situations. For example, if a number-recall strategy is taught to a client, the client should be able to explain how the strategy will be used in situations such as trying to find a date on a calendar, giving change, and remembering one's age. The second type of confirmation involves having clients explain how the strategy results in the desired effect. In our example of the aphasic client, we would also ask the client to explain how a strategy such as sequential counting allows him to arrive at the correct number.

Practice vs. Strategies. There are various ways new behaviors can be learned. The most common method is to focus on practicing the behavior until it is mastered. Although a commonly held belief, there is evidence to show that the use of practice techniques without regard for strategies is an inefficient method of changing behaviors (Carver & Leibert, 1995; Rabinowitz, 1991). There is evidence to suggest that practice alone adds little to the learner's ability to effect change (Kiewra, Mayer, Christensen, Kim et al., 1991). When change occurs within the context of practice, it probably is attributable to the learner's developing a strategy for doing things differently. Although clients may eventually learn how to produce behaviors, they may have had to endure an enormous amount of failure along the way. Additionally, they probably have only learned how to perform a specific behavior. With a new, but similar behavior, the entire process will need to be repeated. By teaching strategies rather than relying on rote practice, new behaviors may be learned faster (Sanchez & Iniguez, 1993).

Classifying Clients by Strategy Use. It would be very useful if clients could be classified in terms of the types of strategies they use to solve problems. Some instruments have been developed which attempt to identify basic features of an individual's learning style (Biggs, 1988). With this type of knowledge, clinicians could easily develop the most efficient procedures and strategies for helping each client. Unfor-

tunately this is currently not possible. Studies have shown that cognitive classification systems used to categorize clients are not reliable (Roberts, Wood, & Gilmore, 1994). Some have maintained that strategy selection may be related to personality types (Matthews and Harley, 1993), learner's feelings of internal control (Dee, Dansereau, Peel, Boatler et al., 1991), or the need for contextual cues (Meng & Patty, 1991). Even though learners differ in terms of their selection of strategies, there is evidence to suggest that each individual learner tends to consistently use a set of strategies (Siegler, 1991). This has significant clinical importance both for clients who appear not to be using any strategies and those who use inappropriate ones. Consistency of usage seems to imply that individuals have a certain cognitive style that they use to solve problems in various areas. If a more efficient strategy for solving a given problem can be taught to a client, it is possible that the strategy might be generalized to other problem areas which would include, but go beyond, their communicative disorders.

Strategies and Performance Speed. Although we are more interested in the accuracy of responses rather than in the speed of their production, there are times when speed may be important. For example, when an aphasic client is attempting to order something at a restaurant, increased processing time may result in annoyance on the part of the server and embarrassment on the part of the client. In cases such as these, increases in processing and response speed are important. The use of strategies can be important in increasing response speed. In one study examining the effect of strategies in learning and producing complex motor behaviors, individuals who were instructed in the use of strategies not only performed more accurately than those who were not provided with strategies, but also performed them more quickly (Singer, Flora, & Abourezk, 1989).

Strategy Examples. Regardless of what strategy will be taught to the client, examples of how to use it should be incorporated within the teaching. Although it is a common practice for clinicians to present the examples, there is evidence to suggest that, when clients are provided with the opportunity to generate their own examples, the acquisition and retention of the strategy is enhanced (Gorrell, Tricou & Graham, 1991). The only problem with allowing clients to generate examples is that they may be too limited and therefore not cover all important generalization situations. Therefore, a good procedure is to first allow clients to generate their own examples, with generalization categories provided by the clinician. For example, in teaching the use of a strategy to reduce vocal tension, clinicians may ask clients to provide examples of how the strategy could be used in a classroom and playing an activity with friends in a public place. Only when the client is unable to provide an example in the category or provides an inappropriate example should the clinician provide one.

Effort, Strategy Selection, and Usage. As with all things in life, strategies can be made very simple or very complex. We know that in trying to grasp an understanding of something, the more detailed it is, the more information will be made available and the more likely a deeper understanding of the phenomenon will be developed. However, the process of developing this deeper understanding requires a greater amount of cognitive effort. When clients are asked to change something about their behavior, sometimes just the process of change can be exhausting. Even when provided with a strategy necessary for change to occur, the transition may still be difficult. Given the overwhelming requirements for change that are placed on clients, strategies should involve as little effort as is necessary for achieving the goal. Research with young children has shown that the less effortful the strategy, the more likely it will be acquired and retained. An example in stuttering therapy involves strategies that can be used with children for developing fluent speech. In one successful therapy program, the four-part strategy used with adults is reduced to one element, prolongation (Goldberg, 1991). By reducing the effort required to use the strategy, it became more acceptable to children and therefore was used. Striving to reduce the effort required to use a strategy should not only be limited to children. It is a maxim that should transcend all age groups. The principle here is analogous to the joke told by audiologists. When asked what the best hearing aid is, audiologists usually respond, "Whatever one the client will wear." The same adage should be applied to the selection of strategies.

General Strategies

In this section, 10 general strategies are provided. Many are appropriate for a variety of disorders while others are appropriate for a very few. Not one of these strategies is a priori better than another. The best strategy for any given client is simply the one that works best. Essentially, this is an empirical question. If the clinician can document that a strategy produces results, then it should be used *with that client*. If it does not work, then it should not be used, regardless of its theoretical rigor or elegance.

Major Life Transitions. Clients who have suffered a major medical change, such as a stroke, often undergo a radical change in lifestyle. These changes can significantly impact on therapy. At the very least, they need to be considered when formulating therapy. The most difficult time for clients is the period of transition, when they are coming to the realization that what they were able to do in the past is no longer possible and different forms of interaction and behaviors will be necessary. An effective method that has been used to ease the transition is to have clients focus on those coping strategies and skills they were able to use for other transitional phases in their life, prior to the major medical event, rather than focusing on the specific behaviors they can no longer perform (Brammer, 1992).

Categorization. Often, a simple strategy involving categorization can significantly increase the client's ability to retrieve information and learn new behaviors (Macrae & Shepherd, 1991). Because the goal of therapy is not just to teach a behavior in the clinic, but to have it generalize, the use of categories as a learning strategy needs to be assessed in terms of its ability to generalize behaviors. The use of categories has been shown to be very effective in the generalization of behaviors (Bock, 1994).Younger children function better with smaller categories, while older children perform better with larger categories (Lange, Griffith, & Nida, 1990). For example, when teaching transportation categorization to young children, it would make more sense to use size as a category rather than places where the object can be operated (e.g., earth, roads, air, etc.). The reverse would be true for older children. When making intervention decisions involving the size of the category for young children, a certain amount of experimentation will be necessary.

It is best not to present more than one categorization strategy for any given task, as individuals will only use one (Thompson, 1994). The introduction of the second strategy will only be confusing. When a second strategy is used, the task or event will be broken into competing units. For example, if, when given a number of objects, clients are instructed to sort them into those that can be used for writing and are made of plastic, two competing schemes will be used: the function of writing and the com-

position of plastic. It appears that learners focus on encoding the training examples as wholes, rather than focusing on individual features (Krascum & Andrews, 1993). Therefore, when using this strategy, it is important that examples of what should be placed in specific categories are easily identifiable. In the above example, clients should be instructed to focus either on function or composition, but not both.

Visualization. Visualization is a relatively new technique in speech-language pathology, but one that has been used extensively in other areas. Musicians frequently visualize themselves playing in front of large audiences, flawlessly performing solos. Many star athletes go through elaborate visualization activities where they slow down a pitcher's fast ball and effortlessly make perfect contact with it, sending it into the furthermost reaches of the centerfield bleachers. In speech-language therapy, clients are asked to visualize anticipated speaking situations in which they are able to produce the desired speech or language behaviors. The technique is similar to that athletes use when they envision a likely event in a game, such as catching a pop fly with the sun shining in their eyes. They not only place themselves in the situation, but they also *see* themselves performing successfully. Visualization is relatively new in the area of speech-language pathology, being used primarily in the area of stuttering therapy (Daly, 1984, 1988). Its use has been reported for a number of years in other health professions (Johnson & Korn, 1980), in self-help literature (Sommer, 1978), sports psychology (Fetz & Landers, 1983; Hird, Landers, Thomas, & Horan, 1991; Vealey, 1986), and in general psychology texts (Paivio, 1971; Richardson, 1969; Samuels & Samuels, 1975). There is evidence to suggest that visualization can strengthen clients' commitment to therapy, because it increases the level of confidence they experience (Pinkard, 1990).

Various studies have attempted to determine if the basic process of visualization could be further strengthened through the use of either written information or graphic representation (Gambrell & Jawitz, 1993). It appears that using an illustration when instructing individuals to visualize an event results in an improvement in performance. In a clinical context, when asking clients to visualize an event, it would be beneficial if a general picture could be simultaneously presented. For example, if stutterers are asked to visualize using their fluency strategies in front of a large group of people, it would be beneficial if the instructions could be accompanied by a large picture of an audience looking directly at the stutterer.

Stress Reduction. At times, clients may experience such a significant amount of anxiety that it becomes difficult or impossible for them to utilize the strategies that are being taught. This occurs most often with stutterers, voice clients, and aphasics who maintain that the anxiety they experience in various speaking situations prevents them from utilizing strategies they know can facilitate the production of target behaviors. Although the effectiveness of behavioral methods for stress reduction has been well documented in children, adolescents, and adults, there appears to be minimal research with elders (Hersen & Van Hasselt, 1992). For that reason, the suggestion has been made that clinicians wishing to use stress reduction techniques with this population view the approach as experimental, and carefully document both the process and outcome measures in order to evaluate its effectiveness. For clients who experience anxiety, two simple strategies which have been shown to reduce its presence can be used.

The first is progressive relaxation. *Progressive relaxation* involves the physical relaxation of the client followed by introduction of various speech situations. Clients are asked to tense one portion of

their bodies and then release the tension. The progression is generally from the head to the feet. As each new area of the body becomes relaxed, the client experiences deeper levels of relaxation. The rationale for using progressive relaxation is that, by producing both a physical and a psychological state of relaxation, the threshold at which it becomes impossible for clients to focus on their strategy is increased. Various audiotapes are available that allow clinicians to use a standardized format, or to learn the sequence and to present instructions to the client in the clinician's voice. A generic program for all clients appears in Table 8–2.

The second strategy for stress reduction is called *systematic desensitization*. This involves the use of hierarchies of stress-inducing experiences. Clients initially devise a list of stress-causing situations, starting from the least anxious to the most anxious situation. With this information, the clinician then constructs clinical experiences which simulate the clients' examples. Starting with the least anxious situation, time is spent engaging in and discussing the activity until clients indicate that they no longer experience any anxiety. Once that occurs, the next simulation is undertaken and the same procedure is employed. For example, if aphasic clients find that it is impossible to use their strategies when they speak in front of small groups of strangers, the first step in the desensitization process would involve having the client speak in front of one individual with whom she felt comfortable. This could be the clinician. With a base comfort level determined, the next step could involve the addition of another individual who is known only slightly. After talking about her anxiety and possibly engaging in relaxation exercises, the client would be asked to speak to the individual only when her level of anxiety was similar to that experienced when only the clinician was present. This process would continue until even a small group of strangers would not trigger

TABLE 8-2
Progressive Relaxation

STEPS	ACTIVITY	DESCRIPTION
1	Assume a relaxing position.	Clients either sit in a comfortable chair or lay in a prone position.
2	Begin easy comfortable breathing	Clients are asked to breathe easily and deeply, completely filling both lungs and then exhaling gently.
3	Relax facial muscles	Clients are asked to visualize the tension in their face, increase it, then release it, visualizing all the tension dissipating.
4	Relax shoulders, neck, chest areas.	Same technique as in step 3.
5	Relax legs, feet areas.	Same technique as in step 3.
6	Relax whole body.	Clients are asked to systematically go through each muscle group and identify any tension. When an area is identified, the procedures outlined in step 3 are applied.
7	Initiate speech in a relaxed position.	Clients are now asked to begin speaking, with their eyes closed, in a relaxed position.
8	Initiate speech in a sitting position with eyes open.	Clients are asked to speak with their eyes open in a more normal position.
9	Initiate speech in a standing position.	While standing, clients are asked to speak with the clinician.
10	Initiate speech while walking.	Clients are asked to remain as relaxed as possible and begin walking. As they walk, they begin talking.
11	Generalization instruction begins.	Clients are taught how to initiate relaxation methods during their daily activities.

the level of anxiety that originally made it difficult for the client to use her strategies. The generic sequence for systematic desensitization appears in Table 8–3.

It should be emphasized that the use of stress-reduction strategies should not be viewed as separate, independent strategies for improving communicative disorders.

TABLE 8–3
Systematic Desensitization

STEPS	ACTIVITY	DESCRIPTION
1	Assume a relaxing position.	Clients are asked to visualize a situation in which they are completely relaxed. This may involve progressive relaxation or visualization techniques. This step may be repeated in the beginning of each new session.
2	Present a nonthreatening stimulus.	A nonthreatening form of a feared stimulus is presented to the client and its effect on the client's level of anxiety is discussed. For example, the client who fears speaking to large groups of people is asked to speak only to the compassionate clinician. When the client feels no anxiety, the next activity begins.
3	Systematic presentation of stimuli with increasing levels of threat.	The stimulus presented in step 2 is slightly modified, possibly resulting in a slight increase in anxiety. For example, instead of having only the clinician in the room with the stutterer, a non-threatening individual may join them. The anxiety-producing level of the stimulus is slowly increased through the use of various steps. Each new step is begun only when the client indicates that no anxiety remains.
4	Presentation of feared stimulus.	The final presentation is of the feared stimulus. In this example, the client may be asked to make a presentation to a group of people.

Rather they should be viewed as an adjunct to therapy, much in the same way psychologists and counselors prefer to use it (Overholser, 1991). Stress reduction allows clients to focus on the use of strategies, it does not remediate communicative disorders.

Post Organizers. During the process of teaching clients to use specific strategies and perform certain behaviors, graphic organizers are often used. For example, when teaching the concepts *food* and *toys*, clinicians may have some graphic representation of each. Clients may then be taught why certain items are classified as toys and others as food. As valuable as the graphic organizer was in teaching the concepts, so is it in the retrieval process. The use of post organizers has been shown to significantly enhance retrieval of concepts and the components of specific behaviors (Spiegel & Barufaldi, 1994).

Different types of post organizers can be used. Two of the main ones are categorical and spatial. Categorical post organizers use categories into which objects, events, or other things are placed. For example, when asked to name everything in her room, a child may think in terms of all of her toys, the furniture, and pictures in the room. Spatial organizers are more global. Instead of thinking in terms of categories, the child may visualize the entire room, ticking off objects as they come into her mind's eye. The types of preferred post organizers, at least for children, may vary with age. One study found that children between the ages of 10 and 12 used categorical post organizers more than spatial organizers. Children between the ages of 12 and 14 preferred the reverse (Spiegel & Barnfield, 1994).

Elaboration. Elaboration is a term used to describe strategies that involve patterns that are connected to the desired behavior (Short, 1992). There are five basic elaboration strategies which differ from each other in terms of sophistication and use. The very simplest, yet very effective strategy, is to have clients verbalize what they are doing as they perform. This procedure appears to have a clarifying and organizing effect on the learner, which produces better results than when no verbalization occurs (Chen, 1990). Verbalization can also be used for self-correction. Following an error, clients are instructed to verbally analyze what they have just done and determine what was done incorrectly. The ability to verbally self-correct, by aphasic clients, has been suggested as a prognostic indicator of language treatment outcomes (Marshall, Neuburger, & Phillips, 1994). Aphasics who were able to use this strategy before therapy began tended to have better outcome results

from therapy than individuals who were unable to use the strategy.

Another simple form of elaboration can be called *expansion,* as it requires clients to expand on the concept that is being learned, such as *transportation.* For example, after explaining what *transportation* refers to, the clinician may say, "Now tell me everything you can about *transportation.* Few parameters are provided to clients, and the responses provided to the clinician are not necessarily related. For example, *everything* may include things that transport, what is transported, experiences with transportation, and so on.

A more complex form of elaboration is known as *elaborative interrogation.* In this strategy, clients are asked to indicate why they chose the answer or were able to engage in a behavior during retrieval activities. For example, during the production of esophageal speech, a client was able to produce an utterance that was significantly longer than another he had previously produced. In response to the question by the clinician of how he was able to do that, the client provided an explanation that became the basis of a new strategy for producing longer utterances. The use of elaborative interrogation appears to result in better retention of information than the use of a more basic elaboration task similar to the one described above (Wood, Miller, Symons, Canough et al., 1993). It forces clients to begin understanding how they were able to accomplish successful behaviors.

A fourth elaborative strategy is known as *functional association,* as it requires clients to develop associations between the target behavior and its functions. This strategy is often used with aphasics when the retrieval of the names of objects is difficult. When learning and retrieving the names of objects, elaborate descriptions of how the object is used may be required. For example, in relearning the names of utensils, aphasic clients upon seeing the object may be required to describe all of its uses before a name is provided. The same procedure would be used for retrieval activities. Clients would first describe an object's functions, then attempt to retrieve its name. This elaborative strategy has been shown to facilitate the recall of linguistic concepts (Best, 1993).

A fifth elaborative strategy is known as *concept mapping*. Clients are asked to describe how *transportation, money*, and *work* are all related. Theoretically, concept mapping is designed to provide learners with a way of developing neural networks that will facilitate the understanding of broader issues. For example, if a goal is to train parents how to teach their child to use strategies, then the concepts of memory retention, associative learning, and generalization may be linked together. Although this elaborative strategy seems intuitively to make more sense than teaching concepts independently, there is still no evidence to suggest that it is significantly better either for learning of concepts or retention of information (Heinze, Fry, & Novak, 1990).

Although elaborative strategies can significantly improve learning, there are some qualifications that clinicians should consider. One study found that not only were appropriate connections activated during the retrieval process, but additional nonhelping connections can be made that interfere with the correct production of the behavior (O'Brien & Albrecht, 1991). Therefore, care should be taken that only relevant connections are accepted when the client is either using basic elaboration or elaborative interrogation.

Active Involvement. Earlier in this text, the features critical in designing activities for children were discussed. One of the critical features mentioned was movement. By having the child actually physically move during an activity, the intrinsic reinforcing values of the activity could be enhanced. The principle of activity movement has been elaborated into a stategy

where learners physically act out whatever is to be learned. The theory behind the use of this strategy is that, by physically being involved in the learning, the individual will be able to learn and retain information better than if the learning was more passive. Research, however, has shown that although this strategy is effective for learning and retaining specific target behaviors, it is not effective for integrating concepts into a whole (Ratner & Hill, 1991).

Visual Cues. Strategies can be visual, tactile, or auditory. Although all are appropriate, the literature suggests that the use of visual cues may result in greater benefits to the client in terms of retention of the strategy and its correct use (Skaggs et al., 1990). Although research indicates that visual cues aid in the learning and retention of information, there is no evidence to suggest that one form of visual cue is better than any other (Dunston, 1992). Clinicians should experiment with various visual cues to determine if there are any differences among cues such as pictures, drawings, static models (e.g., plastic representations of the oral cavity), and active models (e.g., clinician demonstration). It is likely that the effectiveness of various visual cues has less to do with the modality used and more to do with its components, such as figure-ground comparisons and identifying its critical features.

Summary Skills. In an earlier chapter it was noted that telling clients what they will be doing, why it is being performed, and how it will look improve their ability to focus on the activity. A logical extension of this procedure is to use it as a learning strategy. In the literature, this is known as a summary skills strategy. A study was designed to determine its effect on the learning of written text material by minority learning disabled students (Nelson, Smith, & Dodd, 1992). Prior to beginning the reading of a science text, the students were told what they were expected to learn. The results of the study indicated that the use of a summary skills strategy enabled learners not only to acquire information, but also to retain it for an extensive amount of time. This study confirms the importance of providing relevant information to clients about the activities they will be engaging in, *prior to beginning*.

Problem Solving. Earlier in the text, the importance of allowing clients to formulate the goals of therapy was discussed. These goals are usually related to specific problems that have been created by their communicative disorders. By allowing clients to select the goals of therapy, motivation increases. Sensitivity toward client preferences has been expanded into a simple problem-solving strategy. The basic tenet of this strategy is to structure the entire therapy process around the specific problems clients identify as important to them. For example, if a child is having difficulty remembering how to use a new speaking pattern, the clinician and the client together will discuss the reasons why the behavior is not remembered. After identifying the reasons, particular solutions are cooperatively developed. Therapy from this point on is confined to implementing the proposed solutions. Although the use of this strategy may not initially result in as many quick benefits as one that is more clinician-directed, it leads to a greater amount of transfer to new situations and intrinsically is more reinforcing (Norman and Schmidt, 1992).

Areas for Use

In therapy, there are many things we may wish clients to learn. Some are very minor; others involve broad categories. The use of strategies may be more effective for some of these than for others. Below are some of the findings from a study which attempted to determine the appropriate learning areas in which to use strategies (Lonka, Lindblom, & Maury, 1994).

Detailed Information and Behaviors. Most of the behaviors clinicians attempt to teach clients involve details and are specific. This may involve learning the linguistic rule for producing actor + action + object constructions, using specific behavior components of fluent speech, or engaging in conversations according to acceptable social conventions. For behaviors of these types, most strategies are very appropriate.

Central Ideas or Concepts. In therapy, not all goals involve specific behaviors. Some involve central or encompassing concepts such as trying to have stutterers come to the realization that they can exert control over their speech. It appears that the acquisition and acceptance of central ideas and concepts is not dependent on the use of most structured strategies. Rather, there is evidence to suggest that a better way of teaching central ideas and concepts is through the use of elaboration strategies, where various relationships are discussed (Seifert, 1994).

Applications

The selection and application of strategies should be made in relationship to the entire intervention process. It is not an isolated event. Clinicians may elect to present the strategy using a structured format or may apply it in conjunction with other important therapeutic elements.

Methodology. Although the use of strategies significantly increases the probability that clients will learn new behaviors, it was found that by applying a specific methodology for using strategies, even greater improvements resulted (Afflerbach & Walker, 1992). The proposed methodology has three parts. First there should be an explanation of the task to be completed or learned.

Clinician: Now, we are going to work on your ability of having a conversation with your friends.

This is then followed by an acknowledgment of the strategies that will be used.

> *Clinician:* Last week you learned how to follow what someone says with something that is related to it. That's the strategy we will be using today.

Finally, both the strategies and behaviors are monitored.

> *Clinician:* As we talk, I will be pointing to one of the cards that helps you remember to stay on the conversation. If you are doing it correctly, I will shake my head "yes." If you don't do it correctly, I'll shake my head "no."

Combining Strategies. It would be wonderful if one strategy would be effective for all aspects of learning and retrieval. Unfortunately, that is not the case. It appears that the effects of strategies are very specific in terms of content, purpose, and learner abilities. In one study, for example, four strategy conditions were studied: (1) rehearsal, (2) elaboration, (3) rehearsal with elaboration, and (4) no strategy training (Turner, Dofny, & Dutka, 1994). The purpose of the study was to determine which strategy or combination of strategies best enabled clients to retrieve learned behaviors. Subjects in the two groups that used rehearsal outperformed subjects in the other two groups where rehearsal was not used. The implication of this part of the study is that having clients verbally explain what they will be doing enhances the likelihood of correct productions. However, we are not only concerned

with how easily a behavior can be retrieved in one situation, but how well it can be transferred to others. In transfer activities, subjects in the combined rehearsal-elaboration group performed better than subjects in the other three groups.

Combining Strategies with Monitoring. Earlier in this chapter the importance of monitoring was discussed and evidence for its positive effects in therapy were presented. Logically, it makes sense to combine strategies with monitoring. The effects of the combination were studied with 5th and 6th grade students (Delclos & Harrington, 1991). Three training conditions were compared: (1) problem-solving training, (2) problem-solving and self-monitoring training, and (3) no training. The group receiving both problem-solving and self-monitoring training solved more complex problems than either of the other two groups and took less time to solve them. The results of the study present very convincing evidence that, when training clients to use strategies to solve problems or change behavior, an integral part of the training should include methods for self-monitoring.

Strategies and Feedback. Studies have also examined how the combination of strategies with and without feedback affects learner performance. Although both conditions led to more learning than when no strategy-no feedback or feedback-only conditions were used, the combination of a strategy with feedback produced the greatest amount of learning (Schunk & Rice, 1993). Therefore, when using a strategy that enables a client to learn a new behavior, feedback should be provided on a constant and consistent basis. An example for a young child learning to produce /t/ would be, "That was terrific, when you said /t/, you put your tongue right behind your teeth, just like you said you were going to do."

Strategies Within Comprehensive Approaches. One study not only combined strategies with feedback, but also provided the rationale for the strategy's use, encouragement to utilize the strategy in nontrained situations, and extraneous reinforcers for efforts in using the strategy (Lange & Pierce, 1992). The 6- to 8-year olds in the experimental group that used this comprehensive approach had better retention of the target material and more generalization of effective strategies than the subjects in the control group who were not introduced to any of the experimental group's instructional devices. Although the design of the control group does not allow the reader to determine which of the instructional techniques was most beneficial, the idea of combining a variety of successful instructional devices should be of interest to speech-language clinicians. At times it is not possible to determine which of several techniques may be most effective in changing a behavior. In those situations a "shotgun" approach, where a variety of successful approaches are combined in a systematic way, is appropriate. Culatta and Goldberg (1995) found that most of the successful stuttering therapy programs addressed all of the possible variables that might be maintaining the stuttering behavior.

Contrasting Strategies. Another study was conducted to compare how well words learned in two different ways were retrieved (Wright, 1993). One set of severely language impaired children were taught the words using an elaborative approach, in which the various associations were made with the word. A matched group of subjects were taught the words using a more structured approach in which specific learning steps were taught. The group that learned the words through the structured strategy approach performed significantly better than the group using the elaborative approach. The importance of this study to speech-language clinicians is that strategies that are more structured will probably result in better retention and retrieval of information than ones lacking structure.

Another contrasting study compared visualization with elaboration. It was found that the use of visualization as a strategy was more effective than elaboration, when the learners' knowledge base is limited (Willoughby, Wood, & Khan, 1994). In therapy, clinicians are often faced with trying to explain something to clients that may be intricate and difficult to comprehend, either because it is complex or is dependent on clients having a broad knowledge base. For example, it might be difficult to try to explain the concept of a zoo to a child who has a cognitive impairment and has led a very sheltered life. The use of elaboration may be very frustrating, as there would be little on which to elaborate. However, a modified form of visualization, in which toy animals were placed in boxes, could make understanding the concept of zoo significantly easier.

There may be times when either a categorization or a functionality strategy could be used. There are some general guidelines for making this determination (Best, 1993). Functionality as a strategy is found more often in problem solving of older rather than younger children. It seems that categorization is cognitively an easier strategy for younger children to use, possibly because of some features that are more concrete in the objects than in functionality. Categorization is also a better strategy to use than functionality if it is more obvious. For example, Monday, Tuesday, Wednesday, Thursday, Friday, Saturday, and Sunday obviously are better organized using a category strategy than a functionality strategy. Each is a day of the week. The reverse would be true for legs, car, horse, sled, and airplane. For these words, a functionality strategy which involved what each does would be more efficient. They all move.

In Table 8–4, the strategies are grouped according to their appropriateness for different age groups. This should be viewed only as a heuristic device that can be used for making initial decisions with strategies, because the exact matching of strategies to particular learners is highly individualistic and may be related to a wide variety of variables. Most of these strategies can be used with virtually all communication disorders.

GENERALIZATION

Generalization is one of the most important aspects of therapy, and one that is often neglected. It usually occurs at the end of therapy, which is too late. The technical definition of generalization was developed by Stokes and Baer (1977): "The occurrence of a relevant behavior under different, non-training conditions (i.e., across subjects, settings, people, behaviors, and/or time) without the scheduling of the same events in those conditions as had been scheduled in the training condition." Simply put, generalization occurs when the behavior is present outside the clinic, in a variety of situations with a variety of people. Occasionally, the terms *transfer, carryover,* and *generalization* are used interchangeably. Generalization is used here instead of either transfer or carryover, because it has a standard definition.

TABLE 8–4
Suggestions for Age-Appropriate Strategies

AGE	DETAILED INFORMATION AND BEHAVIORS	CENTRAL IDEAS OR CONCEPTS
Children	External Categorization Elaboration Active Involvement Post Organizers Visual Cues	External Elaboration Active Involvement
Adolescents	External Adolescents Categorization Post Organizers Elaboration Active Involvement Visual Cues Problem Solving	External/Internal Elaboration Active Involvement Visualization Summary Skills Problem Solving
Adults	External/Internal Categorization Post Organizers Elaboration Active Involvement Visual Cues Problem Solving	Internal Elaboration Active Involvement Visualization Summary Skills Problem Solving Major Life Transitions Stress Reduction

Timing

Generalization can occur either as a distinct phase of therapy or as a procedure that is incorporated throughout the therapy process. Although most intervention programs have it as the final phase of therapy, a strong argument will be made that it should be an integrated part of all therapy.

A Stage of Therapy. Intervention programs that directly address generalization of behaviors usually describe it as the final stage of therapy (Andrews, 1995; Shames & Florance, 1980). As the final stage of therapy, the established target behaviors are practiced in a variety of nonclinical settings, utilizing self-monitoring techniques and specific activities. Regardless of the behavior that is targeted, the basic generalization procedure is to teach a behavior within a protective environment (the clinic), to establish it, and then to replicate it in a nonclinical setting. For example, some approaches for teaching the production of target phonemes use the following sequence.

1. Sound in isolation in clinic
2. Sound in syllable in clinic
3. Sound in word in clinic
4. Sound in sentences in clinic
5. Sound in sentences in nonclinical settings

In this example, before the sound is generalized it is fully developed in sentences.

An Integrated Part of Therapy. Generalization is also used as an ongoing process in therapy. Van Riper's (1973) early forms of stuttering therapy incorporated generalization within, rather than at the end of, therapy. He emphasized the importance for the stutterer to continually practice new reduced stuttering patterns in social situations. In Webster's Precision Fluency Shaping Program (1974), clients begin generalizing each new step of the flu-ency development from the beginning of therapy. In Goldberg's Behavioral Cognitive Stuttering Therapy Program (1981), clients are required to generalize exaggerated forms of fluency from the first day of therapy.

Sheehan (1978), a strong advocate of immediate generalization applications, maintained that if a separate generalization stage was required, inadequate therapy procedures were probably applied. According to him, if the procedures were appropriate, generalization would be a logical consequence of their mastery, rather than something that required an additional stage. This position finds support in the results of generalization experiments in other areas. In psychotherapy, for example, Ager (1987) found that the degree to which his clients were able to generalize new behaviors was related more to the components of the establishment procedures than to any other variable. This important relationship that exists between establishment procedures and generalization is also found in teaching social communicative behaviors to retarded adolescents (Hunt, Goetz, Alwell, & Sailor, 1986), speech skills in hearing-impaired children (Perigoe and Ling, 1986), and production of new phonemes in misarticulating children (Gierut, Elbert, and Dinnsen, 1987). In these studies it was shown that the procedures used during establishment of new behaviors had a significant effect on the length of time required and the extent to which generalization took place.

Generalization of a new behavior is more complex than it may appear. Clinicians often have difficulty understanding why it is so difficult for clients to continue to display a behavior taught in the clinic. For example, explanations as to why a client cannot maintain the production of a target phoneme in unstructured speech might include distractions not present in the clinic, unavailability of reinforcers, or even a lack of motivation. Regardless of the explanation, the fault is usually seen as unrelated to the establishment procedures used in the clinic. However, studies have clearly indicated that the success or failure of generalizing behaviors is most often a function of the establishment procedures. With appropriate establishment procedures, generalization is possible even with individuals who have been classified as being profoundly cognitively disordered (Fox, 1989).

Stimulus Generalization

Stimulus generalization is a neglected aspect of most therapy. *Stimulus generalization involves the production of a specific behavior under various conditions.* For example, when teaching a child to produce a specific type of utterance, such as wh-questions, the clinician wants the child to ask questions not only in the clinic, but also in the classroom and home. By including activities very early in therapy that focus on stimulus generalization, the likelihood that the child will be able to produce the target behavior in other settings will be enhanced. Often in therapy a new behavior is taught and apparently mastered in the clinic room. Clinicians then are dumbfounded when clients are unable to produce that same behavior when they are standing or during a nonstructured activity. Based on studies which only minimally changed the environment in which a behavior was to be produced, it appears that any changes in the context in which the behavior was learned results in the use of different strategies to retrieve and produce that behavior (Starnes & Loeb, 1993). For example, aphasic clients who are taught to retrieve the names of objects in a quiet, stressless setting may not be able to use these strategies when waiting in line at a fast food restaurant with an annoying cashier demanding to know what they want to order. If clients are to be able to produce the target behavior in many contexts, attention must be paid to the contexts present when the behavior is

taught. A more precise name for the context in which the behavior is taught is stimu-lus configuration.

Stimulus Configurations. A stimulus configuration is a set of stimuli that is present when a specific response is elicited. The configuration may involve only a few critical variables or it may encompass a much greater number.

Training Sequence. Table 8–5 illustrates the sequence for generalizing action + object constructions (e.g., *push ball*). In this illustration, four stimulus configurations result in the same response. Only four steps are used in this example. Complete programs may contain fewer steps or more. The first two steps in the example are training situations, and the last two are untrained situations. A training situation involves teaching a behavior during which as many aspects of the stimulus configuration, response, and consequences are controlled. During the untrained situation, some aspects of the sequence are not controlled. In this illustration, the two training stimulus configurations differ in terms of only one element. In the first step, the clinician prompts the client for the response by tapping on two cards, indicating that there are two units to the response. In the second step, this does not occur.

In step 1, the clinician attempts to facilitate the client's response of "push ball" when the clinician asks, "What should I do?" The client has already been taught a strategy for producing the response. Both the client and the clinician are in a quiet clinic room, facing each other on the floor, and the clinician has a ball in front of her. The clinician says, "What should I do?" followed by tapping on the two cards. In this situation, the desired response is the client saying "push ball." One other form of stimulus generalization occurs if various balls are placed between them and the clinician asks, "What should I do?" The activity may continue over a number of sessions until

TABLE 8-5
Training Sequence for Stimulus Generalization

STEP	SITUATION	STIMULUS CONFIGURATION	RESPONSE
1	Trained	**People:** clinician and client. **Physical situation:** client and clinician sitting on floor in clinic with various toy balls between them. **Utterance:** clinician asks, "What should I do?", followed by prompt (tapping two cards).	Client answers "push ball."
2	Trained	**People:** clinician and client. **Physical situation:** client and clinician sitting on floor in clinic with various toy balls between them. **Utterance:** clinician asks, "What should I do?"	Client answers "push ball."
3	Untrained	**People:** specific individuals (e.g., parents) who have agreed to participate in therapy. **Physical situation:** specific places in house where various toy balls are placed. **Utterance:** parent asks, "What should I do?"	Client answers "push ball."
4	Untrained	**People:** anyone. **Physical situation:** various settings (e.g., school, relatives' houses, etc.). **Utterance:** different people ask, "What should I do?"	Client answers "push ball."

the client is able to respond correctly. With success, the clinician moves on to step 2.

In step 2 the desired response remains the same, but the stimulus configuration changes: this time the prompt is removed. When the client can successfully say "push ball," therapy moves on to a new phase, which is untrained situations. Between sessions, the parents of the client are instructed to place balls on various flat surfaces in the home and ask their daughter, "What should I do?" The client's response remains the same. With success, the stimulus configuration is again changed. This time, other individuals are asked to replicate the parent's interaction in a variety of situations and with various balls.

Rationale. The rationale for designing activities that incorporate stimulus generalization is that it prepares clients to produce a specific desired response in a variety of situations. It is a critical component of generalization.

Response Generalization

Response generalization occurs when a specific stimulus configuration can elicit two or more responses that are similar in some aspects but different in others. During stimulus generalization, the response stayed the same throughout the procedures. During response generalization, the reverse is true: The stimulus remains the same, but the response changes.

Training Sequence.

An example of response generalization appears in Table 8–6. In this example, the stimulus configuration remains the same throughout the interaction. The clinician and the client sit on the clinic floor with various balls in front of them. The client has already added "throw" to her verbal repertoire. This time, it is hoped that the client can say either "throw ball" or "push ball" in response to the question, "What should I do?" The same sequence found in stimulus generalization is used.

Rationale. The rationale for designing activities that incorporate response generalization is that it prepares clients to produce a variety of desired responses to a specific stimulus. Just like stimulus generalization, it is a critical component for the generalization of behaviors.

TABLE 8–6
Training Sequence for Response Generalization

	SITUATION	STIMULUS CONFIGURATION	RESPONSE
1	Trained	**People:** clinician and client. **Physical situation:** client and clinician sitting on floor in clinic with various toy balls between them. **Utterance:** clinician asks, "What should I do?"	Client answers "push ball."
2	Trained	**People:** clinician and client. **Physical situation:** client and clinician sitting on floor in clinic with various toy balls between them. **Utterance:** clinician asks, "What should I do?"	Client answers "throw ball."
3	Untrained	**People:** clinician and client. **Physical situation:** client and clinician sitting on floor in clinic with various toys, including balls between them. **Utterance:** clinician asks, "What should I do?"	Client answers, "give ball" (with the word give being a word the client has produced, but was not present in the training situation).
4	Untrained	**People:** clinician and client. **Physical situation:** client and clinician sitting on floor in clinic with various toys, including balls between them. **Utterance:** clinician asks, "What should I do?"	Client answers, "throw house" (with the word house being a word the client has produced, but was not present in the training situation).

Combinations

There is obvious merit in using both stimulus and response generalization techniques. Each contributes to the ability of the client to generalize new behaviors in untrained situations because the client often encounters new stimulus configurations that require complex response patterns. It is not possible to anticipate all the situations in which clients will be required to produce target behaviors. However, the greater the emphasis in therapy on stimulus and response generalization, the more likely it will be that the critical variables found in nonclinical situations will have been incorporated within the training sequence during therapy.

Activities

Generalization activities usually take the form of *homework*. These are assignments provided to clients or their parents that are designed to facilitate practice of the new behaviors. Studies have shown that when homework activities are practiced, they result in better performance than if no practice is performed (Neimeyer & Feixas, 1990). However, the form and structure of the assignments significantly affected their value during the maintenance phase of therapy. Considerations on how to construct activities which last through the maintenance phase of therapy are provided below.

Scheduling Activities. One of the most critical considerations in the use of extraclinical activities is how they are scheduled. The easiest procedure for the clinician is to give clients and their families the activity and tell them to take so many minutes each day and practice the behaviors. In this case, what is easiest for the clinician is the worst for the client. The purpose of generalization activities is to engage in behaviors in as natural a situation as is possible. Carving out a given

number of minutes each day for *speech and language practice* defeats the purpose of the activity. The activity should be incorporated into the client's everyday activities. For example, if a client is working on the retrieval of number concepts, memory strategy should be used when making change for the bus. The stutterer who has been taught to use a controlled form of fluency should practice the method when ordering food in a restaurant. The child who has learned how to correctly produce the phoneme /d/ should use it while playing with his toys.

Contracts. Generalization activities should include a method for assessing correct or incorrect productions. It may involve something as simple as a checkmark system or as complicated as assessing the correct use of the components of a behavior, such as single ingestion of air during esophageal speech. One of the best ways for assessing performance is the use of contracts. A contract is a commitment that clients make with themselves to perform certain behaviors at prescribed times, with predetermined criteria for assessment. The use of contracts in counseling is widespread and has become infused into a large number of clinical approaches in the helping sciences because of its demonstrated effectiveness (Smith, 1994). In the area of speech-language pathology it has been used primarily in stuttering therapy. Initially used by Shames and Florence (1980), it was expanded and made more formal by Goldberg in the Behavioral Cognitive Stuttering Therapy Program (1981). An example appears in Table 8–7. In this program, specific behaviors are specified, criteria for assessing the accuracy of behaviors are used, and days and times are predetermined for when the behavior is to be performed. The use of contracts that clients make with themselves facilitates the development of self-determination (Parsons & Durst, 1992).

TABLE 8-7

Maintenance Contract Example

Client _____ Date _____

15 continuous minutes each waking hour   Record number of disfluencies off contract

CONT. NUMBER	TIME	SIGNAL 2 PT	RATE 2 PT	WORD 2 PT	FLUENT 4 PT	TOTAL	% CORRECT	OPTIONAL POINTS	DISFLUENCIES
1	7:00								
2	8:00								
3	9:00								
4	10:00								
5	11:00								
6	12:00								
7	1:00								
8	2:00								
9	3:00								
10	4:00								
11	5:00								
12	6:00								
13	7:00								
14	8:00								
15	9:00								
16	10:00								
17	11:00								

Totals

Scoring: Sig./rate/PWC   0 = not at all   1 pt = sometimes   2 pt = always
          Fluent   0 = not fluent   4 pt = fluent

(From *Behavioral Cognitive Stuttering Therapy* by S. A. Goldberg, 1981. San Francisco, CA: IntelliGroup Publishing Company. Reprinted with permission.)

278

Highlighting Stimulus Configurations. Activities which take place in the home often involve specific places, such as bathrooms for training self-help skills for cognitively impaired children or common objects for aphasic clients with memory problems. By highlighting the targeted objects or places in the home, clients may be able to focus better on the generalization activity. Color has been shown to focus attention on the activity, especially for older clients (Cooper, Letts, & Rigby, 1993). This can be as simple as placing a removable color tag on items in the house that the client is expected to use. Additional cues for memory activities could be placing the first letter of the object's name on the color tag, moving all of the objects within one room, or placing all of the objects in one place in a room.

Age Factors. Age is an irrelevant factor in the use of generalization activities. Children as young as 27 months are able to generalize simple matching tasks with minimal training (Brown, Brown, & Poulson, 1995). In fact, if sufficient attention is paid to the construction of the stimulus configurations during the acquisition stage of learning, young children can generalize behaviors even easier than can adolescents or adults. A key component in the successful generalization of behaviors with children and adolescents is the involvement of their parents, caregivers, or available school personnel. Their involvement is critical because children and adolescents require more monitoring and feedback than adults to generalize behaviors.

MAINTENANCE

Maintenance is a phase in therapy that occurs after regular clinic visits cease. Clients have already learned the new behaviors and strategies and are in the process of applying them on their own.

Things to Maintain

During therapy clients were taught how to produce specific behaviors, how to use compensatory strategies or use strategies that result in the production of target behaviors. Each of these three types of things may require different maintenance activities.

Specific Behaviors. In order for behaviors to become a part of a client's behavioral repertoire, they must become automatic. Automaticity is a function of practice. Therefore, for some motor behaviors, regularly scheduled practice activities may be required. Obviously, the more these can be incorporated within the client's everyday activities, the more quickly they will be generalized and maintained. Some clients, however, believe that they require additional concentrated practice time. One client spent 20 minutes every morning practicing a slow rate of speech. He was convinced that it enabled him to maintain the target rate throughout the day.

Compensatory Strategies. There is some evidence to suggest that compensatory strategies are less resistant to decay during maintenance than strategies that were learned to create new behaviors (Pearson, 1993). This may be related to the fact that many of the factors involved in the creation of the old behavior are still active, and while compensatory strategies may be effective in reducing the old behavior, competing influences remain. Therefore, if the strategy taught to clients is a compensatory one, additional maintenance activities may need to be used.

New Behavior Strategies. Although new behavior strategies are more resistant to decay than compensatory strategies, they may require a greater effort to consistently use. The learning of new behaviors may be a difficult process. The strategy may be complex or just take a significant amount of effort to use. The daily application of strategies that were used to learn new behaviors may require a great effort on part of the client.

ERROR ANALYSIS

When clients respond incorrectly to questions, clinicians can merely note the error or analyze it in terms of the cognitive or behavioral processes that caused it. The first procedure provides little feedback to the client other than that the target behavior was not properly executed. The second procedure not only provides more information to the client, but also enables clinicians to understand the process whereby learning is not complete. Errors can be analyzed either in terms of general information or of types.

Identifying Certitude of Answers

The degree to which clients believe they know the correct answer may be partially determined by observing the speed of their answers and the intonation patterns of their speech. In a study examining the certitude of answers provided by undergraduates, it was found that for those answers the subjects rated as being low, there was a correlation with slower response times and rising intonation patterns at the end of the response (Smith & Clark, 1993). Although other aspects of intonation have been examined to determine if they can provide any information on answer certitude, only rising intonation patterns appear to be reliable (Hirschberg & Ward, 1992). When either of these response patterns are apparent in the answers of clients, clinicians should engage clients in a discussion of why they are not sure of their answer. There is obviously something about the answer that the client is unsure about. By de-

termining what this is, the faulty learning process can be corrected.

The use of fillers (uh, um, etc.) and qualifiers (maybe, sort of, I think so, etc.) may also provide information on client answer certitude. These speech insertions were found to be correlated with the answers of subjects where certitude was low (McMullen & Pasloski, 1992; Smith & Clark, 1993).

Types

There are five types of errors clients can make. It is important for clinicians to be able to identify the type of error that occurred because each should result in a different response from clinicians. By knowing the type of errors clients make, appropriate corrective strategies and feedback can be provided.

Unlearned Prerequisites. Many of the behaviors clinicians ask clients to do are complex, with distinct units that are sequentially related. The assumption is that clients have already learned and retained the prior behaviors necessary to produce the current one. Clients do not always retain new behaviors. This might be due either to inadequate learning or few opportunities to practice the behavior. For example, clients cannot use an actor + action construction if they confuse actors and inanimate objects. Errors that are based on unlearned prerequisites, such as this one, require that clinicians go back to teaching the prerequisites. Of even more importance to clinicians is a determination of *why* the client failed. Answers to this question can provide clinicians with information that will allow them to redesign their training procedures.

Systematic Conceptual Errors. Systematic conceptual errors occur when clients consistently apply an inappropriate strategy. For example, a child may have been taught to exaggerate the /r/ sound in order to produce an appropriate target sound in isolation. When moving to produce the sound in words, the exaggerated form of /r/ remains, even though it is no longer necessary for producing the sound. To correct errors of this type it is suggested that clients be asked to go through the decision process with the clinician (Mozdzierz & Greenblatt, 1992). By using this procedure, clinicians can help clients determine the cause for the error and learn how to substitute the correct strategy.

Random. Occasionally there is no easy way to identify why an error occurred other than possible inattention. Errors such as these do not require the type of learning activities necessary in the first two error types. Usually, just refocusing the client's attention on the task is sufficient. Clinicians may try to identify extraneous variables that may have been interfering. These can range from high noise levels to clients focusing on nontherapy activities.

Noncompliance. Errors of noncompliance can be problems of either learning or behavior. It is important that clinicians can make this distinction, because each requires a different modification of the learning activity. Often what may appear as noncompliance is actually a defensive tactic which some children use to hide their inability to produce the requested response. One Down syndrome child would respond to identification requests with, "No, you do it." For several sessions the clinician believed this was a behavioral noncompliance error. With testing, it became apparent that the child did not know how to respond correctly and preferred to appear belligerent rather than incompetent. By simplifying the activities, the child's use of "No, you do it" dramatically decreased. With gains in knowledge, the behavior was eventually eliminated. Noncompliance also can result from clients not finding anything reinforcing about the activity. The appropriate course of action in cases such as these involve restructuring the activity so that it is either intrinsically, extrinsically, or extraneously reinforcing.

Nonvolitional Inattention. Errors of nonvolitional inattention refer to errors that are created due to the introduction of "noise" which interferes with the client's processing of the request. For example, a young man who had a stroke could not comprehend what the clinician was requesting if the rate of the clinician's speech was too rapid. In spite of his desire to attend, his impairment made it impossible to do so in the presence of a rapid auditory signal. When the clinician reduced his rate of speech, the client was able to attend to the auditory signal and consistently responded appropriately. When clients have nonvolitional errors, clinicians should determine the variables that are associated with it. Once identified, a multiple cuing approach that controls the variables should be used. For example, with the young man, the clinician began each request with, "Jim . . ." He then waited for the client to look directly at him, and finally spoke at a very slow rate. Gradually the rate was increased. This was followed by the elimination of "Jim," and eventually the requests were produced when the client was not looking at the clinician.

CORRECT RESPONSE ANALYSIS

When we ask clients to produce specific behaviors, our analysis of their responses usually stops with determining if it was correct or incorrect. Unfortunately, this shortsighted procedure deprives both clinician and client with the opportunity to understand the cognitive processes involved in learning. With incorrect responses clients may be told why the response was incorrect. Rarely are correct responses analyzed. The assumption is that if the behavior is produced correctly, the client obviously understands it components. This may not be entirely true.

Confirmation of Prior Learning

Clients may attribute success to additional factors that are irrelevant to the successful completion of a behavior and detrimental to correctly producing the behavior in other instances. For example, a client had been taught to use a signal that would enable him to concentrate on a steady rate and not to anticipate difficult sounds or words. During clinical activities he was able to produce fluent speech 100% of the time. Unknown to the clinician, the client was also manipulating breath control in a very unnatural way. While the clinician assumed success was related to the use of his three techniques, the client attributed success to the three taught and his breath control. During outside activities the client's fluency decreased with each passing day. When he came for his weekly session the clinician could not understand why he was having so much difficulty. The client explained that during the week, his ability to control his breath was disrupted by a cold. If the clinician knew at the prior week's session that the client was partially attributing success to a technique which was destined to fail, a week of frustration could have been avoided. At least the first time that clients produce successful behaviors, inquire how they accomplished it.

Self-Analysis

When you ask a client to explain how he or she was able to produce a specific behavior or know that an answer is correct, the client is forced to carefully analyze his or her own behavior. This process not only results in the development of a richer knowledge base (Willoughby & Wood, 1994), but also improves the acquisition of problem-solving skills (Chie, deLeeuw, Chie, & LaVancher, 1994). Because most people have their own unique problem-solving strategies, by understanding how clients are able to produce one behavior or solve a specific problem, clinicians can gain insight on how to enable the clients to solve problems in other areas.

CHAPTER

9

Complex Process Skills

*C*omplex process skills might be the most difficult ones to learn. They involve a degree of sophistication, timing, and experience that appear to go beyond all other skills. There are six categories of skills in this chapter that contain 44 techniques and behaviors.

REPHRASING

The use of nondirective rephrasing is a very helpful technique developed by Carl Rogers (1965). It involves taking clients' utterances and rewording them in order that the intent or meaning of the utterance is made clearer. There are various positive effects of rephrasing and methods for achieving them. Four positive benefits can occur by rephrasing clients' utterances. They are that (1) it clearly indicates to clients that clinicians are attending to what they are saying, (2) it provides an opportunity to subtly move the client's orientation towards that of the clinician, (3) it allows for the summation of material, and (4) it can personalize the problem or discussion.

Indicating Clinician Attention

At a very basic level, rephrasing can indicate to clients that clinicians are paying attention to what they just said. Not only were the clinicians listening at a cursory level, but focusing on the clients' communication to such an extent that they were able to take their words and rephrase them into a structure that was even more meaningful or accurate than the message initially communicated. Although not necessarily the most sophisticated use of rephrasing, it is more in line with Rogers' intent of imposing a minimal amount of clinician viewpoint, and can serve as a relatively easy way of refocusing the client. A good analogy can be found in bread making. After kneading the dough into a ball, it has a certain amount of elasticity, yet can hold its shape nicely. If left alone, the dough ball will slowly flatten out slightly. To reshape it back into a sphere, the baker needs only to gently push on its sides. A similar process occurs when rephrasing is used in this manner. As clients begin to get off task, what they are discussing or attempting to perform can be gently "pushed on its sides," so that refocusing takes place.

Restructuring

Rephrasing what the client said can be more than reflection or attempts at refocusing. Often clients will conceptualize a problem or solution in a way that is not necessary conducive to positive change. For example, a client in voice therapy may lament how her voice begins to crack after being exposed to 3 hours of cigarette smoke. Although the description of the causal effects of the smoke is accurate, the phrasing indicates that smoke exposure is something that just happens to her. As part of her therapy, the clinician may believe that it is important for the client to accept responsibility for change. In order to do this she might rephrase the client's statement into one that implicates the client. Take for example, the following statement:

> "My voice begins to crack when it's exposed to cigarette smoke for over three hours.

The clinician may wish to rephrase the client's statement in the following way:

> "Your voice begins to crack when *you decide* to go to a nightclub where cigarettes are smoked.

Rephrasing, when used to restructure clients thoughts, is a very deliberate manipulative technique that can help change how clients conceptualize various aspects of their disorder. It is a very powerful and important clinical technique.

Summation

Often in therapy, complex, difficult, or painful issues are discussed. Rarely are conversations linear. One topic leads to another and soon what started as a well-defined conversation veers in a multitude of directions, most of which are important.

When this occurs, it is very useful for clinicians to rephrase the content of the conversation so that a structure is presented that is logical, simple, and highlights the most significant aspects of the conversation. While this summary process has little effect upon the client's retention of minute, specific facts, it has been shown to facilitate the retention of broader concepts (Nelson, Smith, & Dodd, 1992). There are two times in the session when the use of this technique is particularly useful. The first is at the end of an activity or topic of discussion. Its immediacy in relation to the activity or discussion facilitates its retention and signals closure to the client. The second time it can be effectively used in therapy is at the end of each session. Clients need to leave the session with a concise sense of what was accomplished and what will be done next.

Personalization

At times it is just too painful for some clients to directly accept responsibility for a problem, or even acknowledge that a problem exists. Clients will often depersonalize the problems they are in therapy to correct. Instead of talking about "my stuttering," "stuttering" in general is discussed. For example, instead of saying, "When I stutter," the client may say, "When stuttering occurs." The depersonalization of a problem may occur either because clients find it too painful to accept as part of themselves, or because they do not wish to accept the responsibility for its presence. Regardless of why the problem has been depersonalized, clinicians should rephrase the clients' utterances so that they are personalized. Personalization has been shown to enhance motivation to change and also makes the requirement or change easier to represent mentally (Davis, Ross, & Morrison, 1991). If the depersonalization occurred because the problem was too painful to acknowledge as being a part of the client, rephrasing should include a healthy dose of empathy. For example, "I can understand how hard it must be for you to accept the fact that you will probably always have some problems remembering names." An opposite course of action is taken when depersonalization is used to deny responsibility for the problem. For example, "You say that stuttering just happens. I don't understand. Is there someone or something that forces you not to use your control strategy?"

CONFRONTATION

Usually during a clinical interaction, what clients are saying is both important to them and relevant to therapy. At times, what they are saying may not be conducive to the establishment of clinical goals. They may be presenting faulty assumptions, misrepresentations, or inappropriate perceptions. Many clinicians are reluctant to confront their clients for fear of negatively impacting on the clinical interaction. Yet studies have shown that the selective use of confrontation can facilitate the restructuring of dysfunctional relationships and inappropriate perceptions (Feldman, 1994).

Effectiveness

Confrontation is an integral part of many therapeutic approaches that attempt to radically change certain behaviors such as drug and alcohol addiction (Lowenstein, 1991). Although communicative disorders may not be as dysfunctional as drug or alcohol problems, the judicious use of confrontation may be equally as effective. However, confrontation is not advisable early in the therapy process. Later, after trust has been established, confronting clients when inappropriate statements are made leads to a level of attentiveness and concern that far outweighs the positive benefits of unconditional acceptance. Far from being negative, confrontation is a clinical behavior that has been repeatedly observed in very skilled clinicians.

Methods

Unless careful thought and preparation are given to the confrontation, it may become an impediment to progress, rather than a facilitator. Two procedures have been shown to reduce the potential problems associated with confrontation. They involve enlisting client input and providing a structure for the confrontation.

Enlisting Client Input. It will be easier to confront a client's inappropriate behaviors or attitudes if their own judgments are incorporated into the confrontative dialogue. Take for example, the client who committed to practicing certain behaviors throughout the week. At the next clinic meeting, he informed the clinician that he just did not have any time to practice them. Instead of directly confronting the client's commitment to change, the clinician could ask the client to provide him with the conditions for change to which they had discussed and agreed upon. By using the client's own words, it becomes easier for the clinician to confront the client about his commitment to therapy and change.

Structuring Confrontations. A modification of a procedure used in counseling can provide some structure to the process of soliciting client input for confrontations (Hermans, Fiddelaers, deGroot, & Nauta, 1990). The first step is having clients specify the criteria for making an evaluation. In our example, the clinician might have the client state what conditions would need to prevail for there to be insufficient amount of time to engage in the activity. The second step involves applying the criteria to the occurrence. The client would now have to determine, using the criteria he generated, if his explanation for why the activities were not done was consistent with his criteria. Finally, in the third step, a discussion of the discrepancies occurs. Other reasons than time could be investigated for why the activities were not performed.

Problems

Although confrontation is a very useful and important technique to use in therapy, its use must be judicious and well orchestrated. When someone goes to the boundaries of acceptability, it's often described as "stretching the envelope." It is a very good analogy for understanding the inherent risks and rewards associated with the use of confrontation. There are probably no other counseling techniques with as high a reward-risk ratio. If it is effectively used, few things can so rapidly cut to the to heart of a problem as confrontation. However, if incompetently applied, few things can have as negative effect on the clinical relationship.

Losing Face. When using confrontation with clients, care needs to be taken so clients are not embarrassed. This is especially important in group activities. The "loss of face" can result in negative consequences, including defensive reactions (Eisendrath, 1989). Some studies have shown that confrontative styles that focus on past failures and present conflicts do not do as well as programs that emphasize self-esteem and peer relationships (Kashner, Rodell, Ogden, Guggenheim, et al., 1992). Confrontation, therefore, should be something that is occasionally used, rather than a style of interaction. There is evidence to suggest that the ability of clients to respond nondefensively may be related less to the style of the clinicians' interactions and more to personal needs and problems (Salerno, Farber, McCullough, Winston, et al., 1992).

Cultural Considerations. There are cultural qualifications to the use of confrontation. For Asian American/Pacific Islander clients, there is a tradition of solving problems through negotiation and mediation rather than through direct confrontation (Berg & Jaya, 1993). If these clients present attitudes that are antithetical to therapy, alternative methods of changing them will need to be used. For example, when working with an adult Japanese American who had suffered a stroke, the clinician needed to address the client's negative interpretation of his wife's behavior, which in the eyes of the clinician was exemplary. Instead of directly challenging him, she proceeded to have the client list the many things that she was now required to do following his stroke. After developing a list of over 15 new responsibilities that she had, she reintroduced the client's assessment of her. This time, with a written list of 15 difficult activities that his wife was now performing, his assessment of her was significantly more positive.

Similar problems with confrontation occur when working with Native Americans. Confrontation is not an appropriate technique to be used in counseling. Just as with the Japanese American client, issues that require change need to involve more nondirective methods. Often the use of analogies in a story format can accomplish the same goals as confrontation, but without the negative consequences that would inevitably result from its use.

Aftermath. Much has been written regarding the need for clients to confront beliefs that have negatively affected their lives (Cameron, 1994). Yet little has been written for clinicians in terms of how to deal with their clients after they have confronted them. It is possible that the two-part process that is taught to clients for the aftermath of confrontations is also useful for clinicians. These involve a debriefing and reconfrontation. In this procedure, clinicians and clients discuss the issue that was confronted and any residual negative feelings that the client may have. For example, after confronting a client about his lack of commitment to therapy, the clinician should encourage the client to discuss how he felt when confronted, asking specifically if there was merit in the accusations and assessments made by the clinician.

After a thorough discussion, the clinician's confrontative statements and assessments are again introduced, and clients are asked if they reflect an accurate assessment of his performance.

Clients Deference to Clinicians.

Because of the relationship which exists between clients and clinicians, clients tend to have a deference towards the clinicians' opinions, even if clients intuitively disagree with them (Rennie, 1994). After all, as a professional, the speech-language clinician's viewpoint *must* be correct. The ease at which some clients bend to the viewpoints of clinicians can result in minimizing the effects of confrontation. The purpose of confrontation is to require clients to consciously deal with whatever is being disputed. If clients are overly deferent to clinicians there is a possibility the clinician's position will be accepted without the client fully understanding it. This can be minimized by using a form of confrontation that emphasizes a questioning attitude, rather than one which tells the client what to believe or do.

GROUP THERAPY

Therapy is conducted with clients individually and in group settings. The decision to work individually or a group is dependent on many factors, including work setting, financial resources, disorder, and time commitments. If the group therapy experience is to be beneficial to its members, the group leader needs to be familiar with the clinical behaviors that are related to: (1) the basic group characteristics, (2) interpersonal relationships, (3) management, and (4) functions.

Basic Considerations

Prior to even forming a group, clinicians should know how to prepare its members for the experience and how to incorporate features that are endemic to most types of groups into the intervention plan.

Preparation.

If a group is to work, it should have some degree of cohesion (Lieberman, 1990). Cohesion can be derived from various things such as commonality of nonclinical experiences, disorder characteristics, and mutual interest in a specific group activity. When a natural cohesion is not possible, clinicians need to construct activities which will facilitate its development. It has been found that advance preparation of group members, regardless of the level of commonality of nonclinical experiences, greatly facilities the development of cohesiveness (Bowman & DeLucia, 1993). Preparation should occur both individually and at the very beginning of group therapy. Most of the preparation can involve explanations of the functions of the group, how issues will be addressed, and what are considered to be acceptable and unacceptable patterns of interaction between group members and the group leader. A second method that has been suggested uses a very structured approach (Bergin, 1989). The first thing that should be done is to use an activity that promotes the group process and develops rapport among the group members. The activity should require an extensive amount of communication and collaboration. Additionally, the activity should focus on completing a time-limited task.

Another important aspect of preparing a group involves developing a realistic perception of group membership, with an understanding of the group's purpose. When both are done, groups tend to be more beneficial for their members (Meadow, 1988). When they are not, groups generally fail (Lieberman, 1990).

Group Composition.

Homogeneity appears to be an important feature in the composition of groups, especially for adolescents (Leader, 1991). The closer the ages, interests, and disabilities, the more likely the group will function well. Shared interests and experiences facilitate the group's focusing on topics of discussion and development of behaviors. When groups consist of diverse individuals in terms of cultures and interests, it becomes important for the clinician to develop a focal interest which all clients can adopt. Without at least some commonalities in interest or purpose, group experiences tend to be unsatisfying and unsuccessful.

General Competency. Clinicians should be aware that their attitudes, values, and behaviors may become a model for emulation to clients (Dinkmeyer et al., 1987). Regardless of the orientation used in group therapy, it is critical that the client perceive the clinician as competent. The clinician who is unprepared and disorganized for the group session, presents a very different picture from the clinician whose presentation of activities and topics to a similar group is logically structured, systematic, and clear. Successful management of a group involves balancing individuals with group needs.

Settings. Often one's work setting dictates the parameters of therapy. One-on-one therapy can be expensive and time-consuming. Although the administrators of many settings realize that they are not providing the best of all possible services, financial or time restrictions may limit their options.

Public schools seem to be continually under financial assault. There never seems to be enough money or personnel to provide the best quality service. Traditionally, speech therapy has been carried on in less than ideal circumstances. It is arguable whether the problem is the result of the expense of treating communicative disorders or administrators not realizing the importance of the service speech-language pathol-

ogists provide. Most therapy is conducted in group settings. When possible, children with similar disorders are treated in a group ranging from two to five members. Rarely are more than five children seen together. When children with similar disorders cannot be scheduled together, often they are grouped by age. When this is not possible, children who have time available within their schedule are grouped together.

With the implementation of Public Law 94-142, guaranteeing appropriate services to disabled children, many parents of children with communicative disorders have refused to accept inappropriate grouping of their children. Many administrators are reluctant to require their speech-language pathologists to form inappropriate therapy groups, especially with children whose impairment is moderate or severe.

Senior centers tend to be social organizations where senior citizens can engage in socially or personally rewarding experiences with other individuals of their generation. It is also an ideal setting for aural rehabilitation as the purpose of these classes is to facilitate lip reading by hearing-impaired individuals. In groups where the focus is not aural rehabilitation, such as aphasia, hearing impairments will be found in at least 25% of all group members (Hittner & Bornstein, 1990). Although the purpose of these groups is not to address hearing problems, specific considerations for the hearing impairments of the clients should be made. These include the selection of a quiet room, improved acoustics, hearing rehabilitation referrals, group hearing aids, better placement of group members, and the use of visual aids. Clinicians should also use techniques that will aid the hearing-impaired individual such as repetition, increased loudness, clearer enunciation, special seating, and the use of nonverbal cues.

Preschools often establish speech and language enrichment programs for their children. It usually is a service provided at the expense of the school, and therefore has financial limitations. Most of the preschools' children function within normal limits, and activities within a group setting are very appropriate. In many large cities, an increasing proportion of children are entering the preschool either with limited or no proficiency in English. These children present a special problem to the speech-language clinician who is limited to working with these children in a group setting. An even greater problem are the children whose mothers exposed them to alcohol or drugs prenatally. Even though they may require intensive special services, often the speech-language clinician must provide them with the same amount of attention given to a child who is developing normally.

Community centers can offer the speech-language clinician a unique opportunity to offer services to individuals who either are not aware of services or who could not afford them. These centers tend to be ethnically based and often serve as entry vehicles for immigrants. Often therapy is not only conducted in a group setting, but the speech-language clinician must also rely on the aid of an interpreter. Group therapy in community centers should be viewed as a way of determining appropriate services for new citizens.

Cultural Considerations. Many ethnic cultures express their identity through nonverbal behaviors and language (Gollnick & Chinn, 1990). In a group setting these nonverbal messages are especially prone to misunderstanding. It is easy for the nonverbal behaviors of group members from different ethnic cultures to be misinterpreted. For example, the lack of eye contact, which is a sign of respect in one culture, may be misperceived as disrespectful in another (Cheng, 1987). Other behaviors, such as the physical distance between people, may be misperceived as being sexually suggestive instead of civil and friendly (Saleh, 1986). The group leader needs to become the bridge between cultures. When

it appears that group members are not relating to each other or are becoming segmented because of not understanding the nonverbal behaviors associated with a culture, it is the group leader's responsibility to discuss specific incidents and the way they are being misperceived. By understanding differences, strategies for avoiding future problems within the group can be developed.

In a group setting, language can be used by members of one ethnic group as a form of identification and individuation from other group members. When this occurs, members of other ethnic groups may feel a sense of isolation or may form stereotypical impressions based on the language usage. A good example is contained in a study conducted with 13-year-old English-only speaking and 13-year-old Spanish bilingual students (McKirnan & Hamayan, 1984). The English-only students perceived the Spanish teenagers' style of speech as indicating a desire to remain isolated. English-only students who had little or no contact with Spanish-speaking students also had negative perceptions of the Spanish-speaking students based on their speech. Just as the group leader needs to address the consequences of ethnic-specific nonverbal behaviors, the consequences of linguistic-specific ethnic behaviors should also be discussed.

Group experiences are not perceived as identical in all ethnic cultures. In certain cultures, the exhibition of disordered communicative ability and the discussion of personal problems is desirable, because it offers the individual the support of a community. Studies have shown that individuals from various Hispanic cultures may adapt to group work quite easily (Delgado & Humm-Delgado, 1984; McKinley, 1987). Similar results have been found for African Americans (Higgins & Warner, 1975). For many Asian cultures, though, group therapy may not be desirable for any of the stated group functions, because their cultures minimize the public display of emotions and disabilities (Cheng, 1987).

Besides ethnicity, gender also affects the functioning of groups. With children, both same sex and mixed sex groups display cooperative relationships. However, the style of interaction may be related to the gender composition of the group. In one study of children, it was found that groups of boys tended to be more boisterous than groups of girls, and mixed gender groups functioned more like boy groups than girl groups (Smith & Inder, 1993). The importance of this finding for clinicians relates to issues of control. If the natural inclination of boys is to be involved in more boisterous play, it would seem to make clinical sense to attempt to utilize group activities that capitalize on this natural tendency, rather than choose more passive activities which probably will require clinicians to exert more control mechanisms. The same suggestions would apply to mixed groups.

Competition. There is natural inclination within a group setting to compete. Competition may take various forms, ranging from a desire to win at a game to seeking the approval of the clinician for correct responses. Competition is a natural desire for many children and adolescents. Regardless of the value the clinician places on competition, it is a variable within group settings and as such should not be ignored. It can be used in a positive manner to facilitate the development of new behaviors. Group competitiveness should not be confused with clients' striving to better their own past performance. This characteristic is always positive and should be continually reinforced by the clinician. Group competitiveness relates to an individual's need to better other members of the group, regardless of the quality of his or her own performance. Group competitiveness can be an acceptable behavior of group members as long as it results in improved communicative behavior without negatively affecting the worth of its individual members. The construction of activities that would accomplish both will test the creativity of the clinician. One example of how it can be accomplished is given below.

Group Membership. The group consists of three 7-year-olds, each having an articulation problem. Jim is just beginning to correctly produce /r/ in isolation. Marge had a frontal lisp which has now been corrected and is beginning to generalize her new speech pattern. Elizabeth is beginning to correctly produce /dr/ blends in initial positions.

Group Activity. A board game is being used in which the correct production of a speech behavior will result in movement of the child's piece. What is defined as a *correct production* differs for each child. For this session, Jim is required to produce 10 consecutive /r/ phonemes correctly. During the last session he was required to produce five consecutive /r/ phonemes. Marge must produce two sentences, each containing at least one sound on which she had lisped in the past. During the last session she was required only to produce one sentence. Elizabeth must choose two words containing the /dr/ blends and produce each five times correctly. During the last session she was required only to produce one word five times.

Goals of the Activity. The child who reaches the end of the game first will win an inexpensive toy. Every child who does better this session than they did last session will win a special sticker.

Clinical Orientation. Some orientations are better suited for groups focusing on communication problems than others. For example, many people find the person-centered group therapy orientation of Carl Rogers easily adaptable to communications groups (Frank, 1961). Person-centered therapy is also known as client-centered therapy or nondirective therapy. It involves the therapist reflecting back what the group members have said within a framework that clarifies the individual's thoughts without making any judgments

(Rogers, 1965). The value of this orientation is that it focuses on the unconditional acceptance of the individual by the group. For many of the group members, this is a unique experience, and one which can lead to reinforcing any positive change in their speech or language.

Interpersonal Issues

Group interactions are significantly more complex than those encountered in dyadic relationships. Not only are all of the variables found in one-to-one interactions, but an additional set is added. Some of the most significant variables appear below.

Gender Leadership Issues. Over 90% of speech-language clinicians are female. Therefore the likelihood that group leaders will be female is also overwhelming. Although the evaluation of the leader should be based only on competency, often it is affected by gender. In one study the affective responses given to male and female group leaders were compared (Butler & Geis, 1990). Female leaders received more negative affective responses and fewer positive responses than men offering the same suggestions and arguments. Female leaders also received more negative than positive responses, in contrast to men who received at least as many positive as negative responses. However, when issues are more task oriented, the effects of gender are almost neutralized (Hawkins, 1995). An understanding of the effect of gender upon responses should be factored in by female clinicians when assessing their own effectiveness, but not used as a rationale for inadequate performance.

Ethnicity. The relationship between the ethnicity of the group leader and the members may be quite complex. In one study, it was found that Hispanic university students worked better with an Anglo leader than one who was Hispanic (Garza, Lipton, & Isonio, 1989). It appears that although group members' ethnic identify with the group leader may facilitate therapy, other issues, such as personal characteristics, may be more important. In the same study, members of mixed ethnic groups reported greater motivation when working with leaders who were of the same ethnic background. The issues involved in the effects of the group leader's ethnicity defy simple conclusions. While sensitivity to the ethnic values of group members by the group leader is a necessary ingredient, the importance of a group leader's ethnic identify with group members may be affected by personality issues.

Role Relationships. It is a common misconception that individuals in a group know how to function in a way that facilitates achieving the group's goals. The assumption is not only unwarranted, but can also lead to disastrous effects. Once the purpose of the group is identified, it is incumbent on the group leader to determine if the group members know how to fulfill their roles. With adults, this may involve some simple instructions or a brief demonstration. With children, however, a more structured, lengthy training approach may be required, especially if one of their roles is that of a peer helper (Henriksen, 1991).

In most groups, at least one individual is eventually perceived as a leader. It usually is the individual who is perceived as providing the most facilitative behaviors, suggestions, or insights (French & Stright, 1991). However, the role of leader may shift with changes in group functions (Hare, 1994). For example, individuals who are perceived as leaders in discussion groups because of their supportive persona, may not be leaders in task-oriented projects if they do not possess the competency or knowledge necessary for the completion of the task. Clinicians should not be surprised when leadership roles change with changing group functions.

Member to Member Feedback. Some group activities may require members of the group to give feedback to each other on performance or attitudes. Although these activities promote active participation in the group, they may be the source of inaccurate information being conveyed to the group members. A useful technique for reducing some of the inaccuracies is to delay activities requiring member to member feedback until the group leader has provided a feedback model (Morran, Stockton, & Bond, 1991). Although the members may model some of the leader's behaviors, others are more difficult to change. In a study assessing positive and corrective feedback in groups, it was found that, although members had no problems in providing positive feedback, most expressed difficulties with giving corrective feedback (Morran, Stockton, & Bond, 1991). It appeared that the reluctance to provide corrective feedback involved two fears. The first was that the feedback could be harmful to the recipient. The second was that they would be rejected by the other group members as a result of having delivered corrective feedback. For speech-language clinicians, these findings suggest that care should be taken when relying on group members to provide feedback on performances and attitudes, as there will be a tendency to allow inaccurate behaviors and inappropriate attitudes to go unchallenged.

Group Interactive Styles. Groups tend to develop a dominant style of interaction after a period of time. These have been identified as constructive, passive, or aggressive. One study attempted to determine the effect of each interaction style on the ability of the group to solve problems (Cooke & Szumal, 1994). Constructive styles were found to be positively related with effective problem solving, whereas passive styles were negatively correlated. While aggressive styles showed no relationship with problem solving, they were negatively correlated with acceptance of a solution. The clinical implications of this study are that active, constructive involvement of group members is more likely to result in the development of solutions for individual members than a passive style. And although an aggressive group style may lead to difficulties with individual members accepting solutions, it has no effect on the group's ability to solve problems.

Management

One clinician thought managing groups must be similar to driving a stage coach with four to six independently minded horses. The analogy is appropriate. One of the biggest problems faced by all clinicians who lead groups is management. By understanding how to control the group and use efficient intervention techniques, a large percentage of the problems can be minimized.

Control. Issues of control are different for child, adolescent, and adult groups. Control in groups of children tends to center around appropriateness of behaviors. New clinicians are especially prone to lose control with children, often not recognizing the gradual slippage until it is too late. To maintain control, the speech-language pathologist can use three specific strategies: (1) establish clearly defined parameters of acceptable and nonacceptable behavior, (2) allow choices within established parameters, and (3) establish consequences for both appropriate and inappropriate behavior. Although each of these strategies can be used for both individual and group therapy, they are especially important to use with groups. When using any of these strategies, always strive for consistency.

It is a natural tendency of children to determine the limits of acceptable behaviors. It is the rare child who does not test limits. By clearly establishing what is acceptable and not acceptable, parameters of behavior are given to the child (Fatout, 1995). Usually, the new clinician provides too much freedom for the group, eventually finding it necessary to reduce the parameters of acceptable behavior. A better method of maintaining control is to begin with very narrow parameters and gradually increase them as the behavior of the children warrants it.

The freedom to choose within specified parameters can either develop a cohesiveness for the group or divide it. Avoiding problems with continual splits in voting can be accomplished by allowing the "losing side" to choose the activity for the subsequent session. The imposition of consequences for behaviors establishes a model for behavior within a group. When one child engages in a behavior that he had been previously told was inappropriate and then faced the consequences, a powerful model for the other children is established.

Although some control issues for adolescent and adult groups may be similar to those of child groups, most problems of control involve task orientation. There may be a tendency to stray off the assigned task, or to spend more time than is desired on a given task. In adult stuttering groups, for example, the task may be to require the participants to talk about instances when they were fluent, now using an exaggerated form of fluency called prolongation. Although some members may wish to present instances of disfluency, it is the responsibility of the clinician to keep them on task. The clinician's leadership qualities become important for moving the group in the appropriate direction.

Probably the most successful approach to changing specific, observable behaviors within a group setting is behavioral group therapy (Corey, 1990). In therapy groups of this type, the focus is upon the modification, elimination, and substitution of behaviors, not underlying causes. Some authors, while supporting a behavioral orientation, believe that thoughts are also an acceptable behavior to manipulate within a group setting (Beck, 1976; Meichenbaum, 1977).

Efficiency. One of the most difficult problems encountered when teaching new behaviors within a group setting is the management of time. It goes without saying that when time is spent with one individual, that is time not spent with everyone else. The task for the speech-language clinician is to construct activities for each member of the group that minimizes waiting time. This can be accomplished in three different ways: (1) practicing the newly acquired behaviors, (2) monitoring someone else's production of appropriate behaviors, and (3) engaging in reinforcement activities.

When waiting one's turn, time spent most productively is in the practicing of new behaviors. For example, if a child is working on the production of /r/ in isolation, his task between turns may be to produce the sound a given number of times. If two or more children are working on the same behavior, they could practice together until it is their turn to work with the clinician. An example from an adult stuttering group would be the practice of prolonged speech. *Monitoring* by individuals waiting their turn may be an appropriate use of time, especially if both individuals are working on the same behavior. The role of monitor could be switched, giving each client an opportunity to practice the behavior and also monitor the correct production of the behavior. If it is neither appropriate nor possible to use the time between turns for practice or monitoring, this could be used as an opportunity for the child to be reinforced for correct productions. *Reinforcement* for children and young adolescents should involve an activity that can be continued throughout the session, such as drawing or construction of an object. Reinforcement for adults and older adolescents would not be an appropriate use of time.

With skillful construction of the activity, all participants are constantly involved in therapy. For example, in a group of four children all with a similar phonological problem, while one child is practicing the utterance, all other children could be playing the role of teacher, assessing the correct production and providing suggestions for modifying incorrect productions. Children find peer facilitating roles to be both reinforcing and valuable (Myrick, Highland, & Sabella, 1995). Besides involving all members of the group in the activity, acquisition of the target behavior is facilitated by those assisting in the learning process (Rekrut, 1994).

There are specific strategies that speech-language clinicians can use to maximize the efficiency and effectiveness of the group setting to teach new behaviors. The focus should be on the development of problem-solving strategies. This has been shown to result not only in the acquisition of more behaviors within a group setting, but also resulted in greater retention of learned behaviors after the group ended (McMillon, 1994). Ideally, each individual in the group should have the same disorder of equal severity and be the same age. Rarely, if ever, is the ideal encountered, especially in the public schools. The usual situation is that the group members share a general disorder. It is not unlikely that children with articulation disorders will be grouped together, regardless of what phoneme is misarticulated. A stuttering group may contain individuals whose stuttering ranges from 50% disfluency to monitored normal fluent speech. Voice groups may contain cases of hyper nasality and vocal abuse. The hearing ability of a hearing impaired group may range from a unilateral 40db hearing loss to total deafness. Within school settings, attempts are made to group children not only by disorder, but also by grade. There may be a spread of one grade level within a group.

Structure of Activities

There are various types of activities that can be effectively used in group settings. Usually these are appropriate regardless of the function the group serves. Three large categories of activities are (1) clinician structured, (2) unstructured, and (3) simulations.

Clinician Structured. When a new behavior is learned, clinicians often will wish to have clients produce them in a highly structured activity that would not only result in the best possibility of its correct production, but also begin its generalization. An example would be teaching a child to use the word *in* when any object was placed within a container. During individual therapy, the clinician would hold various objects over a box and ask the child, "Where should it go?" If the child said *in*, the object would be dropped into the box with a loud bang, delighting the child. After consistent production of "in," the clinician introduced the child into a communication-centered group that consisted of six other children, who were at various stages of language therapy. Another child was given an object and asked to hold it over a box until the child said "in" when asked the question. Various clinicians and children could alternate placing objects into different containers.

An adult example would be the generalization of esophageal speech. Once an individual learned how to produce esophageal speech correctly, he or she could enter a communication group consisting of other esophageal speakers. The first activity that he would engage in is to practice producing very short utterances with each member of the group.

Unstructured. As behaviors are learned and consistently produced in clinician-structured activities, the parameters of control should be loosened. The idea is to determine if the behaviors are being generalized, and if not, what factors are preventing it. Although called *unstructured,* control is still exercised by the clinician. In the example given above, instead of directing the other children in a group to ask a where-question, the clinician could merely set up the environment so that the question could be spontaneously asked.

Simulations. Simulations are activities that one engages in that may be similar in the most important respects to real situations. Although they are contrived, they can serve an important function in therapy. They can serve as a bridge between highly structured activities and normal nonclinical activities. An example for a child could involve the development of speech reading skills. A moderately hearing-impaired child has been learning to lip read. Her instructor first taught her individually the skills that she would need. Then, in a group setting, the child practiced reading the lips of the children as they read a sentence or said predetermined words. In preparation for the child entering a non-hearing-impaired class, the speech-language clinician develops a simulation in which she assumes the role of *teacher* and gives instructions to the other group members who pretend to be a class. The key elements of the simulation are that the teacher: (1) modulates her voice, ranging from loud to soft, (2) occasionally turns toward the blackboard when talking, and (3) a few children are talking during the teacher's instruction.

An example for an adult could involve a fluency group. Each member of the group has been taught a form of fluent speech production. Although the speech sounds normal, it requires the client to expend a tremendous amount of energy in its production. An activity is designed to simulate a nonclinical incidence where an individual is placing a food order in a restaurant. Key elements in the simulation are that: (1) the person assuming the role of waiter will interrupt the order if there is any hesitation on the part of the client, (2) everyone at the client's table will be intently listening to the client, and (3) the client will be surrounded by other tables, each filled with people.

Functions

The structure of the group and the skills necessary to run it efficiently and effectively will depend on its function. The techniques used in a group setting depend on the purpose of the group. If the group is to be effective, the leader must be familiar with the skills necessary for each purpose (Polcin, 1991). Quite often, a group has more than one function, alternating between various activities when they are appropriate. Although a group can serve various functions, it is important to realize that the strategies used for each function differ and should not be confused with each other. Groups can serve four functions: (1) teaching of new behaviors, (2) generalization of behaviors, (3) gathering of data, and (4) discussion.

Teaching New Behaviors. The use of a group setting is probably less efficient for teaching a new behavior than is individual therapy (Goldberg, 1993). The argument may be irrelevant if speech-language clinicians find themselves in a setting that only provides service in groups. Due to financial considerations, many public schools provide most of their therapy in small groups. For political, philosophical, and economic reasons, some school districts mandate an inclusion therapy model where all therapy is conducted within the classroom. Regardless of the reasons for teaching new behaviors in a group setting, it is by far significantly more difficult and less efficient than teaching new behaviors in a typical therapy dyad.

Often there is a reliance on the use of various reinforcing contingencies to increase the extent of learning that takes place within a group setting. As was mentioned earlier, it is always important to use intrinsic, extrinsic, and extraneous reinforcement in the design of intervention protocols, whether they involve individual clients or groups. However, reinforcement by itself is not an adequate approach for group learning. A study was conducted that contrasted the learning that occurred in groups that relied only on reinforcement, with ones that combined reinforcement and the use of a well defined strategy. The group using the strategy remained on task significantly more than the groups who were not provided with the strategy (Meloth & Deering, 1994).

Generalization. Groups can serve as safe environments in which new speech and language behaviors can be practiced, under the guidance of a speech-language clinician and with individuals who may be more tolerant of communicative failure than nongroup members. The group can be used to generalize behaviors through the use of unstructured activities. This allows both the clinician and client to assess the degree to which the new behavior is becoming automatic, since during unstructured activities, the careful monitoring of behaviors is less likely to occur. An example with a child could involve correct production of targeted phonemes. After learning how to produce certain sounds in isolation, within words and sentences, and during simulated activities, the children within an articulation group are told that they can engage in a game that requires each to talk. They are not asked to produce any specific words or sounds, just play the game. The clinician, however, notes both the correct and incorrect productions of each child's target phonemes. Children who consistently produce correct productions become candidates for dismissal from therapy.

An adult example would be an aphasic client who has been taught how to structure her language so that it is simplified, direct, and communicative. In the group, she is asked to have a casual conversation with other group members about any topic of interest. The clinician analyzes her verbalizations to see if the response patterns she has been taught are becoming a part of her verbal repertoire.

The end goal of speech and language therapy is the generalization of new behaviors. Once a behavior is learned in a structured setting, it gradually replaces the incorrect behavior. By observing the percentage of time the new behavior is produced, the clinician can begin gauging the extent to which the behavior is becoming a part of the client's behavioral repertoire.

In order for a new behavior to be established, the individual must be given ample opportunity to produce it. If the opportunity is not present, the conditioning, so necessary for the establishment of behaviors, will not occur. For example, although a child may be able to consistently use the question marker, *where,* she may take longer than necessary to generalize it if she is not given any opportunities to practice it. If during the observational group session, the clinician notices that opportunities to ask questions are given to her client, it would become appropriate to structure the sessions so that questions could be asked.

An example for adolescents and adults would be reduction of vocal abuse. During the individual session the goal of therapy could be the modulation of vocal intensity so that vocal nodules would not recur after their surgical removal. The client may have been taught how to engage in conversation at a reduced level, even when the surrounding noises make it difficult. If the level of conversation and the ambient noise levels in the group are low, the client would not have an opportunity to practice her new speaking skills. Based on this type of observation, the clinician could have a radio playing music while the group members engage in unstructured activities.

Gathering Data. Speech-language clinicians are continually gathering data so that client progress can be assessed. Usually, data is gathered prior to therapy, during therapy, and at the end of therapy. The setting most often used in gathering data is the individual session where just the clinician and client are present. A group setting provides a unique opportunity for gathering data. Although contrived in terms of membership and focus, it does offer a more natural environment to observe the client's developing communicative ability. When gathering data, it is important that clinicians not engage in any communicative behavior. Their role is that of an observer. Data can be gathered through the use of check-off forms, audio, or videotapes.

Regardless of the age range of the group, clinicians can focus on some specific areas, most important of which are: (1) correct/incorrect productions of target behaviors, (2) number of correct/incorrect productions of target behaviors, (3) evidence of generalization of the behavior, (4) reaction by the group to correct/incorrect productions, (5) reactions and awareness of the client to correct/incorrect productions of the target behaviors, and (6) extent of communication with other group members as a function of communicative competence.

The use of behaviors in a group structure may be different than how they are presented in a dyadic clinical relationships. Even with sympathetic listeners, common group reactions may be visible. For example, even in the most compassionate group of aphasic clients, members may become impatient when someone is having difficulty retrieving the appropriate linguistic structure, especially if they wish to speak. Clinicians should note how group reactions affect the client's behaviors.

Group settings can either make clients more conscious about their behaviors or oblivious to them. Generally, adults' awareness of their communicative behaviors will be heightened during group experiences. The opposite tends to take place with children. All clients tend to become less aware of new behaviors and strategies in group settings. It appears that the amount of concentration necessary for using the behavior or strategy is difficult to develop when an active group dynamic is occurring. There just are too many competing stimuli. The ways in which clients deal with these problems in a group setting can provide information to the clinician on how the client will perform in nonclinical settings.

Groups provide a wonderful opportunity for clinicians to observe the ability of clients to *communicate*. Of importance is the ability to communicate, not necessarily use the target behaviors. After all, language-disordered children can have many of their disorders corrected, yet because of pragmatic problems, remain unable to communicate their thoughts. In the group, clinicians are provided with an opportunity to observe if what they have been teaching the client will make any difference in improving communication.

Discussion. Speech-language clinicians are not expected to be group counselors competent in leading indepth analyses of the entire spectrum of human emotions and problems. They are, however, expected to enable individuals to examine the relationship a communicative behavior has to their functioning. Counseling courses, both within communicative disorders departments and within other departments, provide the academic knowledge necessary for accomplishing this goal. The purpose of this section is to set the parameters of acceptable goals for speech-language clinician directed groups and to specify some of the basic techniques that can be used to accomplish these objectives. Clinicians who show little regard for the nonspeech concerns of clients also risk alienating clients. Clinicians change many things other than the specific speech-language behaviors they are charged to address. Some of these changes are directed, such as suggesting to a stutterer that he directly confront his parents about their attitude toward his speech. Others are indirect, such as watching a depressed aphasic client modeling the hopefulness seen in her clinician.

Group discussions are often thought by many to be vehicles for individuals to present problems and develop solutions for their remediation or acceptance. During the course of discussions, clients will often self-disclose private and embarrassing information. Contrary to the widely held position that there is a cathartic experience associated with public confession, some research has shown that self-disclosure within group settings can lead to negative consequences for both the individual and the group (Robinson, Stockton, & Morran, 1990). Most of the negative consequences occur when self-disclosure occurs too early, when the group has not yet developed a sense of unity, which is supportive of shocking self-disclosure. In the absence of this feeling of unity, what could have been a supportive response becomes one that may be accusatory or judgmental. Clinicians who wish to use the group for discussions of personal and private problems should prepare the individuals to become supportive by first building a group unity.

The impact that a communicative disorder can have on a child can range from none to devastating. The 5-year-old child, whose /w/ for /r/ misarticulation goes unnoticed by other children, may not even realize that a problem exists. Another 5-year-old child, who is unmercifully teased by his friends about his stuttering, is traumatized daily by his problem. These two very different examples point out the necessity of first determining the extent of impact a communicative disorder has on the children before assuming that they need to discuss it. The old adage, "If it's not broken, don't fix it," is very applicable. Not all children need to talk about their communicative problem. Direct discussion of a child's problem may be too threatening. The use of puppets, stories, or plays is often less threatening and can allow children to openly present and discuss their problem as if it were that of the puppet they are talking about in the story or the character they are portraying in the play.

Adolescence is a difficult developmental stage. The individual is generally affected more by a communicative disorder than the child and has a greater capacity to discuss his or her feelings. Accompanying this greater awareness may be a reluctance to discuss it in the presence of other adolescents. The use of puppets or other indirect methods of talking about their communicative disorder may be inappropriate. Pos-

sibly a less threatening way of discussing feelings may be to focus the discussion on what they are feeling while experiencing communicative successes. Group discussions can function as a very important way for individuals to refocus their attitudes about speech and language. Instead of spending time continually discussing the negative aspects of communicative disorders, clinicians can refocus the group's orientation to discuss members' feelings when they are successful in communicating. The move is positive, reinforces successful communication, and acts as an incentive for continued work, in order that the new successes can be presented to the group and reinforced.

Although it is not essential for clients to be satisfied with a group experience in order for it to be beneficial, it definitely helps. Adults who participated in a 51-hour growth group that lasted 5 months were asked to identify those features of the experience that they valued the most. Openness and participation were rated as most significant, followed by risk taking, decision making, and problem solving (Ponzo, 1991). Given that these five features of the experience were most valued, it would be incumbent upon the group leader to incorporate them within the structure and goals for adult discussion groups.

FEEDBACK

Usually, feedback is thought of as something the clinician provides to the client. Although important, it constitutes only one form of feedback. As teachers, it is important for the clinician to identify not only correct and incorrect responses, but also the reasons each were given. When a client responds correctly or incorrectly and is asked to explain how he or she arrived at that answer or the behavior, the clinician obtains a unique window into the client's thought processes.

Client to Clinician

Requests for Feedback. During learning activities clients often will request feedback from clinicians regarding the correctness of a response, or if the specific requirements of producing the behavior have been met. Rarely do clinicians equate requests for feedback from their clients to anything specific. In one study, however, it was found that the learner's commitment to the activity's goal was correlated with the number of requests made for feedback (Schutz, 1993). In other words, the more feedback requested by learners, the more committed they are in accomplishing the goal of the activity. This finding has important implications for therapy. Although there is no magic number of feedback requests over which we can say that a client is committed to a therapeutic goal, requests for feedback by clients can be used as a general yardstick in assessing commitment to therapy.

Clinician to Client

The feedback provided to clients may serve as the primary way for them to know whether or not they have correctly produced a target behavior. It is a fallacy to believe that clients are capable of differentiating a new desired behavior from one that it is to replace. Often in therapy, changes are minute, or the old behavior is so automatic as to obscure any awareness of the new desired one. Given these parameters, it is important that consistent feedback be provided to clients.

Timing. Often one can see clinicians giving young clients stickers or other extraneous reinforcers at the end of therapy for effort or cooperation. Although well intentioned, it is inappropriate. After engaging in a large number of behaviors for at least 20 minutes and not receiving feedback on their level of cooperation or effort, it is difficult, if not impossible, for children to identify what specific aspects of their behavior were related to the reinforcer. It is not only important that there is a more direct link between desired behaviors and reinforcement, but also there should be immediate feedback to clients regarding all aspects of their behavior or attitudes that the clinician is evaluating. Immediacy of feedback has been shown to significantly improve performance (Miller, Hall, & Heard, 1995).

Specificity. When providing feedback to clients, one usually thinks about telling the client whether or not a response was correct. Although this form of feedback is better than none at all, it may not provide the client with information that may be critical for knowing *why* the response was correct or incorrect. A better procedure is one that has been effectively used with persons with mild disabilities (Cuvo & Klatt, 1992). In this procedure, following each client response, specific feedback is provided to clients which analyzes their performance in behavioral terms. In speech-language therapy, an example would be providing feedback in articulation therapy for the correct production of /l/ by a client who lisps. Instead of just saying "correct" or "great," comments such as the following would be made, "That's perfect, this time you kept the flow of air going out through the front of your mouth and the front of your tongue was up on the ridge." The same type of feedback would be provided when errors are made. For example, "That wasn't perfect, you still are allowing a little bit of air to escape through the sides of your mouth." Feedback with increased amounts of specificity has been shown to produce significantly better results for complex behaviors than less specific forms of feedback (Salas & Dickinson, 1990).

Levels of Acceptability. When providing feedback on the correctness of a response, it is appropriate to speak in terms of acceptability. For example, a response can be:

excellent / on target / perfect

really close / almost on target

not that close, but still it has some correct aspects

not close at all

It may be easier to use a 5-point scale similar to the one provided below to indicate how close the response was.

Perfect	Very Close	Somewhat Close	Not Close	Way Off
1	2	3	4	5

Cultural Considerations. The acceptance of feedback from the clinician may be related to cultural variables. If the communicative style of the feedback is not culturally sensitive to the individual's ethnic values, the insensitivity of the clinician may result in clients disregarding everything the clinician is saying. A more specific problem is gender related. In one study of children, it was found that girls were more adversely affected by negative feedback than were boys (Manolis & Milich, 1993). For clinicians, this translates into softening the negative feedback that is given to girls.

Types

Various types of feedback can be given to clients. Some are more sophisticated than others. Some are more positive than others. Each type of feedback leads to different results. Obviously the choice of feedback type should be dependent on the goals clinicians wish to accomplish.

Levels of Sophistication. When clients engage in activities the clinicians have specified, it is important that they receive feedback using words that are clear and understandable. In the literature on all communicative disorders, virtually all authors emphasize the importance of providing extraneous reinforcement in terms of social praise, especially to children. If during a session, a client is producing 50, 75, or 200 correct responses, it would make sense that there is some alternation in the words chosen by clinicians to convey their approval. Even casual observations to clinicians engaging in this behavior show little variation. After hearing "good" or "good job" a few hundred times during a session, a client may become satiated with the few words that are used. Although this should not be a major concern of clinicians, it can be very easily corrected by substituting equivalent words. The same principle should be used when conveying to clients that what they did was not acceptable.

Positive and Instructional Feedback. Feedback that is given to clients will be perceived as positive if it reinforces the correctness of a performance or expression of an idea. Feedback that is given to clients can be perceived as negative if it is instructive. Instructive feedback can be as simple as suggesting that something is done slightly different, or an outright "no." Although it is important that whatever feedback is provided to clients is honest, the effects of both positive and negative feedback on clients should be understood. It appears that negative feedback will be more acceptable and instructive to individuals who have a high self-esteem, but overgeneralized by individuals with low self-esteem (Kernis, Brockner, & Frankel, 1989). When low self-esteem individuals hear negative feedback, there is a tendency to overgeneralize even constructive criticism to other aspects of their behavior or personality. Because a significant proportion of clients with communicative disorders come to the clinical situation with a low self-esteem associated with failure, negative feedback should be minimized, if possible. The best method of accomplishing this is to use response differentiation, and provide clients with learning and retrieval strategies that result in successful experiences.

The Semantics of Positive and Negative Words. When providing feedback to clients on their performance, it is possible to use either positive or negative words to describe the same event. For example, telling a client that he stuttered on 20% of the words he spoke is identical to saying that he was fluent on 80% of the words. Although both identically describe the same event, they differ in terms of what they denote about the client's efforts. The first focuses on past negative behaviors that the client is in the process of eliminating. Highlighting the presence of these behaviors does little other than to focus on the client's failure at achieving normal fluency. The second focuses on the positive behaviors the client is in the process of learning. It is not only positive but also future oriented. This approach of focusing on the behaviors being learned has been used in the area of drug addiction with very good results (Chandler & Mason, 1995).

PROFESSIONAL COLLABORATION

Speech-language clinicians can no longer work as isolated professionals minimally interacting with professionals from other areas. Whether the work setting is a hospital, rehabilitation center, or public school, speech-language clinicians need to interact with a wide variety of other professionals including physicians, nurses, occupational therapists, physical therapists, special educators, and classroom teachers.

Hospital/Rehabilitation Sites

In hospitals and rehabilitation sites, collaboration tends to be organic, with a team approach used for many clients. Although collaborative in design, often the general direction for intervention is hierarchical, with physicians requesting services (Hegde & Davis, 1995). However, once services are requested, the opinions of speech-language clinicians are generally respected, since few professionals, other than speech-language clinicians, are competent in the area.

Many clients seen in hospital settings have neurological impairments, resulting in behaviors requiring the services of either physical or occupational therapists. Since the speech and language impairments of their clients can significantly interfere with these professionals' ability to provide services, most are eager to work cooperatively with the speech-language clinician. Through collaboration, speech-language clinicians can incorporate activities related to physical and occupational therapy into their therapy, and vice versa.

Although there will always be issues of "turf" in all settings, those in hospital and rehabilitation sites may be more pronounced. These may be related to very practical economic issues, such as who gets paid by Medicare and insurance companies for services provided. It may also be legal, such as which professional assumes legal responsibility to an intervention procedure. Or historical in nature; this is the way it *always* has been done here. Unless speech-language clinicians are aware of these formalities, there is a danger of needlessly antagonizing those individuals with whom they desire to collaborate.

Public Schools

Within the last 10 years the demands placed on speech-language clinicians to function in a collaborative framework have increased substantially. The nature of school-based clinic practice has changed from the treatment of a specific speech or language disorder by a single professional, to a team model where treatment protocols result from the interaction of professionals from various disciplines (Sailor, 1991; Hanson & Lovett, 1992). The resulting service delivery models have been called *collaborative* where there is an equal status among team members (Vandercook & York, 1990), *transdisciplinary* where there is a sharing of general information, informational skills, and performance competencies (Lyon & Lyon, 1980), or *integrated therapy* where intervention occurs in a cooperative manner within the child's natural environment (Giangreco, 1989).

Consultative service delivery models involve the speech-language clinician acting as a consultant to special educators or classroom teachers regarding the speech and language disorders of children, with either more than one disability, or a communication problem that will be treated by another professional (Molyneaux & Lane, 1982). The interdisciplinary model is one that not only requires the speech-language clinician to consult with other professionals, but also has them collaboratively designing and implementing treatment plans that are multidisciplinary.

Advantages of the Collaborative Models. The literature in special education is replete with the advantages of each of these models over purely traditional pull-out service delivery models (Bricker & Campbell, 1980). Some of the most often cited advantages are the diversity of skills brought to solving problems (Johnson & Johnson, 1989), development of a cooperative spirit (Albano, Cox, York, & York, 1981), and possibilities for the cross-disciplinary professional education of special educators (Kruger, 1988).

In the area of speech-language pathology, discussions of treatment models are usually subsumed under three categories: (1) traditional pull-out, (2) interdisciplinary, and (3) consultative (Culatta & Goldberg, 1995). Traditional service delivery models involve the delivery of service by a speech-language clinician, usually operating by him or herself, working on a specific speech or language disorder (Rainforth, York, Macdonald, & Dunn, 1992).

Disadvantages of Collaborative Models. Often, the collaboration involves brief consultative meetings with teachers who wish to have a specific problem addressed. This form of collaboration has resulted in some problems with role relationships between speech-language clinicians and classroom teachers (Prelock, 1995). There are various ways of collaborating, some of which are more productive than others. The speech-language clinician is often asked by the classroom teacher or special educator to provide suggestions for a specific problem or for a specific child. Although collaborating in this manner may be important for establishing a relationship with other school personnel and significantly affecting the life of one child or adolescent, it is rather short-ranged and limited to a specific case. A more beneficial approach is one that promotes the development of the consultees' problem-solving skills so that they are better able to react or respond more effectively to similar problems in the future (Coufal, 1993).

In an attempt to embrace the interdisciplinary and the consultative models, some public school administrators inappropriately have decided that all speech-language therapy, or a significant portion of speech-language therapy, should be performed in the classroom. Although well-meaning in their attempts to ride the wave on inclusion models, many unfortunately do not understand the cognitive and perceptual factors necessary for learning new speech and language behaviors. Some believe that portions of various inclusion models are driven by professional agendas, rather than an understanding of the cognitive requirements for inclusion (Chappell, 1992). Their assumption that pull-out therapy is outmoded tends to rely on theoretical presumptions with little reference to empirical evidence.

Granted, there are problems with a purely pull-out service delivery model: (1) speech-language clinicians tend to become isolated from other school professionals and (2) there is an inadequate generalization of newly taught behaviors. The strength of the pull-out model, however, is that the initial conditions necessary for the development of intricate and complicated behaviors can be controlled and structured in order for the child to attend to the learning stimuli and retain the information (Goldberg, 1993). Given the competing visual and auditory stimuli present in a classroom, it is foolish to believe that the specific components of a behavior can be as effectively and efficiently learned in the classroom as in the controlled environment of the therapy room. Years of research have shown us otherwise (Gagné, 1970).

Combining Pull-out and Inclusion Models. Instructional models that involve teaching specific behaviors through pull-out, individual instruction, and generalization in the classroom have been shown to be effective (McClure, Karge, & Patton, 1995). Their appropriate uses appear in Table 9–1. The strength of the classroom setting is that it provides a wonderful opportunity to generalize and fully develop immature forms of behaviors taught in the relatively controlled environment of the therapy room. Once learned, the behaviors then can be integrated within real-life situations within the classroom. To require the speech-language clinician to teach new communicative behaviors in the classroom may be ideologically correct and economically appropriate, but it is unfair to the child. Children with communicative disorders have a history of failure: failure in understanding basic rules of communication that are automatic to others, failure in having others understand them, and failure in expressing their feelings and ideas. To place an additional hurdle in their path toward normalcy is unwarranted and possibly unethical.

One argument presented for working only in the classroom is that it prevents stigmatizing the child by labeling him or her as needing "special education services." I am reminded of the mother of a 6-year-old child who told me she never used the word *stuttering* in front of her child for fear that it would upset him. The child stuttered severely and had a variety of secondary behaviors. There were no words that could have been used that were more painful than the behaviors he had to face every time he attempted to speak. The child with a communicative disorder is impaired by the disorder, not the label of "special education." It is delusional to believe that by not identifying children as needing special services and only working with them in the classroom we can minimize the problem. Sheehan was fond of talking about his "hippopotamus theory" of stuttering. Pretending it doesn't exist if we don't name it is an exercise in self-deception.

Inclusion. Inclusion refers to the dispensing of therapy within the least restrictive environment within a school. This usually is the classroom. Various types of inclusion activities can be performed in the classroom: (1) teaching of specific behavior, (2) reinforcing the presence of the behavior, and (3) generalization. Each of these functions were addressed under the group therapy section in this chapter. The only function that is not appropriate for classrooms is the teaching of specific behaviors for all of the reasons cited throughout this text. Basically, a classroom consisting of at least 25 students who are engaging in a variety of verbal and nonverbal activities, creating a high ambient noise level, and with a teacher who is attempting to maintain control, is not the most conducive setting for teaching a new communicative behavior to an individual who may also have a cognitive problem. At best, it is a very inefficient procedure, and therefore places children in a position of having to fail a significant number of times before being able to succeed.

PROFESSIONAL AUTHORITY

Clients and their families come to the professional because the professional suppos-

TABLE 9–1
Appropriate Public School Intervention Settings for Various Activities

ACTIVITY		SETTING	
		PULL-OUT	CLASSROOM
TEACHING SPECIFIC BEHAVIORS **Examples** Production of phoneme Auditory attention Vocal quality feature Sequencing Fluency pattern Pragmatic rules Linguistic structure Socialization		YES	NO
OBSERVING INTERACTION PATTERNS **Examples** Client with peers Client with teacher Client with aides, volunteers, etc.		YES	YES
GENERALIZING SPECIFIC BEHAVIORS **Examples** Production of phoneme Auditory attention Vocal quality feature Sequencing Fluency pattern Pragmatic rules Linguistic structure Socialization		YES	YES
FACILITATING PEER SUPPORT **Examples** Teaching facilitative behaviors to peers Teaching pragmatic rules to peers Structuring and engaging in social/academic interactions		YES	NO

edly knows more than they do, or possesses the ability to change behaviors where they have failed. This reliance on authority is a natural phenomena which can be used successfully or abused.

Charisma

Charisma is a difficult concept to define, yet is easily identifiable when it is present. Some have defined it as a perception of an individual that involves the use of expert power (trust in the correctness of an individual's beliefs), referent power (similarity of beliefs, affection for the leader, identifica-

tion with the leader, emulation of the leader), and job involvement, heightened goals, and perceived ability to contribute (Halpert, 1990). The *presence* or personality of the clinician is sufficient in and of itself to effect rapid and often miraculous changes.

Client's Need for Charismatic Clinicians. Although very few clients actively seek charismatic clinical experiences, the needs of individuals of this type should be recognized. It has been hypothesized that clients who seek a charismatic relationship are people who view themselves as powerless to change personal problems (Aberbach,

1995). The clinician is viewed as all knowing and all powerful, able to effect changes without any directed active involvement on the part of the client. Perceptions of these types often occur as a result of client needs, rather than clinician attempts at self-glorification (Woods, 1993). The relationship is both dangerous and ineffective. Even though a clinician may not wish to be viewed as charismatic, often very positive effects in short-term interactions promote it. A personal experience will exemplify this point. When I was doing research on the Flathead Indian Reservation in Montana, a speech-language clinician asked me to do an initial stuttering therapy session with her client. The young woman, whose history I became familiar with only minutes before I began the session, was extremely disfluent, confiding in me that she had never experienced even more than a few minutes of continuous fluency. After asking a number of questions I asked her to begin doing a series of behaviors which I knew from past experience with hundreds of stuttering clients would result in an immediate increase in fluency. For 20 minutes she was able to speak fluently in a variety of settings and during various levels of communicative demand. To the client and the clinician, what I had accomplished in a very short period of time appeared to be miraculous, similar to the laying on of hands by evangelical ministers. My *charisma* could have been dissected into very specific behaviors that have been shown to facilitate clinical success and knowledge of stuttering therapy that I have accumulated over 20 years of practice. Charisma, therefore, is not necessarily a mystical aura possessed by the clinician, but rather a perception the client has of an individual who possesses both knowledge of disorder-specific information and interaction principles.

Minimizing Charismatic Experiences.

In the above example it would have been unethical to leave the client with the belief that I had affected a miraculous change. The concept of personal responsibility for change for all clients should be an important objective. Therapy should not be viewed as magic. It requires the active participation of clients and the acceptance of their responsibility in the change process. Only though the deconstructing of experiences that facilitate the perception of charisma can clients susceptible to the phenomenon begin assuming responsibility for change (Calas, 1993).

Competency

Appropriate Use of Authority. With some cultures, such as Asian American/ Pacific Islanders, the trust granted to professionals may be given more easily than with other cultures, such as African Americans, Native Americans, and Hispanics. The Hmong mother, for example, may find it acceptable to engage in almost any behavior the clinician will suggest even if the suggestion makes no sense to her. Some have argued that recent immigrants from Asia and the Pacific Islands unquestionably accept professional advise more out of fear than respect (McQuaide, 1989). In their native countries individuals who were in positions of authority also had positions of power that would often be used to affect their lives. Within our own country, Ultra-Orthodox Jews expect clinicians to be authoritative, just as Rabbis and other important individuals are within their religious culture (Wieselberg, 1992). This expectation of authority will be found in other fundamental religious societies where religious values are the predominant culture.

Regardless of the reason why clients want to give clinicians ultimate authority, the *a priori* trust that is placed in the clinician merely because of training and title is a heavy responsibility, especially for new clinicians or clinicians with little experience in a specific disorder. So powerful is this aspect of clinical interactions that the clinician should use it very sparingly. The only time clinicians should use their authority as a professional with a client or family is when:

1. the position they are asserting cannot be justified by other means,
2. the client either does not understand or is unwilling to accept the rational justification for the action, or
3. behavior that the client needs to engage in is absolutely crucial for the success of therapy.

Given these three criteria, the use of authority to justify anything in therapy will be judiciously used. It has been my experience that, if the only way I can convince a client to engage in a behavior or examine an emotion is because of who I am, my therapy has been inadequate.

Inappropriate Use of Authority. The belief in someone or something solely out of faith deeply concerned the imminent English philosopher Bertrand Russell. He referred to the use of authority through title as "priestly power" (1961). He was concerned about the amount of influence people had solely because of their position in society. He was concerned that the instructions or pronouncements emanating from a glorified leader were sufficient for some individuals to follow without rational thought. Speech-language clinicians share some of the same role characteristics of Russell's priests. As professionals, clinicians generate respect and power often only because of their position within a societal structure. The ability to influence people and direct their lives may have little to do with one's competence, intelligence, or compassion. Rollin (1987) examined the use of authority in clinical relationships within a Jungian psychoanalytical framework. According to Jung, we all possess a

"shadow side," a part of our personalities that we do not like and try to hide. Because of the nature of clinical interactions, this shadow side often emerges, resulting in specific styles of therapy, each utilizing various degrees of power. Rollin specified five different roles clinicians could assume, depending on their shadow side. Although one may question the relevance of a Jungian perspective, the following clinical roles are easily identifiable to anyone who has supervised clinicians.

The "benign dictator" is one who specifies all action and behaviors for the client. These clinicians assume that they know what is best for the client, and they use their position to intimidate the client into submission. The "benign super-therapist" is one who not only specifies the behaviors that are necessary for the remediation of a communicative disorder, but also intrudes into other areas that are not necessarily related to speech and language. The "sophisticated therapist" is one who may examine very interesting aspects of the client's relationships at the expense of treating the actual communicative disorder. The "benevolent therapist" is one who allows a client to deviate from a prescribed remediation program, often at the expense of the program. Finally, there is the "powerless therapist," a clinician who gives up all power to the client. Rarely does a clinician assume only one of these roles in therapy. Clinicians may assume one role for a specific purpose and then abandon it and substitute another because of other goals. It could be argued that each of these roles has its appropriate and inappropriate uses. It is important that clinicians recognize that each role will probably result in different interaction patterns. This is especially true if the clinician and client are of different ethnic cultures.

Part V

SUMMARY

CHAPTER

10

Qualities of Master Clinicians

*I*n therapy, we often use models for our clients to emulate. Being able to see how something is performed can drastically reduce the amount of time and frustration required to learn a new behavior. The same principle should be applied to learning clinical skills. Unfortunately, student clinicians and new practicing clinicians have limited opportunities to observe excellent therapy being done. In this chapter, qualities of excellent clinicians will be presented with possible associated clinical skills.

THE PROCESS OF PROFESSIONAL DEVELOPMENT

There appears to be a systematic process whereby individuals gain competency in fields of skilled endeavors, whether that field involves the amelioration of communication problems or ones that are more manual such as plumbing, carpentry, or electrical work. A usual designation of three competency levels that are used in counseling are neophyte, mastery, and expert (Hyde & Weinberg, 1991). This can

also apply to the development of competent speech-language clinicians. Usually, the most effective way involves a combination of academic knowledge, experience, and observation of exemplary practice.

Academic Knowledge

Both clinicians and building craftspeople must have a knowledge base before they begin to practice their profession in a structured learning environment. Although there are many ways in which the knowledge can be gained, the purpose is identical: to provide a foundation upon which practice can be based. For craftspeople, there has been a long history of using various methods of acquiring the knowledge necessary for the practice of a profession. These include formal classes, self-directed courses, and literature or oral learning from an experienced craftsperson. Regardless of the vehicle on which knowledge is transported, it is academic. Theories, concepts, and practices are learned by the student in order to eventually practice them. For speech-language pathologists, the primary method of acquiring knowledge is through a multitude of courses at the undergraduate and graduate levels, and a limited amount of guided observation mandated by certification requirements.

Supervised Practice

The purpose of supervised clinical practice is to apply the academic knowledge students have learned and develop the skills necessary for the practice of their profession. Although the purpose is identical, the methodologies used in various professions differ vastly. The work of apprentice craftspeople is closely watched by master craftspeople. Under the guidance of a qualified supervisor, it is hoped that a transformation takes place where academic knowledge becomes practical skills. The same concept applies to the training of medical students. Supervision in both areas, however, involves constant interaction, joint practice, and observation of the master craftsperson or training physicians.

The structure of supervised clinical practicum for speech-language pathology students differs vastly from that of either the building trades or medical training. Supervision tends to involve mostly observation of the student by the supervisor. Only on a few occasions do supervisors engage in demonstration therapy in order to teach a skill to the student. Learning is often by trial and error.

Observation of Exemplary Practice

Throughout history, and still today, the observation of exemplary practice serves an important function in the mastery of skills necessary for the competent practice of a profession. One study compared the gains in skill mastery using various teaching methodologies (Baum & Gray, 1992). The methods that were compared were a lecture, observation of an experienced clinician, and self-observation. Both observations were conducted through the use of videotapes. Although there was an improvement of skills using all three techniques, the most effective method was the observation of the experienced clinician. The least amount of improvement involved self-observations.

During the plumbing student's supervised practice, he or she has daily and constant opportunity to observe how the practice of plumbing should be done. After completion of the learning program, the newly trained craftsperson will undergo an intensely supervised "journey person" experience under the daily tutelage of a master craftsperson that may last for over 2 years. During medical students' one-year internship and throughout their residency, there is the daily opportunity to observe how the practice of medicine should be performed. Students in psychotherapy often must undergo a 2- to 3-year period of their own psychotherapy with an individual who educators in the field believe has exemplary clinical skills, so that students can learn through their own analysis. In our profession, rarely do we have the opportunity to observe and work alongside master clinicians. The closest opportunity we have comes during supervised practicum. During these experiences, the supervisor will occasionally perform demonstration therapy, where the student can actually see how a specific skill should be used. On the completion of graduate training, the students are placed out in the field on their own, with only occasional supervision and minimal opportunities to observe master clinicians. Compare this with the training that occurs in the building professions, medical training, and psychoanalysis. The greatest deficit in our area is the lack of a significant amount of time observing and working with competent master clinicians. The purpose of this chapter is to partially compensate for this problem by identifying the qualities found in exemplary clinicians.

RELATIONSHIP BETWEEN QUALITIES AND SKILLS

The relationship between clinical qualities and clinical skills is similar to that of metalinguistics and linguistics: One is an umbrella for the other. Just as metalinguistics allows us to classify and categorize a multitude of linguistic concepts, so do clinical qualities. A quality is thought to be an attribute possessed by an individual that is discernible through specific observable skills. For example, an *accepting* clinician might be identified as an individual who would be willing to listen to a parent nonjudgmentally and also understand why a client was not able to practice an important assignment. In this section, seven qualities of outstanding clinicians will be presented. For each quality, possible specific skills, behaviors, and procedures necessary for displaying the quality will be listed. These lists have been inferred from clinical experience and limited research. Therefore, they are open for discussion. However, although the selection is debatable, the skills are not. These skills have been selected as important for the practice of speech-language pathology based on many clinical experiments in the health-related sciences. They have been empirically verified as positively affecting therapy. Whether those selected are important for exhibiting a specific quality is open to question. The identification of the qualities is more heuristic than scientific. In other words, the qualities act as organization concepts that allow the reader to see the relationship between various skills. Even if the validity or importance of the characteristics is questioned, the skills should not be.

QUALITIES OF MASTER CLINICIANS

How often have you observed someone doing outstanding therapy and marveled at how everything "clicked"? How the person you observed seemed to do everything right, how they maximized the client's communicative ability or they seemed to accomplish almost a "laying on of hands"? Usually, people walk away from the event holding the person in awe and not quite understanding how the changes were accomplished. If any analysis is done, it is usually limited to the identification of clinician characteristics, or attributes that have been associated with master clinicians.

Past Attempts at Identifying Qualities

There have been various attempts by noted clinicians to identify what they believe are the qualities competent clinicians should possess. Rogers believed that effective counselors needed to be empathetic, accepting, and genuine (Rogers, 1965). By possessing these qualities clinicians could present themselves to their clients as "transparent" individuals who had no agenda other than to facilitate clients in solving their problems. These characteristics embody some of the basic tenents of the *nondirective* therapist. In this form of therapy, the role of the clinician is that of a facilitator who refrains from imposing his or her theories on the problem structure of the client. As intuitively important as these qualities appear to be, their presence in clinicians showed no significant relationship with specific clinical skills (Gallagher & Hargie, 1992). In other words, clinicians who, for example, were transparent were no more or less competent than clinicians who were not.

Satir's list of important qualities for family counselors is similar to that of Rogers. She maintained that those in the helping professions need to possess eight characteristics in order to be effective (Satir, 1967):

1. Reveal yourself clearly to others.
2. Be in touch with your own feelings.

3. Be realistic about yourself and your capabilities.
4. Regard each person as unique.
5. Differences should be viewed as learning experiences, not as a threat or signal for conflict.
6. Understand clients for who they are, not how you wish them to be.
7. Understand that clients are responsible for their own behaviors.
8. Be able to clarify the meaning of a client's utterances.

She believed that clinicians who possessed these eight characteristics would be best positioned to meet the needs of families who were seen for conjoint family therapy.

In the field of speech-language pathology, few attempts have been made to systematically identify the characteristics of competent clinicians. One of the few is Murphy (1982). He believed that competent speech-language pathologists should have an "open" personality system which consists of the following traits:

1. Admit and accept uncertainty
2. Have a spontaneous communicative mode
3. Be somewhat unpredictable
4. Be open to new information
5. Have adaptable behaviors
6. Accept solutions which were assumed to be improbable
7. Be changeable
8. Be pliable and dynamic

Billings (1994) took a different approach in defining the essential features of a good counselor. He believed that the importance of establishing meaningful involvement with the client required that the clinician had to care for the client, function in the present with the client, and be willing to change as needed.

Problems with Characteristics Lists

Although few would argue that clinicians should not strive for any of the character-istics mentioned by the four authors, all present problems both in terms of ease in which they can be operationalized and their necessity in therapy. If a definition or concept is to be clinically useful, it should be able to be operationalized. To be operationalized simply means that whatever it is we are talking about, it has to have some reality within a clinical setting. For example, if the quality *adaptability* is to be useful in the clinic, one is obligated not only to provide examples of its presence, but also to describe the skills necessary to show adaptability. It is difficult to operationalize many of the characteristics found in the above four lists in specific clinic practices. For example, how does one operationalize "regard each person as unique" or "be somewhat unpredictable"?

Characteristics of Exemplary Speech-Language Clinicians

The characteristics espoused by Rogers, Satir, Murphy, and Billings constitute sets of values that each believe should be accepted by all clinicians. Each believes that his or her own set is appropriate and correct. Regardless whether one believes that values are universal, or are merely expressions of belief and preference limited only to the person espousing them, values take the imperative form of *should* or *ought to*. If one believes that values should be universally applied, then all clinicians should be expected to have similar values. The debate regarding what characteristics clinicians should have can be addressed in two ways. The first, and least productive, is to argue the merits of the theories in which the values are germinated. The second is to identify exemplary speech-language clinicians and determine what it is they are doing. In the next section, the second approach is used.

A pilot study conducted for this text examined the therapy of five clinicians who had been identified by their peers as being exemplary. The study, which involved analyses of videotaped therapy sessions, revealed a remarkable similarity in the therapy of the five individuals, even though they were working with clients of various ages and disorders. The results of this study are now being replicated with a larger population. Based on preliminary results, six critical characteristics of exemplary speech-language clinicians have been identified.

Subjectivity of Characteristics

The identification of the characteristics is based on the observation of master clinicians, analysis of their therapy, and extensive interviews. Therefore, even though they appear to have *intuitive* validity, they are open to discussion. The reader may dispute the importance of some or believe that others should be added to the list. For example, what may be identified as "contingency thinking," the reader may call something else, or dispute even if the quality is important in therapy.

Subjectivity of Skill Sets

Regardless of what qualities one ultimately believes a clinician should possess, what is crucial is to identify the behavioral components of the quality. By doing this, the complex behaviors exhibited by master clinicians could be broken down, identified, and used as a basis of learning how to apply specific skills. You will notice that a skill often appears in more than one quality skill list. "Establishes parameters," for example, is identified as a component for *facilitation* and *concentration on acquisition activities.*

The qualities list is probably of less importance than the specific skills list associated with each quality. The lists contain skills that are written in behavioral terms. The importance of this is that they become both trainable and reproducible. In other words, although it may be illuminating to say that a clinician is "compassionate," it is

more valuable to know that by using two or three specific skills, the impression of compassion is conveyed to the client.

COMPASSIONATE SCIENTIST

One characteristic that was prevalent in all the clinicians who were studied was that of a *compassionate scientist.* This refers to an overriding orientation of the clinician which is manifest in individuals who intensely care for the well-being of their clients, and endeavor to meet their needs in the most effective scientific manner. The synthesis of being both caring and scientific may be one of the highest ideals for a clinician to achieve. Usually possessing only one of these qualities results in less than adequate therapy. In a study examining the basis on which clients would like their clinicians to make decisions, it was found that they wanted them to rely on informal successful clinical experiences and research (O'Donohue, Fisher, Plaud, & Link, 1989). This constituted a type of strategy that others have found to be not only effective in treating behaviors, but also perceived by clients to be compassionate (Kleckner, Fran, Bland, Amendt et al., 1992).

The caring but unscientific clinician may falsely believe that compassion is sufficient to effect meaningful behavioral changes. Compassion is important for developing a therapeutic relationship, but without a careful analysis of the client's progress, compassion alone may result in little more than the client's acceptance of him- or herself as a communicatively disordered individual. The reverse problem exists with the uncaring scientific clinician. Although such clinicians may possess substantial knowledge of how to effect behavioral change, the client's perception of the clinician as uncaring may result in rejection of their guidance. Although the clinician may have much to offer to a client, he or she erects a barrier that prevents that knowledge from achieving positive effects.

When the clinician is both scientific and caring, clinical procedures can be developed that are efficient, effective, and facilitative of the client's growth. It is a quality that is considered by many in the health fields as crucial (Kahn & Steeves, 1988). Speech-language clinicians are not merely scientific professionals who mechanistically modify or change one's ability to use speech and language. They are helping professionals who can, and usually do, have a fundamental impact on the lives of their clients and their clients' families. They remediate one the most fundamental of human characteristics: the ability to communicate and be meaningfully involved in the communication process. Often, even the most seemingly insignificant change in a person's speaking pattern can result in lifelong changes, changes to which the clinician needs to be sensitive. Speech-language clinicians obviously do more than merely change tongue positions and teach new linguistic forms. They possess immense power that can be used for either the benefit or detriment of their clients. Whether clinicians like it or not, they possess what Bertrand Russell refers to as "priestly power," or the ability to influence people merely through the office one possesses (Russell, 1961). Clinicians find themselves in unique situations. During a session they might initially be empathetic and compassionate, but then become critical and confrontational. This vacillation may be necessary for the growth of the client. For example, a clinician was attempting to teach his client the proper method of single injections of air to produce short phrases. The program he was using was well thought out and based on the most current clinical research. While he was using the method, the client began talking about a particularly painful experience that was causing him emotional distress. During the discussion, it became very apparent that the single injection method was abandoned in favor of a less productive double injection method. Although the clinician had as his goal for the session to teach the new method,

it became apparent that his client was not able to both use the method and discuss the emotional problem at the same time. Wisely, the clinician decided to temporarily abandon the therapy plan and address the client's emotional distress.

The quality of being a compassionate scientist is probably the most encompassing, most sophisticated, and most laudable quality for a clinician to possess. It is the culmination of learning and utilizing all of the skills that were identified and used throughout this text. It should be used as the ideal to which clinicians should strive.

FACILITATOR

If someone asked you what the primary role of the speech-language clinician is, how would you answer it? A helping professional? Someone who enables a client to improve? An individual who is involved with communicative improvement? All of these answers would be correct, but none captures the essence of the practice of speech-language pathology. Above all else, clinicians are facilitators of change. A facilitator is someone who provides the conditions necessary for a person to develop a new behavior, attitude, or learn new information. A facilitator is basically a teacher. As a teacher, the speech-language clinician needs to exhibit skills that have been shown, both in the clinic and in the classroom, to result in learning. Each of the master clinicians studied displayed this quality. Based on the literature regarding teaching, it appears that there are 33 skills that can be reasonably associated with the quality of being a facilitator. These skills, which are both process oriented and technical, require various levels of sophistication and appear in Table 10–1.

EXQUISITE TIMING

If one examines the comedy sketches of any of the great comedians, one thing they

TABLE 10-1
Facilitator Skills

Foundational

PROCESS	TECHNICAL
Communicates at Client's Level	Age Appropriate Material
Provides Ample Opportunity to Respond	Interesting Material
Flexible	Generalizable Material
Involves Client in Decision Making	Use of Extraneous Reinforcers
	Intrinsically Reinforcing Activities
	Extrinsically Reinforcing Activities
	Reinforces Correct Responses
	Identifies Incorrect Responses
	Uses Modeling

TRANSITIONAL

PROCESS	TECHNICAL
Establishes Parameters	Control Through Materials
Effective Use of Time	Successive Approximations
Matching of Cultural Learning Styles	Multiple-Cuing
	Stages of Learning

COMPLEX

PROCESS	TECHNICAL
Self-Correction	Identifying Client Cognitive Levels (Levels of Learning)
Facilitates Problem Solving	Monitoring
Group Efficiency	Strategies
Feedback	Utilizing Principles of Change
	Stimulus Generalization
	Response Generalization
	Activity Construction Utilizing Critical Features
	Error Analysis
	Correct Response Analysis

all had in common was an incredible sense of timing: Jack Benny's casual look, George Burns' wait until Graci Allen came forth with a ridiculous statement, Charles Chaplin's slapstick movement, and Lou Costello's building of frustration. Just as comedians rely on timing to maximize audience reaction, so do master clinicians use timing to maximize a thought or statement's impact on their clients.

Master clinicians possess an incredible sense of timing, in the sense that they know when to present information and when to withhold it. This ability is beautifully portrayed in an ancient Buddhist story regarding a monk and his young student. One day the student went to a monk and asked him a question of importance. The monk responded with an answer that the student did not understand. The following week, the student asked the monk the same question. This time, the monk responded differently. After 3 years of receiving different answers to the same question, the student finally had the courage to ask the monk why the answer kept changing. The monk responded that he provided answers that the student could understand at the time the question was asked. And that, as the student gained more knowledge, he was able to understand the new answers. The same process exists in therapy. The clinician must continually evaluate when and how much information should be provided to the client.

Timing may involve both decisions on when to provide information and how long to allow a client to attempt to respond appropriately. A clinician was discussing a client's poor record at doing the generalization activities both had agreed to during the preceding session. The client kept repeating a series of excuses for not doing the activities that in fact were weak justifications. In past discussions, the clinician had ascertained that the client had some reluctance toward developing the new communicative behavior, which was fluency. Although the clinician believed that the client's current set of excuses were attempts to retain his current behavior, which in some ways was rewarding, he felt that it was not the time to confront the client. In the past, only when exercises could not be used was the client able to accept his fear of developing a new speaking pattern. Therefore, instead of saying to the client that his excuses were nothing more than rationalizations, the clinician asked the client how they could modify the generalization activities so that they could be practiced for the next week. It is important to allow clients sufficient amount of time to process information, develop answers, and explore alternative responses. As an adult aphasic struggled with retrieving the appropriate phonemes for the production of a specific word, the clinician did not provide any cues until the client had exhausted all

avenues of the strategy he had been taught to retrieve phonetic patterns. It appears that there are 17 skills that play a part in the appropriate use of timing in therapy. These are transitional and complex skills that are both process oriented and technical, and appear in Table 10–2.

CONTINGENCY THINKING

Contingency thinking is the ability to anticipate a client's response before it occurs, and provide the most appropriate response to it. It is an ability that occurs in many professions with individuals who have achieved the pinnacle of expertise in their area. During an interview of Wayne Gretsky, probably one of the greatest hockey players of all time, the interviewer asked him if the reason he was so great was because he was able to consistently get to the puck. He responded, no, it was because he knew where on the ice the puck was going. The same ability was observed in the renowned pool hustler known as Minnesota Fats. While waiting for his "marks" to arrive, he gathered a group of college students around him who had been riveted to his every move and told them he was about to give them a lesson they would never forget. Before even picking up his pool cue, he described every shot he was going to make, not only for the first rack of balls, but also for the next two! Amazingly, every one of his predictions was right on target. As the students gawked in amazement, he explained that the difference between a good and great player was that the good player could call every ball in one rack. The great player could do it for three. Master clinicians view their clients much in the same way that Minnesota Fats viewed his pool balls. This ability is often simplistically identified as clinical intuition. The term "intuition" implies that there is something inherent in the individual that allows him to mystically identify something or provide the correct answer.

TABLE 10–2
Timing Skills

TRANSITIONAL

PROCESS	TECHNICAL
Establishes Parameters	Successive Approximations
Effective Use of Time	Multiple-Cuing
Matching of Cultural Learning Styles	Stages of Learning

COMPLEX

PROCESS	TECHNICAL
Anticipation of Client Responses	Attitude Change Through Goal Attainment
Self-Correction	Identifying Client Cognitive Levels (Levels of Learning)
Facilitates Problem Solving	Monitoring
Feedback	Strategies
	Utilizing Principles of Change
	Error Analysis
	Correct Response Analysis

Supposedly, the ability is something that defies objective analysis. One is either born with it or is not. Nothing could be farther from the truth. Contingency thinking is something that occurs after a vast amount of knowledge and experience has been accumulated. It is the culmination of years of trying various intervention approaches. The decision-making process of the clinician is not apparent. Rather, it appears that no matter what response the client provides, the clinician is ready to respond appropriately. Over a period of years, the skills that the clinician develops have become automatized, a condition that seems to be absent in new clinicians (Patterson, Rak, Chermonte, & Roper, 1992).

An example of this decision-making ability occurs in the following. A clinician was working with a stutterer and when he presented an idea to him, he already knew the full range of responses he could expect. This is based on his experience of working with hundreds of similar clients for thousands of hours. He also knew the way he would respond to any of the client's re-

sponses and all of the possible responses that will follow from him. To an observer, it might appear that the clinician just intuitively knew how to respond to each remark since they were instantaneous. Although it may have appeared that way, he was following a precise decision-making lattice that, after years of practice, was almost automatic to him. The 22 skills necessary for displaying this characteristic appear in Table 10–3. They are both process oriented and technical, and require varying levels of sophistication.

CONSISTENCY

Each of the skills discussed in this text can be found in the therapy of even the newest therapist. The main difference between master clinicians and those with less experience or sophistication involves the consistent use of the skills. In a study conducted with graduate students for this text, most of the advanced clinical skills were noted; however, none was consistently applied by

TABLE 10–3
Contingency Skills

FOUNDATIONAL SKILLS

PROCESS	TECHNICAL
Attentive	Identifies Incorrect Responses
Flexible	
Involves Client in Decision Making	

TRANSITIONAL

PROCESS	TECHNICAL
Effective Use of Time	Successive Approximations
Matching of Cultural Learning Styles	Multiple-Cuing
	Stages of Learning

COMPLEX

PROCESS	TECHNICAL
Anticipation of Client Responses	Attitude Change Through Goal Attainment
Self-Correction	Identifying Client Cognitive Levels (Levels of Learning)
Facilitates Problem Solving	Strategies
Rephrasing	Utilizing Principles of Change
Confrontation	Error Analysis
Minimal Self-Directed Behaviors	Correct Response Analysis
Feedback	

any one individual. Usually, with any given student there was one good example of the skill for every four or five that were poor examples. Consistency in the application of skills is an important feature of master clinicians. It not only results in the dispensing of better therapy, but also allows the client to rely on his expectations. For example, a clinician who is consistently willing to confront a client's inappropriate assessments of her own performance, conveys a picture to the client of someone who will not be unconditionally accepting of her pronouncements. A client with a clinician of this type will be more cautious in cavalierly presenting information or assessments that she may not truly believe. Conversely, a client who has a clinician that is inconsistent, may often present be-

liefs and self-assessments that are not therapeutic. Consistency is as important, if not more so with children. Children, lacking the experiences and intellectual ability of adults, are more dependent on shaping their clinical responses on the behavior of the clinician, than are adults. What is *acceptable* for an adult may be determined by many factors, most of which are based on societal, cultural, and intellectual values. Although a child may base what is acceptable on these areas, with limited experience, hypotheses of what is acceptable will be primarily determined by the clinician's behavior and utterances.

The importance of consistency is exemplified in the following. A clinician was seeing a child for the first time. She had been told that the child had various distracting behaviors and would constantly test and go beyond the prescribed limits of therapy. During the session, whenever the child attempted to get out of his seat the clinician would gently but firmly place him back into it. During the first 10 minutes of therapy, seven attempts were made. During the next 10 minutes, five attempts were made. During the last 10 minutes, only two attempts were made. By being consistent in her responses, the clinician established the parameters under which her interaction with the client were to take place. By being consistent during this session and subsequent ones, the child's disruptive behaviors ceased after the third session. There is no skills list for this quality since the quality should be practiced with each skill.

CONCENTRATION ON ACQUISITION TASKS

In the section on transitional skills, the various levels of learning activities were discussed. In that section you saw that there are various types of learning activities clients can be asked to perform. Those that result in the greatest amount of positive gain involve acquisition tasks. Those that result in minimal gains involve retrieval tasks. An important feature of the therapy of master clinicians is that a significant amount of time is spent on acquisition activities and a minimal amount of time spent on retrieval activities. An acquisition activity involves the teaching of a concept or rule through a strategy that the client can internalize and use for other situations that may be similar in structure, yet different in certain aspects. For example, some approaches to teaching language believe that if children are to learn how to string words together, it should be done using linguistic rules, rather than the use of carrier phrases.

Another example will illustrate the importance of focusing on acquisition tasks. When teaching two word constructions to a

child, a clinician chose a strategy that allowed the child to learn the rule, *action + object*. This was followed by having the child apply the rule to various situations. This was done by physically representing *action + object* through the use of two different blocks or pieces of paper, and then placing action pictures on one piece of paper and object pictures on the other. Given an assortment of action pictures in one pile and object pictures in another pile, he was asked to construct phrases by selecting pictures from each pile, then placing them on the appropriate piece of paper, and finally saying the construction. This would be an example of using a strategy, or an acquisition device to teach the action + object construction. If no strategy was used, and the child was asked to merely model utterances such as "push car," "push airplane," "hold car," and "hold airplane," these would not be acquisition activities. The 30 skills, both process-oriented and technical, and requiring various levels of sophistication, that are required for using acquisition activities appear in Table 10–4.

FOCUSED

After observing a particularly excellent session, someone asked the clinician to describe how he was able to achieve the success he did with the client. After thinking for some time, the clinician said, "When a client comes to see me, he is putting a tremendous amount of trust in me. That's a huge responsibility. Because of this, I owe the client my undivided attention for the entire 50 minute session. It doesn't make any difference what kind of problems I have before the session begins or how preoccupied I may be before the session. During the 50 minutes I am only focused on my client, nothing else exists outside of the clinic room." The ability to focus only on the problems of the client requires clinicians to be prepared and willing to subvert their needs and interests for those of the

TABLE 10–4
Acquisition Activities

FOUNDATIONAL

PROCESS	TECHNICAL
Provides Ample Opportunity to Respond	Generalizable Material
Involves Client in Decision Making	Use of Extraneous Reinforcers
	Reinforces Correct Responses
	Identifies Incorrect Responses
	Intrinsically Reinforcing Activities
	Extrinsically Reinforcing Activities
	Extraneously Reinforcing Activities

TRANSITIONAL

PROCESS	TECHNICAL
Establishes Parameter	Control Through Materials
Effective Use of Time	Successive Approximations
Matching of Cultural Learning Styles	Multiple-Cuing
	Stages of Learning

COMPLEX

PROCESS	TECHNICAL
Anticipation of Client Responses	Identifying Client Cognitive Levels (Levels of Learning)
Self-Correction	Monitoring
Facilitates Problem-Solving	Strategies
Group Efficiency	Utilizing Principles of Change
Feedback	Stimulus Generalization
	Response Generalization
	Activity Construction Utilizing Critical Features
	Error Analysis
	Correct Response Analysis

client. This ability may be dependent upon clinicians' feelings of attentiveness, connectiveness, and integration (Kahn, 1992).

A clinician who just arrived for her session with a client had come from the hospital where her daughter was hospitalized with an internal problem. Although the problem was not life threatening, it was very traumatic for the clinician. In spite of the anxiety she felt, during the 50 minute session with her client, she managed not to think about her daughter. The level of concentration she had on effecting a positive change with her Down syndrome client required her to focus only on the therapy at hand. There appear to be six process skills that are foundational and complex that contribute to the development of being focused. These are process oriented only and appear in Table 10–5.

TABLE 10–5
Focused

FOUNDATIONAL SKILLS

PROCESS
Attentive
Flexible

COMPLEX

PROCESS
Anticipation of Client Responses
Self-Correction
Minimal Self-Directed Behaviors
Professional Collaboration

CHAPTER
11

Self-Evaluation and Summary

Just as it is important for clients to become their own clinicians, so it is important for clinicians to become their own teachers. In this section, two different formats are provided for that purpose. The first form, which appears in Table 11–1, is an abbreviated clinician self-analysis form that can serve as a format for identifying the clinician's own clinical skills and behaviors. Videotape an entire session and analyze it using the checklist. If a behavior is present, first provide an example of it. Then, think about what could have been done differently to have made it more effective. This form of analysis is extremely useful, not only in diagnosing one's own clinical problems, but also solving them.

Tables 11–2 through 11–7 are modified forms that appeared in Chapter 1. They contain each of the clinical behaviors discussed in this text. The clinician or supervisor can use this as an informal check sheet on which occurrences of appropriate behaviors have been demonstrated.

SUMMARY

Much has been covered in this text. Some would say too much. The practice of speech-language therapy is a discipline that requires intellectual rigor, humaneness, and a conviction to the principles that provide our clients with the greatest opportunity to develop communicative normalcy.

Humane Practice Based on Scientific Principles

What many thought were fairly simple, straight forward processes, were presented in this text as complicated procedures with many options. Time-honored approaches that have been used for generations of speech-language clinicians were disregarded as inadequate or inefficient. Instead of therapy being a spontaneous activity where clinicians intuit the *right and humane* thing to do, systematic processes of designing intervention protocols were posited. In an era when cultural sensitivity has become synonymous with ethnic sensitivity, the importance of having a larger conception of culture was emphasized. In a field where research on the effects of clinician skills and behaviors is woefully inadequate, a reliance on interdisciplinary resources was used. And what many clinicians call therapy, was identified using the principles of learning as *assessment*.

Politics, Economics, and Principles

In an era when placements of school children in inclusive settings have become a political and economic issue, it was suggested that decisions should be made on the basis of research data in the areas of learning and instructional design. Politics and economics is also shaping our professional roles. We are in an age when the role of the speech-language clinician is being broadened to include areas only tangentially related to the core of the profession. Sometimes the decisions are based on economics, at other times it is a matter of philosophical conviction. There is an interesting parallel in the world of large corporate enterprises. Large successful companies usually seek to expand their business. Two different approaches are taken. The first is to concentrate on what made them successful. The second is to reach out to new, unrelated, or vaguely related enterprises. Companies of the first type tend to continue their successes, gain more market share, and remain viable entities. A significant number of companies who expand outside of their area become unmanageable and lose the focus of their core business. Other companies infringe on their territory and steal their customers. These are the companies that after sustaining large losses, begin selling off those acquired businesses that were not related to what they did best. Eventually, some of these companies regain their pre-acquisi-

tion stage strength. Others never recover. As a profession, we are dangerously close to venturing into areas that are only tangentially related to our mission: to maximize the communicative capacity of our *speech, language, and hearing disordered* clients. Some would argue that incursions into areas of reading, nonpathological communication enhancement, and medical procedures are only logical extensions of what we do. Although a strong case could be made for these arguments, there is a danger that by providing these additional services, services provided in our core areas suffer. Some would argue that attempts to extend our domain are related to feeling unsuccessful in the areas of our expertise. If that is the case, the appropriate response is to strengthen and improve that which we do best: therapy for communicative disorders. Just like the corporation that refocuses on its core business, speech-language clinicians should focus on how to provide the most efficient and effective therapy for their clients. Hopefully this book contributes to that process.

Clinical Style

The San Francisco community leader, Reverend Cecil Williams, described on a radio program the basis of his style of religious leadership. He stated that it involved *personal risk*. He believed that it was hypocritical to stay behind the podium in the front of his church and preach the goodness of Christianity while refusing to become involved in the problems of his parishioners and the community. Christianity for Reverend Williams was not something to *talked about*, but rather something that needs to be *lived*. There is an analogy to the practice of speech-language pathology. Clinicians need to be willing to risk something in therapy. Therapy is not a distant, objective procedure, where cookbook approaches are mindlessly applied to clients. It is a dynamic process, requiring the commitment of the clinician to the most competent and compassionate practices available. To achieve this, clinical experimentation is necessary. With experimentation comes risk, and the possibility of failure. But with experimentation comes the possibility of substantial benefits, both to the client and the clinician.

The great architect Frank Lloyd Wright was once asked to describe how he designed his buildings. He compared it to what composers do when creating a symphony. The composition contains many component parts, each of which can stand alone, but when put together consitute a harmonious unity. Good therapy in many ways is similar to Wright's concept of good architecture. However, just as each symphony sounds different, although the form is identical, so is the therapy of each clinician. At a music workshop, a participant asked a musician to describe the techniques he used, in order that his rendition of a song would sound identical to that of the musician. The response of the musician was prophetic, and appropriate also for the practice of speech-language therapy.

Music does not come from techniques. It comes from here, your heart and head. Techniques are used to bring out what I feel in my heart and head into what you hear with your ears. Techniques will never create a unique whole sound. Music is not techniques, it is something that's inside you. You can play all of my techniques, even play them better than me, and we will never sound the same. The feelings we have are different.

Just as with music, therapy is a very individual process. The skills, behaviors, and techniques described in this text will hopefully enable you to actualize what you feel about your clients and their communicative problems. With them, you can create clinical *magic*. Without them, well . . .

TABLE 11-1
Clinician Self-Evaluation

Culturally Sensitive Process Skills/Behaviors

SKILL/BEHAVIOR	✓ if present	EXAMPLE	COMMENTS
Acknowledging Feelings and Experiences			
Attitude Change Through Successful Demonstration			
Commonality of Interests			
Concern			
Confrontation			
Conversational Follow-Through			
Flexibility			
Relevant Questions			
Rephrasing			
Respect			
Self-Disclosure			

Designing and implementing intervention protocols

TECHNIQUE	✓ if present	EXAMPLE	COMMENTS
Learning Stages Apprehending ☐% time			
Acquisition ☐% time			
Retention 0 %			
Retrieval ☐% time			
Client Involvement Materials Selection			
Activities Selection			
Conversation Topics			
Control Verbal			
Vocal			
Nonverbal			
Materials/Activities			
Generalization Stimulus			
Response			

(continued)

TABLE 11-1 *(cont.)*

TECHNIQUE	✓ if present	EXAMPLE	COMMENTS
Levels of Learning [rank order in terms of time] Stimulus-Response			
Chaining			
Discrimination			
Concept			
Rule			
Modelling Before using strategy			
After using strategy			
Monitoring Clinician			
Client			
Response Differentiation Successive Approximation			
Multiple-Cuing			
Simplicity Instructions			
Focus			
Strategies Oral			
Graphic			

TECHNIQUE	✓ if present	EXAMPLE	COMMENTS
Face Communicative			
Self-Directive			
Arms/Hands Communicative			
Self-Directive			
Legs/Feet Communicative			
Self-Directive			
Posture Forward			
Backward			
Neutral			

(continued)

TABLE 11-1 *(cont.)*

SKILL/BEHAVIOR	✓ if present	EXAMPLE	COMMENTS
Reinforcing Aspects Intrinsic			
Extrinsic			
Extraneous			
Generalizability			
INTRINSIC CHARACTERISTICS Movement			
Mobility			
Construction			
Destruction			
Completion			
Flexibility			
Excitement			
Mystery			

TABLE 11–2
Preconditions for Successful Therapy

In each of the boxes, place a ✔ checkmark if the skill has been adequately displayed, and an ✗ if a problem was solved.

Ethnicity	Religion	Gender/Age	Age	Exceptionality	Locale	Religion	Class
☐	☐	☐	☐	☐	☐	☐	☐

CLIENT

Responsibility	Motivation	Knowledge
☐	☐	☐

CLINICIAN

Competency in the Disorder	Knowledge Technology of Change	Knowledge of Activity Strategies
☐	☐	☐

331

TABLE 11-3
Planning Intervention

In each of the boxes, place a ✓ checkmark if the skill has been adequately displayed, and an ✗ if a problem was observed.

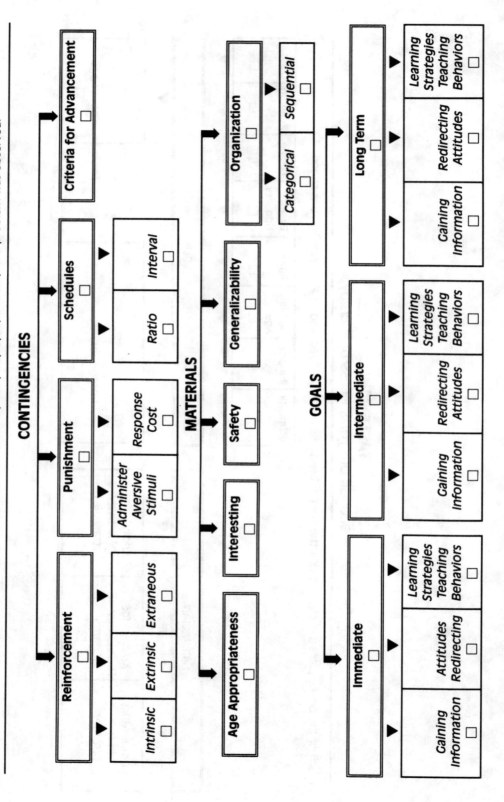

TABLE 11-3 *(continued)*

STIMULUS CONFIGURATIONS

Simplification	Rate	Variation	Visualness	Redundancy	Task Complexity	Context	Figure/Ground
☐	☐	☐	☐	☐	☐	☐	☐

TABLE 11-4

Applying Technical Intervention Skills

In each of the boxes, place a ✓ checkmark if the skill has been adequately displayed, and an ✗ if a problem was observed.

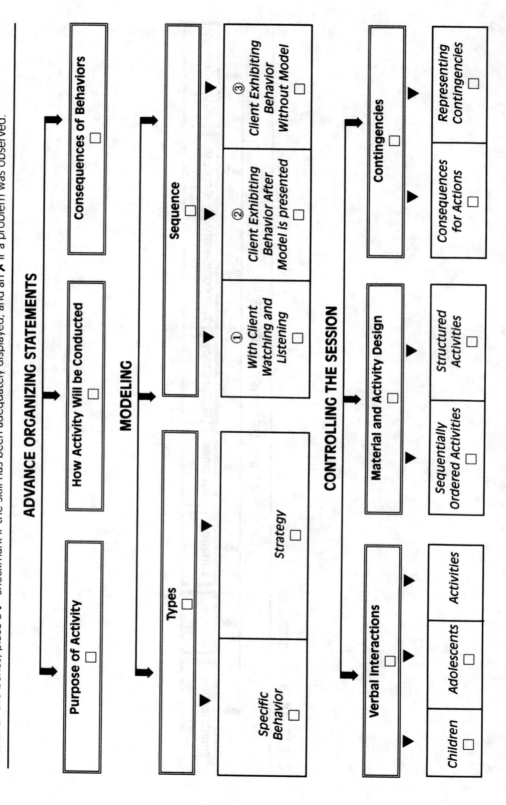

TABLE 11-5

Applying technical intervention skills

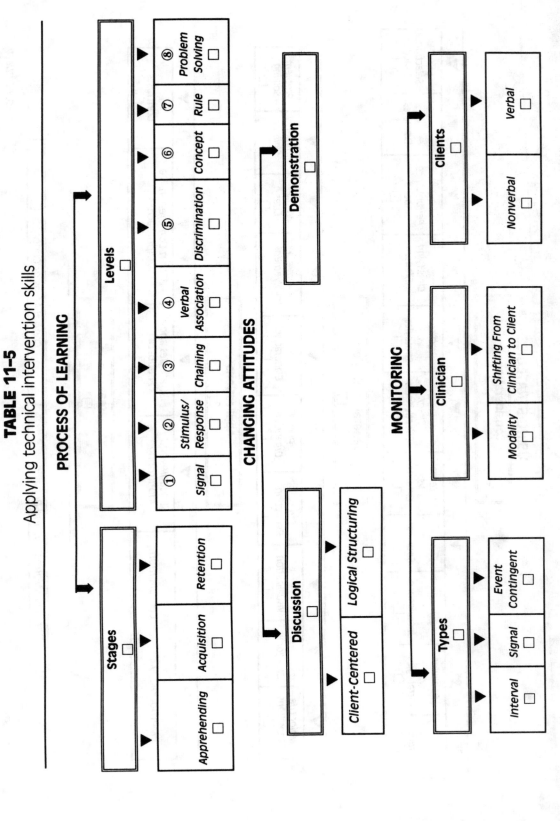

USING STRATEGIES

Considerations ☐

- Criteria ☐
- Behavior vs. Strategies ☐
- Intelligence ☐
- Sources ☐
- Internal vs. External ☐
- Time/Effectiveness ☐
- Practice vs. Strategies ☐
- Classifying Clients ☐
- Performance Speed ☐
- Examples ☐
- Effort Selection Usage ☐

General Strategies ☐

- Major Life Transitions ☐
- Categories ☐
- Visualization ☐
- Stress Reduction ☐
- Post Organizers ☐
- Elaboration ☐
- Active Involvement ☐
- Visual Cues ☐
- Summary Skills ☐
- Problem Solving ☐

Applications ☐

- Methodology ☐
- Combination ☐
- Strategies and Monitoring ☐
- Strategies and Feedback ☐
- Within Comprehensive Approaches ☐
- Contrasts ☐

Areas ☐

- Detailed Information and Behaviors ☐
- Central Areas or Concepts ☐

(continued)

TABLE 11-5 *(continued)*

GENERALIZATIONS

Timing ☐
- State of Therapy ☐
- Part of Therapy ☐

Stimulus ☐
- Configuration ☐
- Training Sequence ☐
- Rationale ☐

Response ☐
- Training Sequence ☐
- Rationale ☐

Combinations ☐
- Scheduling ☐
- Contracts ☐

Activities ☐
- Highlighting ☐
- Age ☐

MAINTENANCE

Things to Maintain ☐
- Specific Behaviors ☐
- Compensatory Strategies ☐
- New Behavior Strategies ☐

ERROR ANALYSIS

Types ☐
- Unlearned Prerequisites ☐
- Systematic Conceptual Errors ☐
- Random ☐
- Non-Compliance ☐
- Non-Volitional Inattention ☐

General Conditions ☐
- Certitude of Answers ☐

TABLE 11-6
Applying Technical Intervention Skills

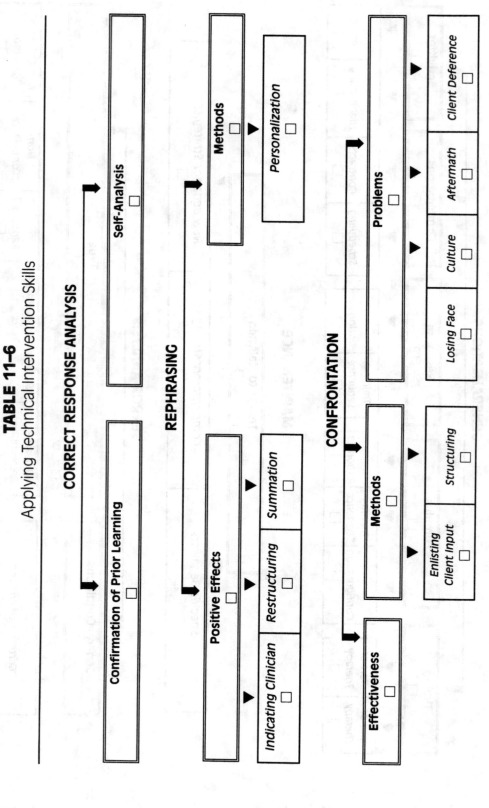

CORRECT RESPONSE ANALYSIS

Confirmation of Prior Learning ☐ ➤ Self-Analysis ☐

REPHRASING

Positive Effects ☐

- ➤ Indicating Clinician ☐
- ➤ Restructuring ☐
- ➤ Summation ☐

Methods ☐ ➤ Personalization ☐

CONFRONTATION

Effectiveness ☐

Methods ☐

- ➤ Enlisting Client Input ☐
- ➤ Structuring ☐

Problems ☐

- ➤ Losing Face ☐
- ➤ Culture ☐
- ➤ Aftermath ☐
- ➤ Client Deference ☐

(continued)

TABLE 11-6 *(continued)*

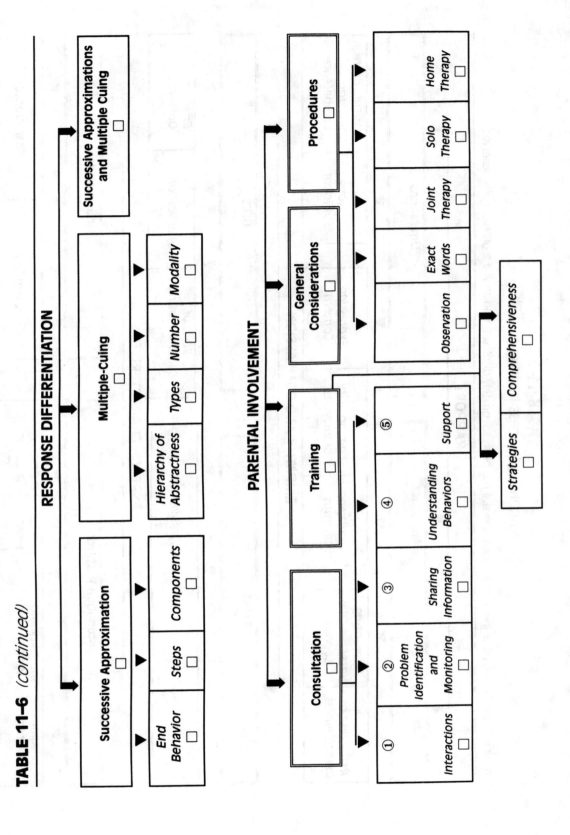

RESPONSE DIFFERENTIATION

Successive Approximation ☐

- End Behavior ☐
- Steps ☐
- Components ☐

Multiple-Cuing ☐

- Hierarchy of Abstractness ☐
- Types ☐
- Number ☐
- Modality ☐

Successive Approximations and Multiple Cuing ☐

PARENTAL INVOLVEMENT

Consultation ☐

- ① Interactions ☐
- ② Problem Identification and Monitoring ☐
- ③ Sharing Information ☐
- ④ Understanding Behaviors ☐
- ⑤ Support ☐

Training ☐

- Strategies ☐
- Comprehensiveness ☐

General Considerations ☐

- Observation ☐
- Exact Words ☐
- Joint Therapy ☐
- Solo Therapy ☐
- Home Therapy ☐

Procedures ☐

TABLE 11-7

Applying Process Intervention Skills

In each of the boxes, place a ✓ checkmark if the skill has been adequately displayed, and an ✗ if a problem was observed.

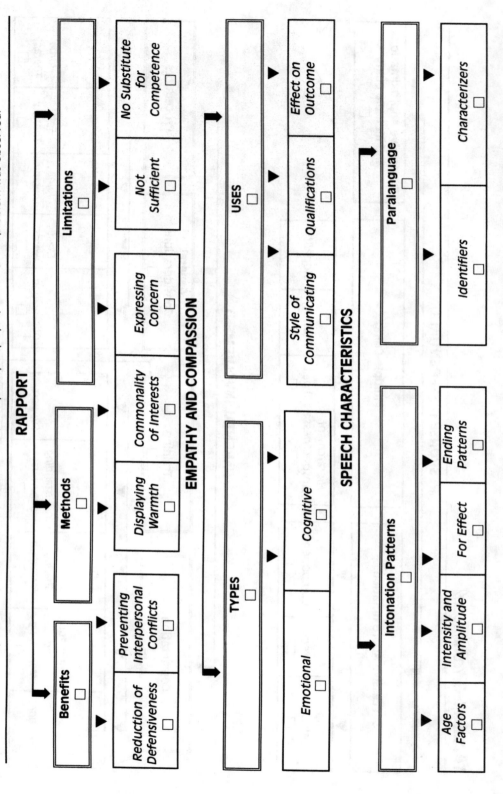

RAPPORT

Benefits ☐
- Reduction of Defensiveness ☐
- Preventing Interpersonal Conflicts ☐

Methods ☐
- Displaying Warmth ☐
- Commonality of Interests ☐
- Expressing Concern ☐

Limitations ☐
- Not Sufficient ☐
- No Substitute for Competence ☐

EMPATHY AND COMPASSION

TYPES ☐
- Emotional ☐
- Cognitive ☐

USES ☐
- Style of Communicating ☐
- Qualifications ☐
- Effect on Outcome ☐

SPEECH CHARACTERISTICS

Intonation Patterns ☐
- Age Factors ☐
- Intensity and Amplitude ☐
- For Effect ☐
- Ending Patterns ☐

Paralanguage ☐
- Identifiers ☐
- Characterizers ☐

TABLE 11-7 *(continued)*

COMMUNICATING AT THE CLIENT'S OWN LEVEL

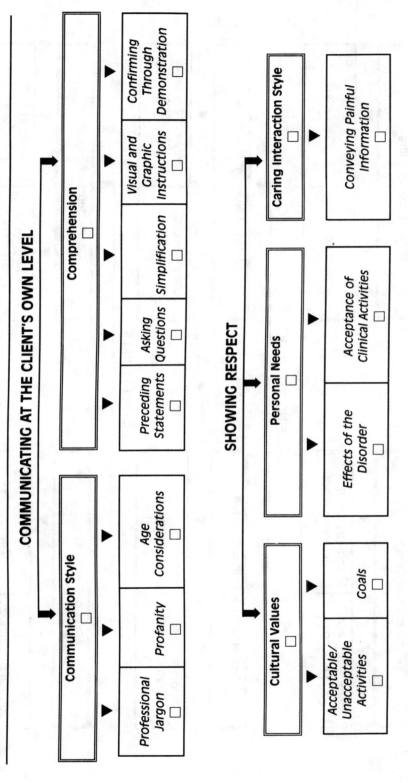

SHOWING RESPECT

MAXIMIZING RESPONSE OPPORTUNTIES

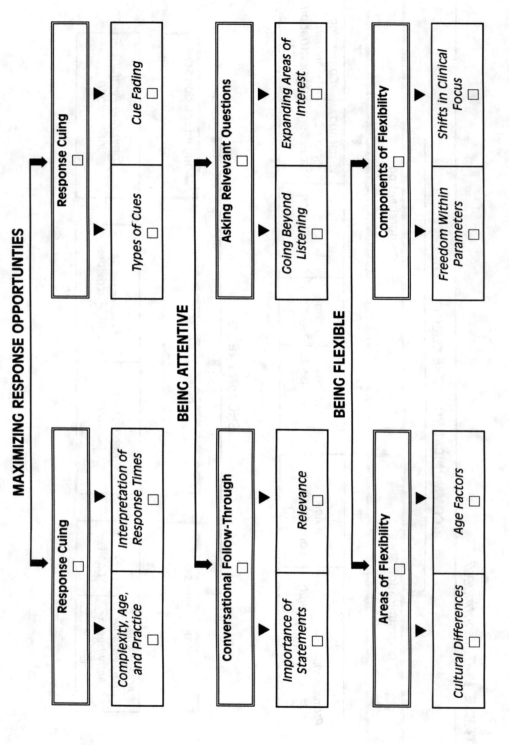

Response Cuing ☐

- **Response Cuing** ☐
  - Cue Fading ☐
  - Types of Cues ☐

- **Response Cuing** ☐
  - Interpretation of Response Times ☐
  - Complexity, Age, and Practice ☐

BEING ATTENTIVE

Asking Relvevant Questions ☐
- Expanding Areas of Interest ☐
- Going Beyond Listening ☐

Conversational Follow-Through ☐
- Relevance ☐
- Importance of Statements ☐

BEING FLEXIBLE

Components of Flexibility ☐
- Shifts in Clinical Focus ☐
- Freedom Within Parameters ☐

Areas of Flexibility ☐
- Age Factors ☐
- Cultural Differences ☐

(continued)

TABLE 11-7 *(continued)*

INVOLVING CLIENTS IN DECISION MAKING

Models for Involvement ☐	Determining Goals ☐	Selecting Methods and Techniques ☐	Selecting Extraneous Reinforcers ☐
Simple ☐	*Children* ☐	*Children* ☐	*Children* ☐
Sophisticated ☐	*Adolescents* ☐	*Adolescents* ☐	
	Adults ☐	*Adults* ☐	

NONVERBAL BEHAVIORS

Client Behaviors ☐	Control ☐	Functions ☐	Clinician Behaviors ☐
Face ☐			*Face* ☐
Arms/ Hands ☐			*Arms/ Hands* ☐
Legs/ Feet ☐			*Legs/ Feet* ☐
Posture ☐			*Posture* ☐

Posture ☐	*Amplify Message* ☐	*Contradict Message* ☐	*Qualify Message* ☐	*Unrelated Message* ☐

343

ACKNOWLEDGMENT

Verbal

- ▶ Conversational Follow-Through □
- ▶ Relevant Goals □
- ▶ Paraphrasing □
- ▶ Client-Centered Techniques □

Vocal □

- ▶ Prosody/ Intonation □
- ▶ Para-language □

Nonverbal □

- ▶ Intentional Messages □
- ▶ Unintentional Messages □

ACCEPTANCE

Withholding Judgments □

- ▶ Effects of Prior Judgments □
- ▶ Developing Trust □

(continued)

TABLE 11-7 *(continued)*

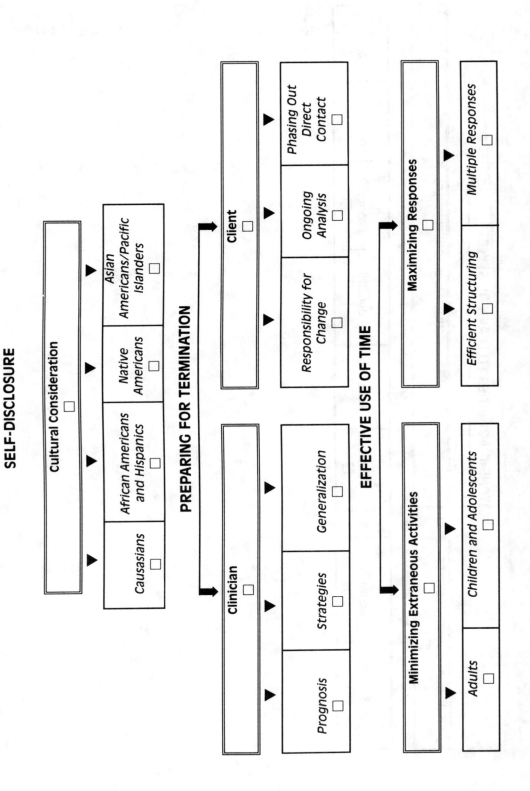

SELF-DISCLOSURE

Cultural Consideration ☐

▶ Causasians ☐

▶ African Americans and Hispanics ☐

▶ Native Americans ☐

▶ Asian Americans/Pacific Islanders ☐

PREPARING FOR TERMINATION

Clinician ☐

▶ Prognosis ☐

▶ Strategies ☐

▶ Generalization ☐

Client ☐

▶ Responsibility for Change ☐

▶ Ongoing Analysis ☐

▶ Phasing Out Direct Contact ☐

EFFECTIVE USE OF TIME

Minimizing Extraneous Activities ☐

▶ Adults ☐

▶ Children and Adolescents ☐

Maximizing Responses ☐

▶ Efficient Structuring ☐

▶ Multiple Responses ☐

MATCHING ACTIVITIES TO LEARNING STYLES

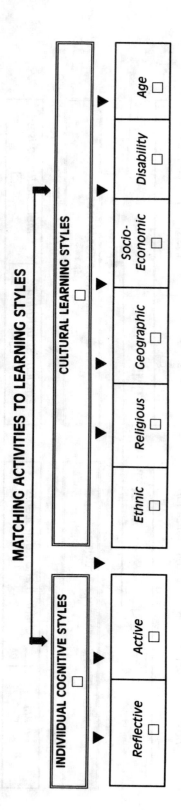

INDIVIIDUAL COGNITIVE STYLES ☐

Reflective ☐	Active ☐

CULTURAL LEARNING STYLES ☐

Ethnic ☐	Religious ☐	Geographic ☐	Socio-Economic ☐	Disability ☐	Age ☐

(continued)

GROUP THERAPY

(continued)

Basic Considerations ☐					
Clinical Orientation ☐	Preparation ☐	Composition ☐	Control ☐	Efficiency ☐	Competition ☐

Settings ☐		
Public Schools ☐	Senior Centers ☐	Preschools ☐

Leadership ☐		
General Competency ☐	Gender ☐	Ethnicity ☐

Interactions ☐				
Styles ☐	Culture ☐	Role Relationships ☐	Member to Member Feedback ☐	Active Involvement ☐

Functions ☐		
Gathering Data ☐	Generalization of Behaviors ☐	Discussion ☐

347

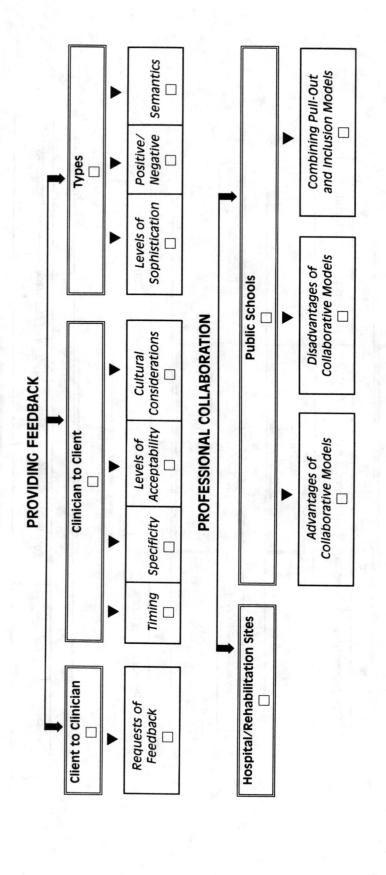

PROVIDING FEEDBACK

Client to Clinician ☐

- Requests of Feedback ☐

Clinician to Client ☐

- Timing ☐
- Specificity ☐
- Levels of Acceptability ☐
- Cultural Considerations ☐

Types ☐

- Levels of Sophistication ☐
- Positive/ Negative ☐
- Semantics ☐

PROFESSIONAL COLLABORATION

Hospital/Rehabilitation Sites ☐

Public Schools ☐

- Advantages of Collaborative Models ☐
- Disadvantages of Collaborative Models ☐
- Combining Pull-Out and Inclusion Models ☐

USE OF PROFESSIONAL AUTHORITY

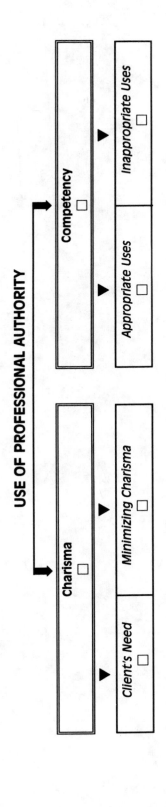

Charisma ☐

Client's Need ☐

Minimizing Charisma ☐

Competency ☐

Appropriate Uses ☐

Inappropriate Uses ☐

(continued)

APPENDIX A

Research Interest Bibliography

The purpose of this bibliography is to provide researchers, clinicians, supervisors, and classroom instructors with a list of references grouped by category. Many of the references are listed in more than one category, because they cover more than one topic. For example, an article that addresses poor elderly attitudes toward therapy would appear in the categories of *Socioeconomic* and *Elderly*. Although most of the articles and books use specific age ranges in their studies, few appear under the categories of *Children, Adolescents* and *Elderly*. If that was done, the size of this bibliography would double. However, an examination of the titles will quickly identify the age group used in the study. References in *Children, Adolescents,* and *Elderly* contain studies on characteristics of the age group. The reference/interest categories that appear in this appendix are in alphabetical order:

Adolescents

African Americans

Asian American/Pacific Islander

Behavioral Management

Children

Clinical Training Issues

Collaboration/Inclusion

Disability Issues

Elderly

Family Therapy/Partent Training

Feedback

Gender/Sexual Orientation

Generalization/Maintenance

Group Therapy

Hispanics

Interaction Variables

Learning/Cognition

Modeling

Monitoring

Motivation

Native Americans

Nonverbal Behaviors

Regional/Geographic

Religion

Socioeconomics

Stimulus Configurations

Strategies

Treatment Efficacy

ADOLESCENTS

Foxx, R. M., Kyle, M. S., Faw, G. D., and Bittle, R. G. (1989). Teaching a problem solving strategy to inpatient adolescents: Social validation, maintenance, and generalization. *Child and Family Behavior Therapy, 11*(3-4), 71–88.

Goldberg, B., and Tidwell, R. (1990). Ethnicity and gender similarity: The effectiveness of counseling for adolescents. *Journal of Youth and Adolescence,* Vol 19(6) 589–603

Johnson, M., and Nelson, T.M. (1978). Game playing with juvenile delinquents. *Simulation and Games, 9* (4), 461–475.

Kottman, T. (1990) Counseling middle school students: Techniques that work. *Elementary School Guidance and Counseling, 25*(2), 138–145

Leader, E. (1991) Why adolescent group therapy? *Journal of Child and Adolescent Group Therapy, 1*(2), 81–93.

LeCroy, C.W. (1986). An analysis of the effects of gender on outcome in group treatment with young adolescents. *Journal of Youth and Adolescence, 15,* 497–508.

Madonna, J. M., and Caswell, P. (1991).The utilization of flexible techniques in group therapy with delinquent adolescent boys. *Journal of Child and Adolescent Group Therapy, 1*(2), 147–157.

Morris, G. B. (1991). Perceptions of leadership traits: Comparison of adolescent and adult school leaders. *Psychological Reports, 69*(3, Pt 1), 723–727.

Nangle, D. W., Carr-Nagle, R. E., and Hansen, D. J. (1994). Enhancing generalization of a contingency-management intervention through the use of family problem-solving training: Evaluation with a severely conduct-disordered adolescent. *Child and Family Behavior Therapy, 16*(2), 65–76.

Sayger, T. V., Szykula, S.A., and Laylander, J.A. (1991). Adolescent-focused family counseling: A comparison of behavioral and strategic approaches. *Journal of Family Psychotherapy, 2*(3), 57–80.

Sykes, D. K. (1987). An approach to working with Black youth in cross cultural therapy. *Clinical Social Work Journal, 15*(3) 260–270.

Zarbatany, L, Ghesquiere, K., and Mohr, K. (1992). A context perspective on early adolescents' friendship expectations. *Journal of Early Adolescence, 12*(1), 111–126.

AFRICAN AMERICANS

Alston, R.J., and Mngadi, S. (1992). The interaction between disability status and the African American experience: Implications for rehabilitation counseling. *Journal of Applied Rehabilitation Counseling, 23*(2), 12–16.

Alston, R., and Mngadi, S. (1992). The interaction between disability status and the African American experience: Implications for rehabilitation counseling. *Journal of Applied Rehabilitation Counseling. Sum 23*(2), 12–16.

Baptiste, D. A. (1990). Therapeutic strategies with Black-Hispanic families: Identify problems of a neglected minority. *Journal of Family Psychotherapy, 1*(3), 15–38.

Berg, J. H., and Wright-Buckley, C. (1988). Effects of racial similarity and interviewer intimacy in a peer counseling analogue. *Journal of Counseling Psychology, 35*(4), 377–384

Blair, C. (1992). Objective: Recruitment-Student Perspective. *Asha, 34*(5), 43–44

Boyd-Franklin, N., and Shenouda, N. T. (1990). A multisystems approach to the treatment of a Black, inner-city family with a schizophrenic mother. *American Journal of Orthopsychiatry, 60*(2), 186–195.

Boyd-Franklin, N. (1989). Five key factors in the treatment of Black families. *Journal of Psychotherapy and the Family, 6* (1–2), 53–69

Brondolo, E., Baruch, C., Conway, E., and Marsh, L. (1994). Aggression among inner-city minority youth: a biopsychosocial model for school-based evaluation and treatment. Special Issue: Multicultural views on domestic violence. *Journal of Social Distress and the Homeless, 3*(1), 53–80.

Campbell, L. R., Brennan, D. G., and Steckol, K. F. (1992). Preservice training to meet the needs of people from diverse cultural backgrounds. *Asha, 35*(12), 29–32.

Chideya, F. (1995). *Don't believe the hype: Fighting cultural misinformation about African Americans.* New York: Penguin Books.

Cole, L. (1989). E pluribus pluribus: Multicultural imperatives for the 1990's and beyond. *ASHA, 31,* 65–70.

Cole, L. (1992). We're Serious. *Asha, 32*(5), 38–39.

Cole, L., and Deal, V. R. (Eds.). (In Press). *Communication disorders in multicultural populations.* Rockville, MD: American Speech-Language-Hearing Association.

Davis, L. E., and Gelsomino, J. (1994). An assessment of practitioner cross-racial treatment experiences. *Social Work, 39*(1), 116–123.

Devereaux, D. (1991). The issue of race and the client-therapist assignment. *Issues in Mental Health Nursing, 12*(3), 283–290.

Dresser, N. (1996). *Multicultural manners.* New York: John Wiley and Sons.

Dunn, R., and Griggs, S. A. (1990). Research on the learning style characteristics of selected racial and ethnic groups. *Journal of Reading, Writing, and Learning Disabilities International, 6*(3), 261–280.

Dunn, R. (1990). Cross-cultural differences in learning styles of elementary-age students from four ethnic backgrounds. *Journal of Multicultural Counseling and Development, 18*(2), 68–93.

Ferraro, K. F. (1993). Are Black older adults health-pessimistic? *Journal of Health and Social Behavior, 34*(3), 201–214.

Flaskerud, J. H. (1986). The effects of culture-compatible intervention on the utilization of mental health services by minority clients. *Community Mental Health Journal, 22*(2), 127–141.

Frankel, S. A. and Frankel, E. B. (1970). Nonverbal behavior in a selected group of Negro and white males. *Psychosomatics, 11*(2), 127–132.

Freed, A. O. (1992). Discussion: Minority elderly. Journal of Geriatric Psychiatry, 25(1), 105–111.

Garza, R. T., Lipton, J. P., and Isonio, S. A. (1989). Group ethnic composition, leader ethnicity, and task performance: An application of social identity theory. *Genetic, Social, and General Psychology Monographs, 115*(3), 295–314.

Goldberg, B., and Tidwell, R. (1990). Ethnicity and gender similarity: The effectiveness of counseling for adolescents. *Journal of Youth and Adolescence, 19*(6) 589–603

Goldstein, G.S. (1974). Behavior modification: Some cultural factors. *Psychological Record, 24*(1), 89–91.

Gollnick, D., and Chinn, P. (1990). *Multicultural education in a pluralistic society* (3rd ed.). NewYork: Merrill/Macmillian.

Goodenough, W. (1987). Multi-culturalism as the normal human experience. In E. M. Effy and W. L. Partridge (Eds.), *Applied anthropology in America* (2nd ed.). New York: Columbia University Press.

Gregory, K., Wells, K. B., and Leake, B. (1987) Medical students' expectations for encounters with minority and nonminority patients. *Journal of the National Medical Association, 79*(4), 403–408.

Griffith, E. E. (1986) Blacks and American psychiatry. *Hospital and Community Psychiatry, 37*(1), 5.

Hines, P. M., Garcia-Preto, N., McGoldrick, M., Almeida, R., et al. (1992). Intergenerational relationships across cultures. Special Issue: Multicultural practice. *Families in Society, 73*(6), 323–338.

Hains, A. A. and Fouad, N. A. (1994). The best laid plans . . . : Assessment in an inner-city high school. Special Issue: Multicultural assessment. *Measurement and Evaluation in Counseling and Development, 27*(2), 116–124.

Hall, L. E. and Tucker, C. M. (1985) Relationships between ethnicity, conceptions of mental illness, and attitudes associated with seeking psychological help. *Psychological Reports, 57*(3, Pt. 1), 907–916.

Harel, Z. (1986). Older Americans act related homebound aged: What difference does racial background make? Special Issue: Ethnicity and gerontological social work. *Journal of Gerontological Social Work, 9*(4), 133–143.

Haynes, N. M., and Gebreyesus, S. (1992). Cooperative learning: A case for African-American students. *School Psychology Review, 21*(4), 577–585.

Hector, M. A., and Fray, J. S. (1987). The counseling process, client expectations, and cultural influences: A review. *International Journal for the Advancement of Counselling, 10*(4) 237–247.

Herbert, J. T., and Cheatham, H. E. (1988). Africentricity and the Black disability experience: A theoretical orientation for rehabilitation counselors. *Journal of Applied Rehabilitation Counseling, 19*(4, Special Issue), 50–54.

Higgins, E., and Warner, R. (1975). Counseling blacks. *Personnel and Guidance Journal, 53,* 383–386.

Hoffman, L. W. (1988). Cross-cultural differences in childrearing goals. *New Directions for Child Development, 40,* 99–122.

Hunt, P. L. (1987). Black clients: Implications for supervision of trainees. Psychotherapy, 24(1), 114–119.

Jones, N. S. (1990). Black/White issues in psychotherapy: A framework for clinical practice. *Journal of Social Behavior and Personality, 5*(5), 305–322.

Kalyanpur, M., and Rao, S. S. (1991). Empowering low-income Black families of handicapped children. *American Journal of Orthopsychiatry, 61*(4), 523–532.

McNair, L. D. (1992). African American women in therapy: An Afrocentric and feminist synthesis. Special Issue: Finding voice: Writing by new authors. *Women and Therapy, 12*(1–2), 5–19.

Meadows, J. L. (1991). Multicultural communication. *Physical and Occupational Therapy in Pediatrics, 11*(4) 31–42.

Miller, S. D. (1993) Increasing the adjustment success of the disabled African American. *Journal of Health and Social Policy, 5* (2), 87–104

Nikelly, A. G., and Majors, R. G. (1986). Techniques for counseling Black students. *Techniques, 2*(1) 48–54.

O'Sullivan, M. J., Peterson, P. D., Cox, G. B., and Kirkeby, J. (1989). Ethnic populations: Community mental health services ten years later. *American Journal of Community Psychology, 17*(1), 17–30.

Screen, R. M. and Anderson, N. B. (1994). *Multicultural perspectives in communication disorders.* San Diego, CA: Singular Publishing Group.

Seymour, H. N., Ashton, N., and Wheeler, L. (1986). The effect of race on language elicitation. *Language, Speech, and Hearing Services in Schools, 17*(3), 146–151.

Spaights, E. (1990). The therapeutic implications of working with the Black family. *Journal of Instructional Psychology, 17*(4), 183–189.

Spolsky, B. (1972). The language education of minority children. In B. Spolsky (Ed.), *The language education of minority children* [pp. 1–10]. Rowley, MA: Newbury House.

Stevenson, H. C., and Renard, G. (1993). Trusting ole' wise owls: Therapeutic use of cultural strengths in African American families. 23rd Annual Mid-Winter Convention of Division 29 (Psychotherapy), 42 (Independent Practice), and 43 (Family Psychology) of the American Psychological Association (1992, Amelia Island Plantation, Florida). *Professional Psychology Research and Practice, 24*(4), 433–442.

Sykes, D. K. (1987). An approach to working with Black youth in cross cultural therapy. *Clinical Social Work Journal, 15*(3) 260–270.

Tien, J. L., and Johnson, H. L. (1985). Black mental health client's preference for therapists: A new look at an old issue. *International Journal of Social Psychiatry, 31*(4), 258–266.

Todisco, M., and Salomone, P. R. (1991). Facilitating effective cross-cultural relationships: The White counselor and the Black client. *Journal of Multicultural Counseling and Development, 19*(4), 146–157.

Vontress, C. E. (1974). Barriers in cross-cultural counseling. Counseling and Values, 18(3), 160-165.

Wade, P., and Bernstein, B. L. (1991). Culture sensitivity training and counselor's race: Effects on Black female clients' perceptions and attrition. *Journal of Counseling Psychology, 38*(1) 9–15.

Watkins, C. E., and Terrell, F. (1988). Mistrust level and its effects on counseling expectations in Black client-White counselor relationships: An analogue study. *Journal of Counseling Psychology, 35*(2), 194–197.

Watkins, C. E., Terrell, F., Miller, F. S., and Terrell, S. L. (1989). Cultural mistrust and its effects on expectational variables in Black client-White counselor relationships. *Journal of Counseling Psychology, 36*(4), 447–450.

Westermeyer, J. (1987). Cultural factors in clinical assessment. *Journal of Consulting and Clinical Psychology, 55*(4), 471–478.

Wetzel, C. G., and Wright-Buckley, C. (1988). Reciprocity of self-disclosure: Breakdowns of trust in cross-racial dyads. *Basic and Applied Social Psychology, 9*(4), 277–288.

Willis, J. T. (1988). An effective counseling model for treating the Black family. *Family Therapy, 15*(2), 185–194.

Wilson, L. L., and Stith, S. M. (1991). Culturally sensitive therapy with Black clients. *Journal of Multicultural Counseling and Development, 19*(1) 32–43

Yetman, N. R. (Ed.). (1985). *Majority and minority: The dynamics of race and ethnicity in American life* (4th ed.). Boston: Allyn and Bacon.

Ziter, M. L. (1987). Culturally sensitive treatment of Black alcoholic families. *Social Work, 32*(2), 130-135.

ASIAN AMERICANS/PACIFIC ISLANDERS

Agbayani-Stewart, P. (1994). Filipino American culture and family: Guidelines for practitioners. *Families in Society, 75*(7), 429–438.

Berg, J. H., and Wright-Buckley, C. (1988). Effects of racial similarity and interviewer intimacy in a peer counseling analogue. *Journal of Counseling Psychology, 35*(4), 377–384

Berg, I. K., and Miller, S. P. (1992). Working with Asian American clients: One person at a time. Special issue: Multicultural practice. *Families in Society, 73*(6), 356–363.

Berg, I. K., and Jaya, A. (1993). Different and same: Family therapy with Asian-American families. *Journal of Marital and Family Therapy, 19*(1), 31–38.

Chan, F., Hedl, J. J., Parker, H. J., Lam, C. S., et al. (1988). Differential attitudes of Chinese students toward people with disabilities: A cross-cultural perspective. *International Journal of Social Psychiatry, 34*(4) 267–273.

Chan, F, Lam, C. S., Wong, D., Leung, P., et al. (1988). Counseling Chinese Americans with disabilities. *Journal of Applied Rehabilitation Counseling, 19*(4, Spec Issue), 21–25.

Cheng, L. L. (1992). Objective: Recruitment-Asians and Pacific Islanders. *Asha, 34*, 41–42

Cheng, L. R. I. (1987). Cross cultural and linguistic considerations in working with Asian populations. *Asha, 29*, 33–37.

Cole, L., and Deal, V. R. (Eds.). (In Press). *Communication disorders in multicultural populations.* Rockville, MD: American Speech-Language-Hearing Association.

Cole, L. (1989). E pluribus pluribus: Multicultural imperatives for the 1990's and beyond. *Asha, 31*, 65–70.

Cole, L. (1992). We're serious. *Asha, 32*, 38–39.

Davis, L. E. and Gelsomino, J. (1994). An assessment of practitioner cross-racial treatment experiences. Social Work, 39(1), 116–123.

Devereaux, D. (1991). The issue of race and the client-therapist assignment. *Issues in Mental Health Nursing, 12*(3), 283–290.

Dresser, N. (1996). *Multicultural manners.* New York: John Wiley and Sons.

Dunn, R., and Griggs, S. A. (1990). Research on the learning style characteristics of selected racial and ethnic groups. *Journal of Reading, Writing, and Learning Disabilities International, 6*(3), 261–280.

Durvasula, R. S., and Mylvaganam, G. A. (1994) Mental health of Asian Indians: Relevant issues and community implications. Special Issue: Asian-American mental health. *Journal of Community Psychology, 22*(2), 97–108

Exum, H. A., and Lau, E. (1988). Counseling style preference of Chinese college students. *Journal of Multicultural Counseling and Development, 16*(2), 84–92.

Farver, J. A., and Howes, C. (1988). Cross-cultural differences in social interaction: A comparison of American and Indonesian children. *Journal of Cross-Cultural Psychology, 19*(2), 203–215.

Flaskerud, J. H. (1986). The effects of culture-compatible intervention on the utilization of mental health services by minority clients. *Community Mental Health Journal, 22*(2), 127–141.

Freed, A. O. (1992). Discussion: Minority elderly. *Journal of Geriatric Psychiatry, 25*(1), 105–111.

Garza, R. T., Lipton, J. P., and Isonio, S. A. (1989). Group ethnic composition, leader ethnicity, and task performance: An application of social identity theory. *Genetic, Social, and General Psychology Monographs, 115*(3), 295–314.

Gim, R. H., Atkinson, D. R., and Whiteley, S. (1990). Asian-American acculturation, severity of concerns, and willingness to see a counselor. *Journal of Counseling Psychology, 37*(3), 281–285.

Goldberg, B., and Tidwell, R. (1990). Ethnicity and gender similarity: The effectiveness of counseling for *adolescents. Journal of Youth and Adolescence, 19*(6) 589–603

Goldstein, G. S. (1974). Behavior modification: Some cultural factors. *Psychological Record, 24*(1), 89–91.

Gollnick, D., and Chinn, P. (1990). *Multicultural education in a pluralistic society* (3rd ed.). New York: Merrill/Macmillian.

Goodenough, W. (1987). Multi-culturalism as the normal human experience. In E. M. Effy and W. L. Partridge (Eds.), *Applied anthropology in America* (2nd ed.). New York: Columbia University Press.

Gregory, K., Wells, K. B., and Leake, B. (1987) Medical students' expectations for encounters with minority and nonminority patients. *Journal of the National Medical Association, 79*(4), 403–408.

Hains, A. A., and Fouad, N. A. (1994). The best laid plans . . . : Assessment in an inner-city high school. Special Issue: Multicultural assessment. *Measurement and Evaluation in Counseling and Development, 27*(2), 116–124.

Hall, L. E. and Tucker, C. M. (1985) Relationships between ethnicity, conceptions of mental illness, and attitudes associated with seeking psychological help. *Psychological Reports, 57*(3, Pt. 1), 907–916.

Harel, Z. (1986). Older Americans act related homebound aged: What difference does racial background make? Special Issue: Ethnicity and gerontological social work. *Journal of Gerontological Social Work, 9*(4), 133–143.

Hector, M. A., and Fray, J. S. (1987). The counseling process, client expectations, and cultural influences: A review. *International Journal for the Advancement of Counselling, 10*(4) 237–247.

Hines, P. M., Garcia-Preto, N., McGoldrick, M., Almeida, R., et al. (1992). Intergenerational relationships across cultures. Special Issue: Multicultural practice. *Families in Society, 73*(6), 323–338.

Hoffman, L. W. (1988). Cross-cultural differences in childrearing goals. *New Directions for Child Development, 40,* 99–122.

Kinzie, J. D., Leung, P., Bui, A., Ben, R., et al. (1988). Group therapy with Southeast Asian refugees. *Community Mental Health Journal, 24*(2), 157–166.

McQuaide, S. (1989). Working with Southeast Asian refugees. *Clinical Social Work Journal, 17*(2), 165–176.

Meadows, J. L. (1991). Multicultural communication. *Physical and Occupational Therapy in Pediatrics, 11*(4) 31–42.

O'Sullivan, M. J., Peterson, P. D., Cox, G. B., and Kirkeby, J. (1989). Ethnic populations: Community mental health services ten years later. *American Journal of Community Psychology, 17*(1), 17–30.

Screen, R. M., and Anderson, N. B. (1994). *Multicultural perspectives in communication disorders.* San Diego, CA: Singular Publishing Group.

Seymour, H. N., Ashton, N., and Wheeler, L. (1986). The effect of race on language elicitation. *Language, Speech, and Hearing Services in Schools, 17*(3), 146–151.

Spolsky, B. (1972). The language education of minority children. In B. Spolsky (Ed.), *The language education of minority children* (pp. 1–10). Rowley, MA: Newbury House.

Sue, S., Fujino, D. C., Hu, L. , Takeuchi, D.T., et al. (1991). Community mental health services for ethnic minority groups: A test of the cultural responsiveness hypothesis. *Journal of Consulting and Clinical Psychology, 59*(4), 533–540.

Takeuchi, D. T., Mokuau, N., and Chun, C. A. (1992). Mental health services for Asian Americans and Pacific Islanders. Special Issue: Multicultural mental health and substance abuse services. *Journal of Mental Health Administration, 19*(3), 237–245.

Tamura, T., and Lau, A. (1992). Connectedness versus separateness: Applicability of family therapy to Japanese families. *Family Process, 31*(4), 319-340.

Tedeschi, G. J., and Willis, F. N. (1993). Attitudes toward counseling among Asian international and native Caucasian students. *Journal of College Student Psychotherapy 7*(4), 43–54.

Vontress, C. E. (1974). Barriers in cross-cultural counseling. *Counseling and Values, 18*(3), 160–165.

Watkins, D., and Ismail, M. (1994). Is the Asian learner a rote learner? A Malaysian perspective. *Contemporary Educational Psychology, 19*(4), 483–488.

Westermeyer, J. (1987). Cultural factors in clinical assessment. *Journal of Consulting and Clinical Psychology, 55*(4), 471–478.

Wetzel, C. G., and Wright-Buckley, C. (1988). Reciprocity of self-disclosure: Breakdowns of trust in cross-racial dyads. *Basic and Applied Social Psychology, 9*(4), 277–288.

Yetman, N. R. (Ed.). (1985). *Majority and minority: The dynamics of race and ethnicity in American life* (4th ed.). Boston: Allyn and Bacon.

Dunn, R. (1990). Cross-cultural differences in learning styles of elementary-age students from four ethnic backgrounds. *Journal of Multicultural Counseling and Development, 18*(2), 68–93.

BEHAVIORAL MANAGEMENT

Bandura, A. (1969). *Principles of behavior modification*. New York: Holt, Rinehart and Winston.

Barnes, D., and Keenan, M. (1993). Concurrent activities and instructed human fixed-interval performance. *Journal of the Experimental Analysis of Behavior, 59*(3), 501–520.

Baroff, G. S. (1976). On the use of aversive techniques in controlling self-injurious behavior. *American Psychologist, 31*(8), 616.

Costello, J. M. (1980). Operant conditioning and the treatment of stuttering. Seminars in Speech, *Language and Hearing, 1*, 311–325.

Costello, J. (1982). Techniques of therapy based on operant conditioning. In W. Perkins (Ed.), *General principles of therapy*. New York: Thieme-Stratton.

Costello, J., and Ingham, R. J. (1984). Stuttering as an operant disorder. In R. Curlee and W. Perkins (Eds.), *Nature and treatment of stuttering*. San Diego, CA: College-Hill Press.

Durdic, S. (1983). Odnos izmedu terapeuta I pacijenta u bihejvior psihoterapiji [The therapist-patient relationship in behavioral psychotherapy]. *Psihijatrija Danas, 15*(2–3), 265–269

Ferster, C. B. (1957). Withdrawal of positive reinforcement as punishment. *Science, 126*, 509.

Goldstein, G. S. (1974). Behavior modification: Some cultural factors. *Psychological Record, 24*(1), 89–91.

Holland, A. L. (1967). Some applications of behavioral principles to clinical speech problems. *Journal of Speech and Hearing Disorders, 32*, 11–18.

Hollander, M., and Kazaoka, K. (1988). Behavior therapy groups. In S. Long (Ed.), *Six group therapies* (pp. 257–326). New York: Plenum.

Ingham, R. J. (1984). Stuttering and behavior therapy: Current status and experimental foundations. San Diego, CA: College-Hill Press.

Jochums, B. L. (1989). Behavioral versus insight-oriented marital therapy: Labels can be misleading. Counseling and curriculum opportunities in the training of disadvantaged adults. *College Student Journal, 23*(3), 243–250

Kendall, P. C. (1984). Cognitive processes and procedures in behavior therapy. *Annual Review of Behavior Therapy Theory and Practice, 9*, 132–179.

Koocher, G. P. (1976). Civil liberties and aversive conditioning for children. *American Psychologist, 31*(1), 94–95.

Lovaas, O. I., Freitag, G., Gold, V. J. and Kassorla, I. C. (1965). Experimental studies in childhood schizophrenia: Analysis of self-destructive behavior. *Journal of Experimental Child Psychology, 2*, 67–84.

Lovaas, O. I. (1966). A program for the establishment of speech in psychotic children. In J.K. Wing (Ed.), *Early childhood autism*. New York: Pergamon.

Meichenbaum, D. (1977). *Cognitive-behavior modification*. New York: Plenum Press.

Shames, G. H., and Sherrick, C. E., Jr. (1963). A discussion of nonfluency and stuttering as operant behavior. *Journal of Speech and Hearing Disorders, 28*, 13–18.

Skinner, B. F. (1953). *Science and human behavior*. New York: MacMillan.

Sloane, H. N., Jr., and MacAulay, B. D., (Eds.). (1968). *Operant procedures in remedial speech and language training*. New York: Houghton Mifflin Co.

Wilson, G. T. (1989). Behavior therapy. In R. J. Corsini and D. Wedding (Eds.), *Current psychotherapies,* (4th ed., pp. 241–282). Itasca, IL: Peacock.

Wilson, G. T. (1984). Clinical issues and strategies in the practice of behavior therapy. *Annual Review of Behavior Therapy Theory and Practice, 10*, 291–320.

CHILDREN

Forlin, C., and Cole, P. (1994). Attributions of the social acceptance and integration of children with mild intellectual disability. *Australia and New Zealand Journal of Developmental Disabilities, 19*(1), 11–23

Gardner, R. A. (1982). *Psychotherapeutic approaches to the resistant child*. New York: Aronson.

Silverman, W. K., La Greca, A. M., and Wasserstein, S. (1995) What do children worry about? Worries and their relation to anxiety. *Child Development, 66*(3), 671–686

Walker, H. M. (1979). *The acting-out child*. Boston: Allyn and Bacon.

Walsh, M. E., and Buckley, M. A. (1994). Children's experiences of homelessness: Implications for school counselors. *Elementary School Guidance and Counseling, 29*(1) 9–15.

Williams, C., and Bybee, J. (1994). What do children feel guilty about? Developmental and gender differences. *Developmental Psychology, 30*(5) ,617–623.

CLINICAL TRAINING ISSUES

Barnes, H. N., O'Neill, S. F., Aronson, M. D., and Delbanco, T. L. (1984). Early detection and outpatient management of alcoholism: a curriculum for medical residents. *Journal of Medical Education, 59*(11, Pt 1), 904–906

Baum, B. E., and Gray, J. (1992). Expert modeling, self-observation using videotape, and acquisition of basic therapy skills. *Professional Psychology Research and Practice, 23*(3) 220–225.

Berger, M. M. (1978). *Videotape techniques in psychiatric training and treatment*. New York: Brunner/Mazel.

Chevron, E. S., Rounsaville, B. J., Rothblum, E. D., and Weissman, M. M. (1983). Selecting psychotherapists to participate in psychotherapy outcome studies: Relationship between psychotherapist characteristics and assessment of clinical skills. *Journal of Nervous and Mental Disease, 171*(6), 348–353.

Cohn, E. S. (1989). Fieldwork education: Shaping a foundation for clinical reasoning. *American Journal of Occupational Therapy, 43*(4), 240–244.

Das, A. K., and Littrell, J. M. (1989). Multicultural education for counseling: A reply to Lloyd. *Counselor Education and Supervision, 29*(1), 7–15.

Dorpat, T. L. (1993). Clinical education: 1: Response. *Journal of Clinical Psychoanalysis, 2*(3), 318–320

Dowling, S. (1986). Supervisory training: Impetus for clinical supervision. *Clinical Supervisor, 4*(4), 27–34.

Dreyfus, H. L., and Dreyfus, S. E. (1986). *Mind over machine*. New York: The Free Press.

Sharf, R. S., and Lucas, M. (1993). An assessment of a computerized simulation of counseling skills. *Counselor Education and Supervision, 32*(4), 254–266.

Durlak, J. A. (1979). Comparative effectiveness of paraprofessional and professional helpers. *Psychological Bulletin, 86*(1), 80–92.

Gallant, J. P., Thyer, B. A., and Bailey, J. S. (1991). Using bug-in-the-ear feedback in clinical supervision: Preliminary evaluations. *Research on Social Work Practice, 1*(2), 175–187

Goldberg, S. A. (1990 November). *Identification of clinical skills and their relationship to clinical training*. Presented at the *American Speech-Language-Hearing Association Annual Convention*. Seattle, WA.

Goldstein, M. D., Hopkins, J. R., and Strube, M. J. (1994). The eye of the beholder: A classroom demonstration of observer bias. *Teaching of Psychology, 21*(3), 154–157.

Hanser, S. B., and Furman, C. E. (1980). The effect of videotape-based feedback vs. field-based feedback on the development of applied clinical skills. *Journal of Music Therapy, 17*(3) 103–112.

Hunt, P. L. (1987). Black clients: Implications for supervision of trainees. *Psychotherapy, 24*(1), 114–119.

Hynan, M. T. (1981). On the advantages of assuming that the techniques of psychotherapy are ineffective. *Psychotherapy Theory, Research and Practice, 18*(1), 11–13.

Jackson, E. (1985). Peer rated therapeutic talent and affective sensitivity: A multiple regression approach. *Psychology: A Quarterly Journal of Human Behavior, 22*(3-4), 28–35.

Klitzke, M. J., and Lombardo, T. W. (1991). A "bug-in-the-eye" can be better than a "bug-in-the-ear": A teleprompter technique for online therapy skills training, *Behavior Modification, 15*(1), 113–117.

Levy, L. H. (1983). Evaluation of students in clinical psychology programs: A program evaluation perspective. *Professional Psychology Research and Practice, 14*(4), 497–503

Loschen, E. L. (1993). Using the objective structured clinical examination in a psychiatry residency. *Academic Psychiatry, 17*(2) 95–104.

Marek, L. I., Sandifer, D. M., Beach, A., Coward, R. L., et al. (1994). Supervision without the problem: A model of solution-focused supervision. *Journal of Family Psychotherapy, 5*(2), 57–64

Mayadas, N. S., and Duehn, W. D. (1977). The effects of training formats and interpersonal discriminations in education for clinical social work practice. *Journal of Social Service Research, 1*(2) 147–161

Mir, M. A., Evans, R. W., Marshall, R. J., Newcombe, R. G., et al. (1989). The use of video recordings of medical postgraduates in improving clinical skills. *Medical Education, 23*(3), 276–281

Neufeldt, S. A. (1994). Use of a manual to train supervisors. *Counselor Education and Supervision, 33*(4) 327–336.

Patterson, L. E., Rak, C. F., Chermonte, J., and Roper, W. (1992). Automaticity as a factor in counselor skills acquisition. *Canadian Journal of Counseling, 26*(3), 189–200.

Pletts, M. (1981). Principles and practice of clinical teaching—a need for structure. *British Journal of Disorders of Communication, 16*(2), 129–134

Powell, T. W., Gospel, M. D., and Williams, A. L. (1991). Attitudes toward the clinical supervisory model: Results from in service training. *Clinical Supervisor, 9*(2) 53–62.

Rosenkrantz, A. L. and Holmes, G. R. (1974). A pilot study of clinical internship training at the William S. Hall Psychiatric Institute. *Journal of Clinical Psychology, 30*(3), 417–419.

Seymour, C. M. (1992). Objective: Recruitment-mentoring fosters leadership. *Asha 34*, 45–46.

Shames, G. H. (1989). Stuttering: An RFP for a cultural perspective. *Journal of Fluency Disorders, 14*, 67–77.

Shapiro, D. A., and Anderson, J. L. (1988). An analysis of commitments made by student clinicians in speech-language pathology and audiology. *Journal of Speech and Hearing Disorders, 53*(2), 202–210.

Shapiro, D. A., and Anderson, J. L. (1989). One measure of supervisory effectiveness in speech-language pathology and audiology. *Journal of Speech and Hearing Disorders, 54*(4), 549–557.

Sommers-Flanagan, J., and Sommers-Flanagan, R. (1989). A categorization of pitfalls common to beginning interviews. *Journal of Training and Practice in Professional Psychology, 3*(1), 58–71.

Sriram, T. G., Chandrashekar, C. R., Isaac, M. K., and Srinivasa-Murthy, R. (1990). Development of case vignettes to assess the mental health training of primary care medical officers. *Acta Psychiatrica Scandinavica, 82*(2), 174—177.

Stackhouse, J., and Furnham, A. (1983). A student-centered approach to the evaluation of clinical skills. *British Journal of Disorders of Communication 18*(3), 171–179.

Stillman, P. L., Regan, M. B., Swanson, D. B., and Case, S., et al. (1990). An assessment of the clinical skills of fourth-year students at four New England medical schools. *Academic Medicine, 65*(5), 320–326.

Swanson, D. B., and Stillman, P. L. (1990). Use of standardized patients for teaching and assessing clinical skills. Special Issue: Reflections on research in medical problem solving. *Evaluation and the Health Professions, 13*(1), 79–103.

Taylor, O. (1989). Old wine and new bottles: Some things change yet remain the same, *Asha, 31*(9), 72–73.

Tuters, E. (1988). The relevance of infant observation to clinical training and practice: An interpretation. *Infant Mental Health Journal, 9*(1), 93–104.

Tyler, J. D., and Clar, J. A. (1985). Promoting clinical expertise in academic faculty supervisors. *Professional Psychology Research and Practice, 16*(6), 902–904.

Uhlemann, M. R., Lee, D. Y., and Martin, J. (1993). Perceptions of counselors' intentions with high versus low quality counselor responses. *Canadian Journal of Counseling, 27*(2), 104–112.

Van der Vleuten, C. P., and Swanson, D. B. (1990). Assessment of clinical skills with standardized patients: State of the art. *Teaching and Learning in Medicine, 2*(2), 58–76

Volz, H. B., Klevans, D. R., Norton, S. J., and Putens, D. L. (1978) Interpersonal communication skills of speech-language pathology undergraduates: The effects of training. *Journal of Speech and Hearing Disorders, 43*(4), 524–541.

Vrugt, A. (1990). Negative attitudes, nonverbal behavior and self-fulfilling prophecy in simulated therapy interviews. *Journal of Nonverbal Behavior, 14*(2), 77–86.

Vu, N. V., Barrows, H. S., Marcy, M. L., and Verhulst, S. J., et al. (1992). Six years of comprehensive, clinical, performance-based assessment using standardized patients at the Southern Illinois University School of Medicine. *Academic Medicine, 67*(1), 42–50.

Wade, P., and Bernstein, B. L. (1991). Culture sensitivity training and counselor's race: Effects on Black female clients' perceptions and attrition. *Journal of Counseling Psychology, 38*(1) 9–15.

Weiss, S. J. (1984). The effect of transition modules on new graduate adaptation. Research in *Nursing and Health, 7*(1), 51–59.

COLLABORATION/INCLUSION

Albano, M., Cox, B., York, J., and York, R. (1981). Educational teams for students with severe and multiple handicaps. In R. York, W. K. Schofield, D. J. Donder, D. L. Ryndak, and B. Reguly (Eds.), *Organizing and implementing services for students with severe and multiple handicaps*, (pp. 23–24). Springfield: Illinois State Board of Education.

Bricker, W .A., and Campbell, P. (1980). Interdisciplinary assessment and programming for multihandicapped students. In W. Sailor, B. Wilcox, and L. Brown (Eds.), *Methods of instruction for severely handicapped students* (pp. 3–45). Baltimore: Paul H. Brookes.

Coufal, K. L. (1993). Collaborative consultation for speech-language pathologists. *Topics in Language Disorders, 14*(1), 1–14.

Fine, M. J., and Gardner, A. (1994). Collaborative consultation with families of children with special needs: Why bother? *Journal of Educational and Psychological Consultation, 5*(4), 283–308.

Fox, L. (1989). Stimulus generalization of skills and persons with profound mental handicaps. *Education and Training in Mental Retardation 24*(3), 219–229

Giangreco, M. (1989). Making related service decisions for students with severe handicaps in public schools: Roles, criteria, and authority. *Dissertation Abstracts International, 50*, 1624A. (University Microfilms No. DA8919516)

Griener, T. (1992). Objective: Recruitment—Public schools. *Asha, 34*, 40–41

Hanson, M. J., and Lovett, D. (1992). Personnel preparation for early interventionists: A cross-disciplinary survey. *Journal of Early Intervention, 16*(2), 123–135.

Henriksen, E. M. (1991). A peer helping program for the middle school. *Canadian Journal of Counselling, 25*(1), 12–18.

Karge, B. D., McClure, M., and Patton, P. L. (1995). The success of collaboration resource programs for students with disabilities in Grades 6 through 8. *Remedial and Special Education, 16*(2), 79–89.

Lyon, S., and Lyon, G. (1980). Team functioning and staff development: A role release approach to providing integrated educational services for severely handicapped students. *Journal of the Association for the Severely Handicapped, 5*(3), 250–263.

Myrick, R. D., Highland, W. H., and Sabella, R. A. (1995). Peer helpers and perceived effectiveness. *Elementary School Guidance and Counseling, 29*(4), 278–288

Prelock, P. A. (1995). Rethinking collaboration: A speech-language pathology perspective. *Journal of Educational and Psychological Consultation, 6*(1), 95–99.

Rainforth, B., York, J., Macdonald, C., and Dunn, R. (1992). Collaborative Assessment. In Rainforth, B., York, J., and Macdonald C. (Eds.), *Collaborative teams for students with severe disabilities*. Baltimore: Paul H. Brookes.

Sailor, W. S. (1991). Special education in the restructured school. *Remedial and Special Education, 12*(6), 8–22.

Vandercook, T., and York, J. (1990). A team approach to program development and support. In W. Stainback, and S. Stainback (Eds.), *Support networks for inclusive schooling: Interdependent integrated education* (pp. 95–122). Baltimore: Paul H. Brookes.

DISABILITY ISSUES

Beckwith, J. B. (1994). Prejudice, reverse prejudice, and positive attitude towards differences among people with intellectual disabilities. *Psychological Reports, 74*(3, Pt. 1), 938.

Darrow, A. A., and Johnson, C. M. (1994). Junior and senior high school music student's attitudes toward individuals with a disability. *Journal of Music Therapy, 31*(4), 266–279.

Esten, G., and Willmott, L. (1993) Double bind messages: The effects of attitude towards disability on therapy. *Special Issue: Women with disabilities: Found voices Women and Therapy 14*(3-4), 29–41.

Forlin, C., and Cole, P. (1994). Attributions of the social acceptance and integration of children with mild intellectual disability. *Australia and New Zealand Journal of Developmental Disabilities, 19*(1), 11–23

Keany, K. C., and Glueckauf, R. L. (1993). Disability and value change: An overview and reanalysis of acceptance of loss theory. *Rehabilitation Psychology, 38*(3), 199–210

Law, M., and Dunn, W. (1993) Perspectives on understanding and changing the environments of children with disabilities. *Physical and Occupational Therapy in Pediatrics, 13*(3), 1–17.

Lee, T. M. C., and Rodda, M. (1994) Modification of attitudes toward people with disabilities. *Canadian Journal of Rehabilitation, 7*(4), 229–238

Lindstrom, B., and Kohler, L. (1991). Youth, disability and quality of life. *Pediatrician, 18*(2), 121–128

McKirnan, D. J., and Hamayan, E. V. (1984). Speech norms and attitudes toward outgroup members: A test of a model in a bicultural context. *Journal of Language and Social Psychology, 3,* 21–38.

Nosek, M. A., Fuhrer, M. J., and Hughes, S. O. (1991). Perceived counselor credibility bypersons with physical disability: Influence of counselor disability status, professional status, and the counseling content. Rehabilitation *Psychology, 36*(3), 153–161.

Smart, J. F., and Smart, D. W. (1991). Acceptance of disability and the Mexican American culture. *Rehabilitation Counseling Bulletin, 34*(4) 357–367.

Heller, T., Markwardt, R., Rowitz, L., and Farber, B. (1994). Adaptation of Hispanic families to a member with mental retardation. *American Journal on Mental Retardation, 99*(3), 289–300

Szivos, S. E., and Griffiths, E. (1990). Group processes involved in coming to terms with a mentally retarded identity. *Mental Retardation; 28*(6) 333–341.

Weisel, A., and Florian, V. (1990). Same- and cross-gender attitudes toward persons with physical disabilities. *Rehabilitation Psychology, 35*(4), 229–238.

Westbrook, M. T., and Legge, V. (1993). Health practitioners' perceptions of family attitudes toward children with disabilities: A comparison of six communities in a multicultural society. *Rehabilitation Psychology, 38*(3), 177–185.

ELDERLY

Florsheim, M. J., and Herr, J. J. (1990). Family counseling with elders. Special Issue: Counseling and therapy for elders. *Generations, 14*(1), 40–42.

Freed, A. O. (1992). Discussion: Minority elderly. *Journal of Geriatric Psychiatry, 25*(1), 105–111.

Gross, D. (1990). Communication and the elderly. *Physical and Occupational Therapy in Geriatrics, 9*(1), 49–64.

Harel, Z. (1986). Older Americans act related homebound aged: What difference does racial background make? Special Issue: Ethnicity and gerontological social work. *Journal of Gerontological Social Work, 9*(4), 133–143.

Hawkins, K. W. (1995). Effects of gender and communication content of leadership emergence in small task-oriented groups. *Small Group Research, 26*(2), 234–249.

Hersen, M., and Van Hasselt, V. B. (1992). Behavioral assessment and treatment of anxiety in the elderly. *Clinical Psychology Review, 12*(6), 619–640.

Hines, P. M., Garcia-Preto, N., McGoldrick, M., Almeida, R., et al. (1992). Intergenerational relationships across cultures. Special Issue: Multicultural practice. *Families in Society, 73*(6), 323–338.

Hittner, A., and Bornstein, H. (1990). Group counseling with older adults: Coping with late-onset hearing impairment. Special Issue: Techniques for counseling older persons. *Journal of Mental Health Counseling, 12*(3), 332–341.

Newbern, V. B. (1992). Failure to thrive: A growing concern in the elderly. *Journal of Gerontological Nursing, 18*(8), 21–25.

Rogers, W. A., and Fisk, A. D. (1990). A reconsideration of age-related reaction time slowing from a learning perspective: Age-related slowing is not just complexity-based. Special Issue: Frontiers of learning and individual differences: Paradigms in transition. *Learning and Individual Differences, 2*(2) 161–179.

Ryan, E. B., Hamilton, J. M., and See, S. K. (1994). Patronizing the old: How do younger and older adults respond to baby talk in the nursing home? Special Issue: Intergenerational communication. *International Journal of Aging and Human Development, 39*(1) 21–32.

Weeks, J. R., and Cuellar, J. B. (1983). Isolation of older persons; The influence of immigration and length of residence. *Research on Aging, 5*(3), 369–388.

FAMILY THERAPY/PARENT TRAINING AND THERAPY

Alexander, J. F. and Newberry, A.M. (1988) The interview process in functional family therapy. *Family Therapy Collections, Sum, 24,* 33–48.

Andrews, J. A., and Andrews, M. (1990). *Family based treatment in communicative disorders—a systemic approach.* Sandwich, IL: Janelle Publications.

Christenson, S. L., and Cleary, M. (1990). Consultation and the parent-educator partnership: A perspective. *Journal of Educational and Psychological Consultation, 1*(3) 219–241.

Crais, E. (1991). Moving from "parent involvement" to family-centered services. *American Journal of Speech-Language Pathology, 1,* 5–8.

Donahue-Kilburg, G. (1992). *Family-centered early intervention for communication disorders,* Gaithersburg, MD: Aspen Publishers.

Ellinwood, C. (1989). The young child in person-centered family therapy. Special Issue: Person-centered ability, affective states, and psychological distress. *Journal of Counseling Psychology, 42*(1), 105–115.

Feldman, P. (1994). The use of therapeutic questions to restructure dysfunctional triangles in marital therapy: A psychodynamic family therapy approach. *Journal of Family Psychotherapy, 5*(3) 55–67.

Florsheim, M. J., and Herr, J. J. (1990). Family counseling with elders. Special Issue: Counseling and therapy for elders. *Generations, 14*(1), 40–42.

Franklin, A. J. (1992). Therapy with African American men. Special Issue: Multicultural practice. *Families in Society, 73*(6), 350–355.

Gesuelle-Hart, S., Kaplan, L. W., and Kikoski, C. (1990). Assessing the family in context. Special Issue: Working with the urban poor. *Journal of Strategic and Systemic Therapies, 9*(3), 1–13.

Knafl, K., Breitmayer, B., Gallo, A., and Zoeller, L. (1992). Parents' views of health care providers: An exploration of the components of a positive working relationship. *Children's Health Care, 21*(2) 90–95.

Nangle, D. W., Carr-Nagle, R. E., and Hansen, D. J. (1994). Enhancing generalization of a contingency-management intervention through the use of family problem-solving training: Evaluation with a severely conduct-disordered adolescent. *Child and Family Behav-ior Therapy, 16*(2), 65–76.

Pfiffner, L. J., Jouriles, E. N., Brown, M. M., Etscheidt, M. A., et al. (1990). Effects of prob-lem-solving therapy on outcomes of parent training for single-parent families. *Child and Family Behavior Therapy, 12*(1), 1–11.

Piercy, F., and Sprenkle, D. (1986). *Family therapy source book.* New York: Guilford.

Rettig, K. D. (1993). Problem-solving and decision-making as central processes of family life: An ecological framework for family relations and family resource management. *Marriage and Family Review, 18*(304), 187–222.

Rueter, M. A., and Conger, R. D. (1995). Interaction style, problem-solving behavior, and family problem-solving effectiveness. *Child Development. 66*(1) 98–115.

Satir, V. (1967). *Conjoint family therapy* (rev. ed.). Palo Alto, CA: Science and Behavior Books.

Sayger, T. V., Szykula, S. A., and Laylander, J. A. (1991). Adolescent-focused family counseling: A comparison of behavioral and strategic approaches. *Journal of Family Psychotherapy, 2*(3), 57–80.

Schultz, C. L., Kemm, M. A., Bruce, E. J., and Smyrnios, K. X. (1992). Caring for fathers and mothers of children with intellectual disability: A pilot study. *Australia and New Zealand Journal of Developmental Disabilities, 18*(1), 45–56.

Smith, S. E. (1994). Parent-initiated contracts: An intervention for school-related behaviors. *Elementary School Guidance and Counseling, 28*(3), 182–187.

Spaights, E. (1990). The therapeutic implications of working with the Black family. *Journal of Instructional Psychology, 17*(4), 183–189.

Tamura, T., and Lau, A. (1992). Connectedness versus separateness: Applicability of family therapy to Japanese families. *Family Process, 31*(4), 319–340.

Webster-Stratton, C., and Herbert, M. (1993). What really happens in parent training? *Behavior Modification, 17*(4), 407–456.

Wieselberg, H. (1992). Family therapy and ultra-orthodox Jewish families: A structural approach. *Journal of Family Therapy, 14*(3), 305–329.

Wilkinson, W. K., Parrish, J. M., and Wilson, F. E. (1994) Training parents to observe and record: A data-based outcome evaluation of a pilot curriculum. *Research in Developmental Disabilities, 15*(5), 343–354.

Willis, J. T. (1988). An effective counseling model for treating the Black family. *Family Therapy, 15*(2), 185–194.

Zeskind, P. S. (1983). Cross-cultural differences in maternal perceptions of cries of low- and high-risk infants. *Child Development, 54*(5), 1119–1128.

Ziter, M. L. (1987). Culturally sensitive treatment of Black alcoholic families. *Social Work, 32*(2), 130–135.

FEEDBACK

Chen, L. C. (1990). The effects of attributional feedback and strategy training on achievement behaviors with mathematical learning disabled students. *Bulletin of Educational Psychology, 23*, 143–158.

Hatfield, E., Hsee, C. K., Costello, J., Weisman, M. S., and et al. (1995). The impact of vocal feedback on emotional experience and expression. *Journal of Social Behavior and Personality, 10*(2), 293–312.

Miller, A. D., Hall, S. W., and Heard, W. L. (1995). Effects of sequential 1-minute time trials with and without inter-trial feedback and self-correlation on general and special education students' fluency with math facts. *Journal of Behavioral Education 5*(3), 319–345.

Morran, D. K., Stockton, R., and Bond, L. (1991) Delivery of positive and corrective feedback in counseling groups. *Journal of Counseling Psychology, 38*(4), 410–414.

Salas, S. B., and Dickinson, D. J. (1990). The effect of feedback and three different types of corrections on student learning. *Journal of Human Behavior and Learning, 7*(2), 13–19.

Schunk, D. H., and Rice, J. M. (1993). Strategy fading and progress feedback: Effects on self-efficacy and comprehension among students receiving remedial reading services. *Journal of Special Education, 27*(3), 257–276.

Schutz, P. A. (1993). Additional influences on response certitude and feedback requests. *Contemporary Educational Psychology, 18*(4), 427–441.

Smith, V. L., and Clark, H. H. (1993). On the course of answering questions. *Journal of Memory and Language, 32*(1), 25–38.

GENDER/SEXUAL ORIENTATION

Barfield, J. (1976). Biological influences on sex differences in behavior. In M. S. Teitelbaum (Ed.), *Sex differences: Social and biological*

perspectives (pp. 62–121). Garden City, NY: Anchor Press.

Buenting, J. A. (1992). Health life-styles of lesbian and heterosexual women. Special issue: Lesbian health: What are the issues? *Health Care for Women International, 13*(2), 165–171.

Cameron, C. (1994). Women survivors confronting their abusers: Issues, decisions, and outcomes. *Journal of Child Sexual Abuse, 3*(1), 7–35.

Carter, R. T., and Helms, J. E. (1992) The counseling process as defined by relationship types: A test of Helms's interactional model. Special Issue: Gender and relationships. *Journal of Multicultural Counseling and Development, 20*(4), 181–201

Clutton-Brock, T. H., and Parker, G. A. (1995). Sexual coercion in animal societies. *Animal Behaviour, 49*(5), 1345–1365.

Cramer, P., and Skidd, J. E. (1992). Correlates of self-worth in preschoolers: The role of gender-stereotyped styles of behavior. *Sex Role, 26*(9–10), 369–390.

Frazier, N., and Sadker, M. (1973). *Sexism in school and society.* New York: Harper and Row.

Galea, L. A., and Kimura, D. (1993). Sex differences in route-learning. *Personality and Individual Differences, 14*(1), 53–65.

Giles, S., and Dryden, W. (1991). Fears about seeking therapeutic help: The effect of sex on subjects, sex of professional, and title of professional. *British Journal of Guidance and Counseling, 19*(1) 81–92.

Goldberg, B., and Tidwell, R. (1990). Ethnicity and gender similarity: The effectiveness of counseling for adolescents. *Journal of Youth and Adolescence, 19*(6), 589–603

Kratz, N. A., and Marshall, L. L. (1988). First impressions: Analog experiment on counselor behavior and gender. *Representative Research in Social Psychology, 18*(1), 41–50

LeCroy, C. W. (1986). An analysis of the effects of gender on outcome in group treatment with young adolescents. *Journal of Youth and Adolescence, 15*, 497–508.

Lundberg, M. A., Fox, P. W., and Punccohar, J. (1994). Highly confident but wrong: Gender differences and similarities in confidence judgments. *Journal of Educational Psychology, 86*(1) 114–121.

Maccoby, E. E. (1990). Gender and relationships: A developmental account. American Psychological Association: Distinguished

Scientific Contributions Award Address (1989, New Orleans, LA). *American Psychologist, 45*(4), 513–520.

Manolis, M. B. and Milich, R. (1993). Gender differences in social persistence. *Journal of Social and Clinical Psychology, 12*(4), 385–405.

Martinez, M. E. (1992). Interest enhancements to science experiments: Interactions with student gender. *Journal of Research in Science Teaching, 29*(2), 167–177.

McMullen, L. M., and Pasloski, D. D. (1992). Effects of communication apprehension, familiarityof partner, and topic on selected "women's language" features. Annual Convention of the Canadian Psychological Association (1990, Ottawa, Canada). *Journal of Psycholinguistic Research, 21*(1), 17–30.

McNair, L. D. (1992). African American women in therapy: An Afrocentric and feminist synthesis. Special Issue: Finding voice: Writing by new authors. *Women and Therapy, 12*(1–2), 5–19.

Meyer, S. L., Murphy, C. M., Cascardi, M., and Birns, B. (1991). Gender and relationships: Beyond the peer group. *American Psychologist, 46*(5), 537.

Miller, D. L., and Kelley, M. L. (1992). Treatment acceptability: The effects of parent gender, marital adjustment, and child behavior. *Child and Family Behavior Therapy, 14*(1), 11–23.

Moran, M. R. (1992). Effects of sexual orientation similarity and counselor experience level on gay men's and lesbians' perceptions of counselors. *Journal of Counseling Psychology. 39*(2) 247–251.

Murphy, L. O., and Ross, S. M. (1990). Protagonist gender as a design variable in adapting mathematics story problems to learner interests. *Educational Technology Research and Development, 38*(3), 27–37.

Sadker, M., Sadker, D., and Steindam, S. (1989). Gender equity and educational reform. *Educational Leadership, 46*(6), 44–47.

Smith, A. B., and Inder, P. M. (1993). Social interaction in same and cross gender preschool peer groups: A participant observation study. *Educational Psychology, 13*(1), 29–42.

Stockard, J., and Johnson, M. M. (1980). *Sex roles: Sex inequality and sex role development.* Englewood Cliffs, NJ: Prentice-Hall.

Weisel, A., and Florian, V. (1990). Same- and cross-gender attitudes toward persons with physical disabilities. *Rehabilitation Psychology, 35*(4), 229–238.

Williams, C., and Bybee, J. (1994). What do children feel guilty about? Developmental and gender differences. *Developmental Psychology, 30*(5) ,617–623.

Wittmer, D. S., and Honig, A. S. (1991). Convergent or divergent? Teacher questions to three-year-old children in day care. Special Issue: Varieties of early child care research. *Early Child Development and Care, 68*, 141–147.

GENERALIZATION/MAINTENANCE

Ager, A. (1987). Minimal intervention: a strategy for generalized behavior change with mentally handicapped individuals. *Behavioral Psychotherapy, 15*(1), 16–30.

Bock, M. A. (1994). Acquisition, maintenance, and generalization of a categorization strategy by children with autism. *Journal of Autism and Developmental Disorders, 24*(1), 39–51.

Brown, A. K., Brown, J. L., and Poulson, C. L. (1995). Generalization of children's identity matching-to-sample performances to novel stimuli. *Psychological Record, 45*(1), 29–43

Chan-ho, M. W. (1988, July-January). From classroom to clinic: Promoting the transfer of knowledge and clinical skills: A personal view. *Bulletin of the Hong Kong Psychological Society,* pp. 78–86.

Elbert, M. (1989). Generalization in the treatment of phonological disorders. In L. V. McReynolds and J. E. Spradlin (Eds.), *Generalization strategies in the treatment of communication disorders* (pp. 31–43). Philadelphia: B. C. Decker.

Gierut, J. E. M., and Dinnsen, D. (1987). A functional analysis of phonological knowledge and generalization learning in misarticulating children. *Journal of Speech and Hearing Research, 30*(4), 462–479.

Haring, T. G., and Lovinger, L. (1989). Promoting social interaction through teaching generalized play initiation responses to preschool children with autism. *Journal of the Association for Persons with Severe Handicaps, 14*(1), 58–67.

Lowman, J. (1990). Failure of laboratory evaluation of CAI to generalize to classroom settings: The SuperShrink interview simulation. *Be-*

havior *Research Methods, Instruments, and Computers, 22*(5), 429–432.

Nangle, D. W., Carr-Nagle, R. E., and Hansen, D. J. (1994). Enhancing generalization of a contingency-management intervention through the use of family problem-solving training: Evaluation with a severely conduct-disordered adolescent. *Child and Family Behavior Therapy, 16*(2), 65–76.

Perigoe, C., and Ling, D. (1986). Generalization of speech skills in hearing-impaired children. *Volta Review, 8*(7), 351–366.

Stokes, T., and Baer, D. (1978). An implicit technology of generalization. *Journal of Applied Behavior Analyst, 11,* 285–303.

Turner, L. A., Dofny, E. M., and Dutka, S. (1994). Effect of strategy and attribution training on strategy maintenance and transfer. *American Journal on Mental Retardation, 98*(4), 445–454.

GROUP THERAPY

Albertini, J. A., Smith, J. M., and Metz, D. E. (1983). Small group versus individual speech therapy with hearing-impaired young adults. *Volta-Review, 85,* 83–89.

Bergin, J. J. (1989). Building group cohesiveness through cooperation activities. Special Issue: preventive and developmental counseling. *Elementary School Guidance and Counseling, 24*(1), 90–94.

Berne, E. (1966). *Principles of group treatment.* New York: Oxford University Press.

Bowman, V. E., and DeLucia, J. L. (1993). Preparation for group therapy: The effects of preparer and modality on group process and individual functioning. *Journal for Specialists in Group Work, 18*(2), 67–79.

Butler, D., and Geis, F. L. (1990). Nonverbal affect responses to male and female leaders: Implications for leadership evaluations. *Journal of Personality and Social Psychology, 58*(1), 48–59.

Calas, M. B. (1993). Deconstructing charismatic leadership: Re-reading Weber from the darkerside. *Special Issue: Charismatic leadership: Neo Weberian Perspectives, 4*(3–4), 305–328.

Cooke, R. A., and Szumal, J. L. (1994). The impact of group interaction styles on problem-solving effectiveness. *Journal of Applied Behavioral Science, 30*(4) 415–437.

Corey, G. (1990). *Theory and practice of group counseling* (3rd ed.). Pacific Grove, CA: Brooks/Cole.

Delgado, M., and Humm-Delgado, D. (1984). Hispanics and group work: A review of the literature. *Social Work Groups, 7*(3), 85–96.

Deutsch, M. (1949). An experimental study of the effects of cooperation and competition upon group process. *Human Relations, 2,* 199–231.

Edwards, E. D., and Edwards, M. E. (1984). Group work practice with American Indians. *Social Work with Groups, 7*(3), 7–21.

Fatout, M. F. (1995). Using limits and structures for empowerment of children in groups. *Social Work with Groups, 17*(4), 55–69.

French, D. C., and Stright, A. L.(1991). Emergent leadership in children's small groups. *Small Group Research, 22*(2), 187-199.

Garza, R. T., Lipton, J. P., and Isonio, S. A. (1989). Group ethnic composition, leader ethnicity, and task performance: An application of social identity theory. *Genetic, Social, and General Psychology Monographs, 115*(3), 295–314.

George, R. L., and Dustin D. (1988). Group counseling: *Theory and practice.* Englewood Cliffs, NJ: Prentice-Hall.

Gladding, S. T. (1991). *Group work: A counseling specialty.* New York: Merrill.

Hare, A. P. (1994). Types of roles in small groups: A bit of history and a current perspective. *Small Group Research, 25*(3), 433–448.

Hawkins, K. W. (1995). Effects of gender and communication content of leadership emergence in small task-oriented groups. *Small Group Research, 26*(2), 234–249.

Hill, J., and Carper, M. (1985). Group therapeutic approaches with the head injured. *Cognitive-Rehabilitation, 3,* 18–29.

Hittner, A., and Bornstein, H. (1990). Group counseling with older adults: Coping with late-onset hearing impairment. Special Issue: Techniques for counseling older persons. *Journal of Mental Health Counseling, 12*(3), 332–341.

Hollander, M., and Kazaoka, K. (1988). Behavior therapy groups. In S. Long (Ed.), Six group therapies (pp. 257–326). New York: Plenum.

Johnson, D. W. and Johnson, R. T. (1989). *Cooperation and competition: Theory and research.* Edina, MN: Interaction Book Company.

Kinzie, J. D., Leung, P., Bui, A., Ben, R., et. al. (1988). Group therapy with Southeast Asian refugees. *Community Mental Health Journal, 24*(2), 157–166.

Kivlighan, D. M., Mullison, D. D., Flohr, D. F., Proudman, S., et al. (1992) The interpersonal structure of "good" versus "bad" group counseling sessions: A multiple-case study. *Psychotherapy, 29*(3), 500–508.

Leader, E. (1991) Why adolescent group therapy? *Journal of Child and Adolescent Group Therapy, 1*(2), 81–93.

LeCroy, C. W. (1986). An analysis of the effects of gender on outcome in group treatment with young adolescents. *Journal of Youth and Adolescence, 15*, 497–508.

Lieberman, M. A. (1990). Understanding how groups work: A study of homogeneous peer group failures. *International Journal of Group Psychotherapy, 40*(1), 31–52.

Long, S. (1988). The six group therapies compared. In S. Long (Ed.), Six group therapies (pp. 327–338). New York: Plenum.

Madonna, J.M. and Caswell, P. (1991).The utilization of flexible techniques in group therapy with delinquent adolescent boys. *Journal of Child and Adolescent Group Therapy, 1*(2), 147–157.

Mckinley, V. (1987). Group therapy as a treatment modality of special value for Hispanic patients. *International Journal of Group Psychotherapy. 37*(2), 255–268.

McMillon, H. G. (1994). Developing problem solving and interpersonal communication skills through intentionally structured groups. *Journal for Specialists in Group Work, 19*(1), 43–47.

Meadow, D. (1988). Preparation of individuals for participation in a treatment group: Development and empirical testing of a model. *International Journal of Group Psychotherapy, 38*(3), 367–385

Neimeyer, R. A., and Feixas, G. (1990). The role of homework and skill acquisition in the outcome of group cognitive therapy for depression. *Behavior Therapy, 21*(3), 281–292.

Polcin, D. L. (1991). Prescriptive group leadership. *Journal for Specialists in Group Work, 16*(1), 8–15.

Ponzo, Z. (1991). Critical factors in group work: Clients' perceptions. *Journal for Specialists in Group Work, 16*(1) 16–23.

Rosenberg, P.P. (1984). Support groups: A special therapeutic entity. *Small Group Behavior, 15*(2), 173–186.

Szivos, S. E., and Griffiths, E. (1990). Group processes involved in coming to terms with a mentally retarded identity. *Mental Retardation; 28*(6), 333–341.

Wolf, A. (1963). The psychoanalysis of groups. In M. Rosembaum and M. Berger (Eds.), *Group psychotherapy and group function.* New York: Hawthorn.

HISPANICS

Baptiste, D. A. (1990). Therapeutic strategies with Black-Hispanic families: Identify problems of a neglected minority. *Journal of Family Psychotherapy, 1*(3), 15–38.

Berg, J. H., and Wright-Buckley, C. (1988). Effects of racial similarity and interviewer intimacy in a peer counseling analogue. *Journal of Counseling Psychology, 35*(4), 377–384

Brondolo, E., Baruch, C., Conway, E., and Marsh, L. (1994). Aggression among inner-city minority youth: a biopsychosocial model for school-based evaluation and treatment. Special Issue: Multicultural views on domestic violence. *Journal of Social Distress and the Homeless, 3*(1), 53–80.

Campbell, L. R., Brennan, D. G., and Steckol, K. F. (1992). *Preservice training to meet the needs of people from diverse cultural backgrounds. Asha, 35*, 29–32.

Cole, L., and Deal, V. R. (Eds.). (In Press). *Communication disorders in multicultural populations.* Rockville, MD: American Speech-Language-Hearing Association

Cole, L. (1989). E pluribus pluribus: Multicultural imperatives for the 1990's and beyond. *Asha, 31*, 65–70.

Cole, L. (1992). We're serious. *Asha, 32*, 38–39.

Davis, L. E. and Gelsomino, J. (1994). An assessment of practitioner cross-racial treatment experiences. *Social Work, 39*(1), 116–123.

Delgado, M., and Humm-Delgado, D. (1984). Hispanics and group work: A review of the literature. *Social Work Groups, 7*(3), 85–96.

Devereaux, D. (1991). The issue of race and the client-therapist assignment. *Issues in Mental Health Nursing, 12*(3), 283–290.

Dresser, N. (1996). *Multicultural manners.* New York: John Wiley and Sons.

Dunn, R., and Griggs, S. A. (1990). Research on the learning style characteristics of selected racial and ethnic groups. *Journal of Reading, Writing, and Learning Disabilities International, 6*(3), 261–280.

Dunn, R. (1990). Cross-cultural differences in learning styles of elementary-age students from four ethnic backgrounds. *Journal of Multicultural Counseling and Development, 18*(2), 68–93.

Flaskerud, J. H. (1986). The effects of culture-compatible intervention on the utilization of mental health services by minority clients. *Community Mental Health Journal, 22*(2), 127–141.

Freed, A. O. (1992). Discussion: Minority elderly. *Journal of Geriatric Psychiatry, 25*(1), 105–111.

Garza, R. T., Lipton, J. P., and Isonio, S. A. (1989). Group ethnic composition, leader ethnicity, and task performance: An application of social identity theory. *Genetic, Social, and General Psychology Monographs, 115*(3), 295–314.

Goldberg, B., and Tidwell, R. (1990). Ethnicity and gender similarity: The effectiveness of counseling for adolescents. *Journal of Youth and Adolescence, 19*(6) 589–603

Goldstein, G. S. (1974). Behavior modification: Some cultural factors. *Psychological Record, 24*(1), 89–91.

Gollnick, D., and Chinn, P. (1990). *Multicultural education in a pluralistic society* (3rd ed.). NewYork: Merrill/Macmillian.

Goodenough, W. (1987). Multi-culturalism as the normal human experience. In E. M. Effy and W. L. Partridge (Eds.), *Applied anthropology in America* (2nd ed.). New York: Columbia University Press.

Gregory, K., Wells, K. B., and Leake, B. (1987) Medical students' expectations for encounters with minority and nonminority patients. *Journal of the National Medical Association, 79*(4), 403–408.

Hains, A. A., and Fouad, N. A. (1994). The best laid plans . . . : Assessment in an inner-city high school. Special Issue: Multicultural assessment. *Measurement and Evaluation in Counseling and Development, 27*(2), 116–124.

Hall, L. E., and Tucker, C. M. (1985). Relationships between ethnicity, conceptions of mental illness, and attitudes associated with seeking psychological help. *Psychological Reports, 57*(3, Pt. 1), 907–916.

Harel, Z. (1986). Older Americans act related homebound aged: What difference does racial background make? Special Issue: Ethnicity and gerontological social work. *Journal of Gerontological Social Work, 9*(4), 133–143.

Hector, M. A., and Fray, J. S. (1987). The counseling process, client expectations, and cultural influences: A review. *International Journal for the Advancement of Counselling, 10*(4) 237–247.

Heller, T., Markwardt, R., Rowitz, L., and Farber, B. (1994). Adaptation of Hispanic families to a member with mental retardation. *American Journal on Mental Retardation, 99*(3), 289–300

Hines, P. M., Garcia-Preto, N., McGoldrick, M., Almeida, R., et al. (1992). Intergenerational relationships across cultures. Special Issue: Multicultural practice. *Families in Society, 73*(6), 323–338.

Hoffman, L. W. (1988). Cross-cultural differences in childrearing goals. *New Directions for Child Development, 40,* 99–122.

Kayser, H. (Ed.). (1995). *Bilingual speech-language pathology: An Hispanic focus.* San Diego, CA: Singular Publishing Group.

Malgady, R. G., Rogler, L. H., and Costantino, G. (1990). Culturally sensitive psychotherapy for Puerto Rican children and adolescents: A program of treatment outcome research. *Journal of Consulting and Clinical Psychology, 58*(6), 704–712.

Mckinley, V. (1987). Group therapy as a treatment modality of special value for Hispanic patients. *International Journal of Group Psychotherapy. 37*(2), 255–268.

Meadows, J. L. (1991). Multicultural communication. *Physical and Occupational Therapy in Pediatrics, 11*(4), 31–42.

O'Sullivan, M. J., Peterson, P. D., Cox, G. B., and Kirkeby, J. (1989). Ethnic populations: Community mental health services ten years later. *American Journal of Community Psychology, 17*(1), 17–30.

Resendiz, P. S., and Fox, R. A. (1985). Reflection-impulsivity in Mexican children: Cross-cultural relationships. *Journal of General Psychology, 112*(3), 285–290.

Screen, R. M., and Anderson, N. B. (1994). *Multicultural perspectives in communication disorders*. San Diego, CA : Singular Publishing Group.

Seymour, H. N., Ashton, N., and Wheeler, L. (1986). The effect of race on language elicitation. *Language, Speech, and Hearing Services in Schools, 17*(3), 146–151.

Smart, J. F., and Smart, D. W. (1991). Acceptance of disability and the Mexican American culture. *Rehabilitation Counseling Bulletin, 34*(4) 357–367.

Spolsky, B. (1972). The language education of minority children. In B. Spolsky (Ed.), *The language education of minority children* (pp. 1–10). Rowley, MA: Newbury House.

Vontress, C. E. (1974). Barriers in cross-cultural counseling. *Counseling and Values, 18*(3), 160–165.

Westermeyer, J. (1987). Cultural factors in clinical assessment. *Journal of Consulting and Clinical Psychology, 55*(4), 471–478.

Wetzel, C. G. and Wright-Buckley, C. (1988). Reciprocity of self-disclosure: Breakdowns of trust in cross-racial dyads. *Basic and Applied Social Psychology, 9*(4), 277–288.

Yetman, N. R. (Ed.). (1985). *Majority and minority: The dynamics of race and ethnicity in American life* (4th ed.). Boston: Allyn and Bacon.

INTERACTION VARIABLES

Aberbach, D. (1995). Charisma and attachment theory: a cross disciplinary interpretation. *International Journal of Psycho Analysis, 76*(4), 845–855.

Wetzel, C. G., and Wright-Buckley, C. (1988). Reciprocity of self-disclosure: Breakdowns of trust in cross-racial dyads. *Basic and Applied Social Psychology, 9*(4), 277–288.

Bales, R. F. (1950). *Interaction process analysis*. Cambridge, England: Addison-Wesley.

Billings, B. P. (1994). The importance of involvement in counseling. *Journal of Reality Therapy, 13*(2), 26–30.

Bolton, B., Bonge, D., and Marr, J. (1979). Ratings of instruction, examination performance, and subsequent enrollment in psychology courses. *Teaching of Psychology, 6*(2), 82–85.

Borus, J. F., et- al. (1979). Psychotherapy in the goldfish bowl. *Archives of General Psychiatry, 36*(2), 187–190.

Chang, P. (1994). Effects of interviewer questions and response type on compliance: An analogue study. *Journal of Counseling Psychology, 41*(1), 74–82.

Cheng, A. H. H. (1973). Rapport in initial counseling interview and its impact on effectiveness. *Acta Psychologica Taiwanica, 15*, 31–40

Cornett, B. S. ,and Chabon, S. S. (1988). *The clinical practice of speech-language pathology*. Columbus, OH: Merrill.

Eisendrath, S. J. (1989). Factitious physical disorders: Treatment without confrontation. 34th Annual Meeting of the Academy of Psychometric Medicine, (1987, Las Vegas, NV). *Psychosomatics, 30*(4), 383–387.

Fromm-Reichmann, F. (1963). Psychiatric aspects of anxiety. In M. R. Stein, A. J. Vidich, and D. M. White (Eds.), *Identity and anxiety* (pp. 129–144). New York: The Free Press,

Goodare, H. (1994). Counseling people with cancer: Questions and possibilities. *Advances, 10*(2), 4–17.

Gross, P. R. (1994). A pilot study of the contribution of empathy to burnout in Salvation Army officers. *Work and Stress. 8*(1) 68–74.

Halpert, J. A. (1990). The dimensionality of charisma. *Journal of Business and Psychology, 4*(4), 399–410.

Janowsky, D. S., Kraft, A., Clopton, P., and Huey, L. (1984). Relationships of mood and interpersonal perceptions. *Comprehensive Psychiatry, 25*(6), 546–551

Molyneaux, D., and Lane, V.W. (1982). *Effective interviewing*. Boston: Allyn and Bacon.

Morse, J. M., Anderson, G., Bottorff, J. L., Yonge, O., et al. (1992). Exploring empathy: A conceptual fit for nursing practice? *IMAGE Journal of Nursing Scholarship, 24*(4) 273–280.

Orleans, C. S., Houpt, J. L., and Larson, D. B. (1980). Interpersonal factors in the psychiatry clerkship: New findings. *American Journal of Psychiatry, 137*(9), 1101–1103.

Poston, W. C., Craine, M., and Atkinson, D. R. (1991). Counselor dissimilarity confrontation, client cultural mistrust, and willingness to self-disclose. *Journal of Multicultural Counseling and Development, 19*(2) 65–73.

Redfern, S., Dancey, C. P., and Dryden, W. (1993).Empathy: Its effect on how counselors are perceived. *British Journal of Guidance and Counseling, 21*(3), 300–309.

Roberts, S. D. and Bouchard, K. R. (1989). Establishing rapport in rehabilitative audiology. *Journal of the Academy of Rehabilitative Audiology, 22* 67–73.

Robinson, D. D., Stockton, R., and Moran, D. K. (1990). Anticipated consequences of self-disclosure during early therapeutic group development. *Journal of Group Psychotherapy Psychodrama and Sociometry, 43*(1) 3–18.

Rollin, W. J. (1987). *The psychology of communication disorders in individuals and their families.* Englewood Cliffs, NJ: Prentice-Hall.

Salerno, M., Farber, B. A., McCullough, L., Winston, A., et al. (1992). The effects of confrontation and clarification on patient affective and defensive responding. *Psychotherapy Research, 2*(3) 181–192.

Scheuerle, J. (1992). *Counseling in speech-language pathology and audiology.* Columbus, OH: Merrill.

Semmes, C. E. (1991). Developing trust: Patient-practitioner encounters in natural health care. *Journal of Contemporary Ethnography, 19*(4), 450–470.

Shipley, K. G. (1992). *Interviewing and counseling in communicative disorders.* New York: Merrill.

Thompson, B. M., Hearn, G. N., and Collins, M. J. (1992). Patient perceptions of health professional interpersonal skills. *Australian Psychologist, 27*(2), 91–95

Tickle-Degnen, L., and Rosenthal, R. (1990). The behavioral and cognitive response of brain-damaged patients to therapist instructional style. *Occupational Therapy Journal of Research, 10*(6), 345–359.

Van Galen, J. A. (1993). Caring in community: The limitations of compassion in facilitating diversity. Special Issue: Caring across educational boundaries: Redefinitions of caring within and by historically marginalized groups. *Urban Review 25*(1), 5–24.

Woods, P. (1993). The charisma of the critical other: Enhancing the role of the teacher. *Teaching and Teacher Education, 9*(5–6), 545–557.

LEARNING/COGNITION

Afflerbach, P., and Walker, B. (1992). Main idea instruction: An analysis of three basal reader series. *Reading Research and Instruction, 32*(1), 11–28.

Ausubel, D. P. (1968). Educational psychology: a cognitive view. New York: Holt, Rinehart, and Winston.

Balajthy, E., and Weisberg, R. (1990). Transfer effects of prior knowledge and use of graphic organizers on college developmental readers' summarization and comprehension of expository text. *National Reading Conference Yearbook, 39,* 339–345.

Balluerka, N. (1995). The influence of instructions, outlines, and illustrations on the comprehension and recall of scientific texts. *Contemporary Educational Psychology, 20*(3), 369–375.

Barksdale-Ladd, M. A., and Thomas, K. F. (1993). Eight teachers' reported pedagogical dependency on basal readers. *Elementary School Journa, 94*(1), 49–72.

Beck, A. T. (1976). *Cognitive therapy and the emotional disorders.* New York: International Universities Press.

Beckwith, J. B. (1994). Prejudice, reverse prejudice, and positive attitude towards differences among people with intellectual disabilities. *Psychological Reports, 7*(3, Pt. 1), 938.

Berry, D. C. (1991). The role of action in implicit learning. *Quarterly Journal of Experimental Psychology Human Experimental Psychology, 43A*(4), 881–906.

Best, D. L. (1993). Inducing children to generate mnemonic organizational strategies: An examination of long-term retention and materials. *Developmental Psychology, 29*(2), 324–336.

Biggs, J. B. (1988). Assessing student approaches to learning. *Australian Psychologist. 23*(2), 197–206.

Borkowski, J. G., and Buchel, F. P. (1981). Learning and memory strategies in the mentally retarded. In M. Pressley and J. R. Levin (Eds.), *Cognitive strategy research: Psychological foundations.* (pp. 103—128). New York: Springer-Verlag.

Brooke, M., Uomoto, J. M., Mclean, A. Jr., and Fraser, R. T. (1991). *Rehabilitation of persons with traumatic brain injury: A continuum of care.* Austin, TX: Pro-Ed.

Brown, A. L., Smiley, S. S., and Lawton, S. C. (1978). The effects of experience on the selection of suitable retrieval cues for studying text. *Child Development, 49,* 829–835.

Capelli, C., Nakagawa, N., and Madden, C. M. (1990). How children understand sarcasm: The role of context and intonation. *Child Development, 61*(6), 1824–1841.

Carver, R. P., and Leibert, R. E. (1995). The effect of reading library books at different levels of difficulty upon gain in reading ability. *Reading Research Quarterly, 30*(1), 26–48.

Chan, L. K. S. (1994). Relationship of motivation, strategic learning, and reading achievement in Grades 5, 7, and 9. *Journal of Experimental Education, 62*(4), 319–339.

Crowder, R. G. (1976). Principles of learning and memory. Hillsdale, NJ: Lawrence Erlbaum.

Davis, I. P. (1938). The speech aspects of reading readiness. Newer practices in reading in the elementary school, 17th yearbook of the department of elementary school principals, *NEA, 17*(7), 282–289.

Dent, V., and Seligman, S. (1993).The dynamic functions of the act of reading. *International Journal of Psycho Analysis, 74*(6), 1253–1267.

Dortch, H. L., and Trombly, C. A. (1990). The effects of education on hand use with industrial workers in repetitive jobs. *American Journal of Occupational Therapy, 44*(9), 777–782.

Egan, V. (1993). Can specific inspection time strategies be inferred by their latency? *Irish Journal of Psychology, 14*(2), 253–269.

Dunlap, G., and Plienis, A. J. (1991). The influence of task size on the unsupervised task performance of students with developmental disabilities. *Education and Treatment of Children, 14*(2), 85–95.

Dunn, R., and Griggs, S. A. (1990). Research on the learning style characteristics of selected racial and ethnic groups. *Journal of Reading, Writing, and Learning Disabilities International, 6*(3), 261–280.

Dunn, R., (1990). Cross-cultural differences in learning styles of elementary-age students from four ethnic backgrounds. *Journal of Multicultural Counseling and Development, 18*(2), 68–93.

Frensch, P. A., and Miner, C. S. (1994). Effects of presentation rate and individual differences in short-term memory capacity on an indirect measure of serial learning. *Memory and Cognition, 22*(1), 95–110.

Frensch, P.A., Buchner, A., and Lin, J. (1994). Implicit learning of unique and ambiguous serial transitions in the presence and absence of a distractor task. *Journal of Experimental Psychology Learning, Memory, and Cognition, 20*(3), 567–584.

Gagné, R. M. (1970). *The conditions of learning.* New York: Holt, Rinehart and Winston.

Gagné, R. M., Briggs, L. J., and Wager, W. W. (1988). *Principles of instructional design.* New York: Holt, Rinehart, and Winston.

Galea, L. A., and Kimura, D. (1993). Sex differences in route-learning. *Personality and Individual Differences, 14*(1), 53–65.

Hartley, L. L. (1995). *Cognitive-communicative abilities following brain injury.* San Diego, CA: Singular Publishing Group.

Kausler, D. (1974). *Psychology of verbal learning and memory.* New York: Academic Press.

Mayer, R. E. (1987). Instructional variables that influence cognitive processes during reading.In B. K. Britton and S. M. Glynn (Eds.), *Historical foundations of educational psychology* (pp. 327–347). New York: Plenum Press.

McCarthey, S. J., Hoffman, J. V., Christian, C., and, Corman, L., et al. (1994). Engaging the newbasal readers. *Reading Research and Instruction, 33*(3), 233–256.

Oakhill, J. (1993). Children's difficulties in reading comprehension. Special Issue: European educational psychology. *Educational Psychology Review, 5*(3), 223–237.

Ramsay, J. E., and Oatley, K. (1992). Designing minimal computer manuals from scratch. Special Issue: Computers and writing: Issues and implementations. *Instructional Science, 21*(1–3), 85–98.

Ratner, H. H., and Hill, L. (1991). The development of children's action memory: When do actions speak louder than words? *Psychological Research Psychologische Forschung, 53*(3), 195–202.

Resnick, L., and Ford, W. (1981). *The psychology of mathematics for instruction.* Hillsdale, NJ: Lawrence Erlbaum.

Smith, J. A. (1993). Content learning: A third reason for using literature in teaching reading. *Reading Research and Instruction, 32*(3), 64–71.

Rogers, W. A., and Fisk, A. D. (1990). A reconsideration of age-related reaction time slowing from a learning perspective: Age-related slowing is not just complexity-based. Special Issue: Frontiers of learning and individual differences: Paradigms in transition. *Learning and Individual Differences, 2*(2) 161–179.

Rudd, R. E., and Comings, J. P. (1994). Learner developed materials: An empowering product. Special Issue: Community empowerment, participatory education, and health: II. *Health Education Quarterly. 21*(3) 313–327.

Shefelbine, J. L. (1990). Student factors related to variability in learning word meanings from context. *Journal of Reading Behavior, 22*(1), 71–97.

Stock, W. A., Winston, K. S., Behrens, J. T., and Harper-Marinick, M. (1989). The effects of performance expectation and question difficulty on text study time, response certitude, and correct responding. *Bulletin of the Psychonomic Society, 27*(6), 567–569.

Sweller, J., and Chandler, P. (1994).Why some material is difficult to learn. *Cognition and Instruction, 12*(3), 185–233.

Vitz, P. C. (1974). Learning numerical progressions. *Memory and Cognition, 2*(1–A), 121–126.

Zabrucky, K., and Commander, N. (1993). Rereading to understand: The role of text coherence and reader proficiency. *Contemporary Educational Psychology, 18*(4), 442–452.

MODELING

Denis, M. (1974). Religious education among North American Indian peoples. *Religious Education, 69*(3), 343–354.

Katz, P. (1981). Psychotherapy with native adolescents. *Canadian Journal of Psychiatry, 26*(7), 455–459.

Norris, D. (1994). A quantitative multiple-levels model of reading aloud. Special Section: Modeling visual word recognition. *Journal of Experimental Psychology Human Perception and Performance, 20*(6), 1212–1232.

MONITORING

Belfiore, P. J., and Browder, D. M. (1992). The effects of self-monitoring on teacher's data-based decisions and on the performance of adults with severe mental retardation. *Education and Training in Mental Retardation, 27*(1), 60–67.

Bielaczyc, K., Pirolli, P. L., and Brown, A. L. (1995). Training in self-explanation and self-regulation strategies: Investigating the effects of knowledge acquisition activities on problem solving. *Cognition and Instruction, 13*(2), 221–252.

Chi, M. T., de Leeuw, N., Chie, M. H., and LaVancher, C. (1994). Eliciting self-explanations improves understanding. *Cognitive Science, 18*(3) 439–477.

Delclos, V. R., and Harrington, C. (1991). Effects of strategy monitoring and proactive instruction on children's problem-solving performance. *Journal of Educational Psychology, 83*(1), 35–42.

Elliott, R. T., Sherwin, E., Harkins, S. W., and Marmarosh, C. (1995). Self-appraised problem-solving ability, affective states, and psychological distress. *Journal of Counseling Psychology, 42*(1), 105–115.

Harre, R. (1988). The social context of self-deception. In B. P. McLaughlin and A. O. Rorty (Eds.), *Perspectives on self-deception* (pp 364–379). Berkeley, CA: University of California Press.

Hermans, H. J., Fiddelaers, R., de-Groot, R., and Nauta, J. F. (1990). Self-confrontation as a method for assessment and intervention in counseling. *Journal of Counseling and Development, 69*(2), 156—162

King, A. (1994). Autonomy and question asking: The role of personal control in guided student-generated questioning. Special Issue: Individual differences in question asking and strategic listening processes, *Learning and Individual Differences, 6*(2), 163–185.

Kinnunen, R., and Vauras, M. (1995). Comprehension monitoring and the level of comprehension in high- and low-achieving primary school children's reading. *Learning and Instruction, 5*(2), 143–165.

Lloyd, J. W., Bateman, D. F., Landrum, Y. J., and Hallahan, D. P. (1989). Self-recording of attention versus productivity. *Journal of Applied Behavior Analysis, 22*(3), 315–323.

Marshall, R. C., Neuburger, S. I., and Phillips, D. S. (1994). Verbal self-correction and improvement in treated aphasic clients. *Aphasiology, 8*(6), 535–547

Matthews, G. A., and Harley, T. A. (1993). Effects of extroversion and self-report arousal on semantic priming: A connectionist approach. *Journal of Personality and Social Psychology, 65*(4), 735–756.

Meloth, M. S., and Deering, P. D. (1994). Task talk and task awareness under different cooperative learning conditions. *American Educational Research Journal, 31*(1), 138–165.

Wheeler, L., and Reis, H. T. (1991). Self-recording of everyday life events: Origins, types, and uses. Special Issue: Personality and daily experience. *Journal of Personality, 59*(3), 339–354.

Whitney, J. L., and Goldstein, H. (1989).Using self-monitoring to reduce disfluencies in speakers with mild aphasia. *Journal of Speech and Hearing Disorders, 54*(4), 576–586.

Zimmerman, B. J. (1990). Self-regulating academic learning and achievement: The emergence of a social cognitive perspective. *Educational Psychology Review, 2*(2), 173–201.

MOTIVATION

Archer, J. (1994). Achievement goals as a measure of motivation in university students. *Contemporary Educational Psychology, 19*(4) 430–446.

Brackney, B. E., and Karabenick, S. A. (1995). Psychopathology and academic performance: The role of motivation and learning strategies. *Journal of Counseling Psychology, 42*(4), 456–465.

de Luca, R. V., and Holborn, S. W. (1992). Effects of a variable-ratio reinforcement schedule with changing criteria on exercise in obese and nonobese boys. *Journal of Applied Behavior Analysis, 25*(3), 671–679.

Dickinson, A. M. (1989). The detrimental effects of extrinsic reinforcement on "intrinsic motivation." *Behavior Analyst, 12*(1), 1–15.

Flora, S. R. (1990). Undermining intrinsic interest from the standpoint of a behaviorist. *Psychological Record, 40*(3), 323–346.

Gotlib, I. H. (1982). Self-reinforcement and depression in interpersonal interaction: The role of performance level. *Journal of Abnormal Psychology, 91*, 3–13.

Klein, J. D., and Freitag, E. (1991). Effects of using an instructional game on motivation and performance. *Journal of Educational Research, 84*(5), 303–308.

McClean, A. P. (1995). Contrast and reallocation of extraneous reinforcers as a function of component duration and baseline rate of reinforcement. *Journal of the Experimental Analysis of Behavior, 36*(2), 203–224.

Sansone, C., and Morgan, C. (1992). Intrinsic motivation and education: Competence in context. Special Issue: Perspectives on intrinsic motivation. *Motivation and Emotion, 16*(3) 249–270.

NATIVE AMERICANS

Berg, J. H., and Wright-Buckley, C. (1988). Effects of racial similarity and interviewer intimacy in a peer counseling analogue. *Journal of Counseling Psychology, 35*(4), 377–384

Cole, L. (1992). We're Serious. *Asha, 32*, 38–39.

Cole, L., and Deal, V. R. (Eds.). (In Press). *Communication disorders in multicultural populations.* Rockville, MD: American Speech-Language-Hearing Association.

Cole, L. (1989). E pluribus pluribus: Multicultural imperatives for the 1990's and beyond. *Asha, 31*, 65–70.

Darou, W. G. (1987). Counseling and the northern native. *Canadian Journal of Counseling, 21*(1), 33–41.

Devereaux, D. (1991). The issue of race and the client-therapist assignment. *Issues in Mental Health Nursing, 12*(3), 283–290.

Yetman, N. R. (Ed.). (1985). Majority and minority: *The dynamics of race and ethnicity in American life* (4th ed.). Boston: Allyn and Bacon.

Dresser, N. (1996). *Multicultural manners.* New York: John Wiley and Sons.

DuBray, W. H. (1985). American Indian values: Critical factor in casework. *Social Casework, 66*(1), 30–37.

Edwards, E. D., and Edwards, M. E. (1984). Group work practice with American Indians. *Social Work with Groups, 7*(3), 7–21.

Eldredge, N., and Carrigan, J. (1992). Where do my kindred dwell? Using art and storytelling to understand the transition of young Indian men who are deaf. *Arts in Psychotherapy, 19*(1), 29–38.

Flaskerud, J. H. (1986). The effects of culture-compatible intervention on the utilization of mental health services by minority clients. *Community Mental Health Journal, 22*(2), 127–141.

Freed, A. O. (1992). Discussion: Minority elderly. *Journal of Geriatric Psychiatry, 25*(1), 105–111.

Friedlander, R. (1993). BHSM comes to the Flathead Indian Reservation. *Asha, 35*, 29–30.

Garza, R. T., Lipton, J. P., and Isonio, S. A. (1989). Group ethnic composition, leader ethnicity, and task performance: An application of social identity theory. *Genetic, Social, and General Psychology Monographs, 115*(3), 295–314.

Goldberg, B., and Tidwell, R. (1990). Ethnicity and gender similarity: The effectiveness of counseling for adolescents. *Journal of Youth and Adolescence, 19*(6) 589–603

Goldstein, G. S. (1974). Behavior modification: Some cultural factors. *Psychological Record, 24*(1), 89–91.

Gollnick, D., and Chinn, P. (1990). *Multicultural education in a pluralistic society* (3rd ed.). NewYork: Merrill/Macmillian.

Goodenough, W. (1987). Multi-culturalism as the normal human experience. In E. M. Effy and W. L. Partridge (Eds.), *Applied anthropology in America* (2nd ed.). New York: Columbia University Press.

Gregory, K., Wells, K. B., and Leake, B. (1987) Medical students' expectations for encounters with minority and nonminority patients. *Journal of the National Medical Association, 79*(4), 403–408.

Hains, A. A., and Fouad, N. A. (1994). The best laid plans . . . : Assessment in an inner-city high school. Special Issue: Multicultural assessment. *Measurement and Evaluation in Counseling and Development, 27*(2), 116–124.

Hall, L. E. and Tucker, C. M. (1985) Relationships between ethnicity, conceptions of mental illness, and attitudes associated with seeking psychological help. *Psychological Reports, 57*(3, Pt. 1), 907–916.

Harel, Z. (1986). Older Americans act related homebound aged: What difference does racial background make? Special Issue: Ethnicity and gerontological social work. *Journal of Gerontological Social Work, 9*(4), 133–143.

Hector, M. A., and Fray, J. S. (1987). The counseling process, client expectations, and cultural influences: A review. *International Journal for the Advancement of Counselling, 10*(4) 237–247.

Herring, R. D.(1992). Seeking a new paradigm: Counseling Native Americans. *Journal of Multicultural Counseling and Development, 20*(1), 35–43

Hines, P. M., Garcia-Preto, N., McGoldrick, M., Almeida, R., et al. (1992). Intergenerational relationships across cultures. Special Issue: Multicultural practice. *Families in Society, 73*(6), 323–338.

Hoffman, L. W. (1988). Cross-cultural differences in childrearing goals. *New Directions for Child Development, 40,* 99–122.

Katz, P. (1981). Psychotherapy with native adolescents. *Canadian Journal of Psychiatry, 26*(7), 455–459.

LaFromboise, T. D. (1992). An interpersonal analysis of affinity, clarification, and helpful responses with American Indians. *Professional Psychology Research and Practice, 23*(4) 281–286.

Levy, J. E. (1988). The effects of labeling on health behavior and treatment programs among North American Indians. *American Indian and Alaska Native Mental health Research, 1*(Mono1) 211–231.

Little Soldier, L. (1985). To soar with the eagles: Enculturation and acculturation of Indian children. *Childhood Education, 61*(3), 185–191.

Lockhart, B. (1981). Historic distrust and the counseling of American Indians and Alaskan Natives. *White Cloud Journal, 2*(3), 31–34.

Marshall, C. A.; Martin, W. W.; Thomason, T. C., and Johnson, J. J. (1991). Multiculturalism and rehabilitation counselor training: Recommendations for providing culturally appropriate counseling services to American Indians with disabilities. Special Issue: Multiculturalism as a fourth force in counseling. *Journal of Counseling and Development, 70*(1), 225–234.

McCarty, T. L.; Wallace, S., Lynch, R. H., and Benally, A. (1991). Classroom inquiry and Navajo learning styles: A call for reassessment. *Anthropology and Education Quarterl, 22*(1), 42–59.

McShane, D. (1987). Mental health and North American Indian/Native communities: Cultural transactions, education, and regulation. *American Journal of Community Psychology, 15*(1), 95–116.

Meadows, J. L. (1991). Multicultural communication. *Physical and Occupational Therapy in Pediatrics, 11*(4) 31–42.

O'Sullivan, M. J., Peterson, P. D., Cox, G. B., and Kirkeby, J. (1989). Ethnic populations: Community mental health services ten years later. *American Journal of Community Psychology, 17*(1), 17–30.

Screen, R. M., and Anderson, N. B. (1994). *Multicultural perspectives in communication disorders.* San Diego, CA: Singular Publishing Group.

Seymour, H. N., Ashton, N., and Wheeler, L. (1986). The effect of race on language elicitation. *Language, Speech, and Hearing Services in Schools, 17*(3), 146–151.

Spolsky, B. (1972). The language education of minority children. In B. Spolsky (Ed.), *The language education of minority children* (pp. 1–10). Rowley, MA: Newbury House.

Stewart, J. L. (1992). Native American populations. *Asha, 34,* 40–42.

Sullivan, T. (1983). Native children in treatment: Clinical, social, and cultural issues. *Journal of Child Care, 1*(4), 75–94.

Tafoya, T. (1989). Circles and cedar: Native Americans and family therapy. *Journal of Psychotherapy and the Family, 6*(1–2), 71–98

Vontress, C. E. (1974). Barriers in cross-cultural counseling. *Counseling and Values, 18*(3), 160–165.

Westermeyer, J. (1987). Cultural factors in clinical assessment. *Journal of Consulting and Clinical Psychology, 55*(4), 471–478.

Wetzel, C. G., and Wright-Buckley, C. (1988). Reciprocity of self-disclosure: Breakdowns of trust in cross-racial dyads. *Basic and Applied Social Psychology, 9*(4), 277–288.

NONVERBAL BEHAVIORS

Astrom, J., Thorell, L. H., and D'Elia, G. (1993). Attitudes towards and observations of nonverbal communication in a psychotherapeutic greeting situation: III. An interview study of outpatients. *Psychological Reports, 73*(1), 151–168

Baxter, J. C., Winters, E. P., and Hammer, R. E. (1968). Gestural behavior during a brief interview as a function of cognitive variables. *Journal of Personality and Social Psychology, 8,* 303–307.

Blanck, P. D., Rosenthal, R., Vannicelli, M., and Lee, T. D. (1986) Therapists' tone of voice: Descriptive, psychometric, interactional, and competence analyses. *Journal of Social and Clinical Psychology, 4*(2), 154–178

Brennan, S. E., and Williams, M. (1995). The feeling of another's knowing: Prosody and filled pauses as cues to listeners about the metacognitive states of speakers. *Journal of Memory and Language. 34*(3), 383–398.

Bull, P. E. (1987). *Posture and gesture.* New York: Pergamon Press.

Butler, D., and Geis, F. L. (1990). Nonverbal affect responses to male and female leaders: Implications for leadership evaluations. *Journal of Personality and Social Psychology, 58*(1), 48–59,

Eisenberg, A. M., and Smith, R. R., Jr. (1971). *Nonverbal communication.* New York: Bobbs-Merrill.

Ekman, P., and Friesen, W. (1974). Detecting deception from the body or face. *Journal of Personality and Social Psychology, 29,* 288–298.

Ekman, P. (1964). Body position, facial expression, and verbal behavior during interviews. *Journal of Abnormal and Social Psychology, 68*(3), 295–301.

Ekman, P., and Friesen, W. (1971). *Emotion in the human face.* New York: Bobbs-Merrill.

Ekman, P., and Friesen, W. (1968). "Nonverbal behavior in psychotherapy research. *Research in Psychotherapy, 3,* 179–215.

Ekman, P (1985). *Telling lies.* New York: Norton.

Feyereisen, P., and de Lannoy, J. (1991). *Gestures and speech: Psychological investigations.* New York: Cambridge Press.

Frankel, S. A., and Frankel, E. B. (1970). Nonverbal behavior in a selected group of Negro and white males. *Psychosomatics, 11*(2), 127–132.

Frankish, C. (1995). Intonation and auditory grouping in immediate serial recall. Special Issue: Donald Broadbent and Applied Cognitive Psychology. *Applied Cognitive Psychology, 9*(Special Issue), S5–S22.

Gelinas-Chebat, C., and Chebat, J. C. (1992). Effects of two voice characteristics on the attitudes toward advertising messages. *Journal of Social Psychology, 132*(4), 447–459.

Hirschberg, J., and Ward, G. (1992). The influence of pitch range, duration, amplitude, and spectral features on the interpretation of the rise-fall-rise intonation contour in English. *Journal of Phonetics, 20*(2), 241–251.

Grant, E. C. (1968). An ethological description of non-verbal behavior during interview. British *Journal of Medical Psychology, 4*(2), 177–184.

Hall, T., and Lloyd, C. (1990). Non-verbal communication in a health care setting. British *Journal of Occupational Therapy, 53*(9) 383–386.

Hall, E. T. (1959). The silent language. Garden City, NY: Doubleday.

Hewes, G. W. (1957). World distribution of certain postural habits. *American Anthropologist, 57,* 231–244.

Hill, C. E., and Stephany, A. (1990). Relation of nonverbal behavior to client reactions. *Journal of Counseling Psychology, 37*(1), 22–26

Kinseth, L. M. (1989). Nonverbal training for psychotherapy: Overcoming barriers to clinical work with client nonverbal behavior. *Clinical Supervisor, 7*(1), 5–25.

Lee, D. Y., and Hallberg, E. T. (1982). Nonverbal behaviors of "good" and "poor" counselors. *Journal of Counseling Psychology, 29*(4), 414-417.

Rossberg-Bempton, I., and Poole, G. D. (1993). The effects of open and closed postures on pleasant and unpleasant emotions. Special Issue: Research in the creative arts therapies. *Arts in Psychotherapy, 20*(1), 75–82.

Rubin, S. S., and Niemeier, D. L. (1992). Nonverbal affective communication as a factor in psychotherapy. *Psychotherapy, 29*(4) 596–602

Scheflen, A. E. (1967). On the structuring of human communication. *American Behavioral Scientist, 10*(8), 8–12.

Sherer, M., and Rogers, R. W. (1980). Effects of therapists' nonverbal communication on rated skill and effectiveness. *Journal of Clinical Psychology, 36*(3), 696–700.

Siegel, S. M., Friedlander, M. L., and Heatherington, L. (1992). Nonverbal relational control in family communication. *Journal of Nonverbal Behavior, 16*(2), 117–139

Wiener, M., Budney, S., Wood, L., and Russell, R.L. (1989). Nonverbal events in psychotherapy. Special Issue: Psychotherapy process research. *Clinical Psychology Review, 9*(4), 487-504.

Yarczower, M., Kilbride, J. E., and Beck, A. T. (1991) Changes in nonverbal behavior of therapists and depressed patients during cognitive therapy. *Psychological Reports, 69*(3, Pt 1), 915–919.

REGIONAL/GEOGRAPHIC

Fiene, J. I. and Taylor, P. A. (1991). Serving rural families of developmentally disabled children: A case management model. *Social Work, 36*(4), 323–327.

RELIGION

Denis, M. (1974). Religious education among North American Indian peoples. *Religious Education, 69*(3), 343–354.

Georgia, R. T. (1994). Preparing to counsel clients of different religious backgrounds: A phenomenological approach. *Counseling and Values, 38*(2), 143–151.

Markowitz, J. C. (1994). Religiosity and psychopathology. *Journal of Clinical Psychiatry, 55*(9), 414–415.

Morrow, D., Worthington, E. L., and McCullough, M. E. (1993). Observers' perceptions of a counselor's treatment of a religious issue. *Journal of Counseling and Development, 71*(4), 452–456.

Presley, D. B. (1992). Three approaches to religious issues in counseling. *Journal of Psychology and Theology, 20*(1), 39–46.

Sazar, L., and Kassinove, H. (1991). Effects of counselor's profanity and subject's religiosity on content acquisition of a counseling lecture and behavioral compliance. *Psychological Reports, 69*(3, pt. 2 Special Issue), 1059–1070.

SOCIOECONOMIC FACTORS

Campbell, L. R., Brennan, D. G., and Steckol, K. F. (1992). Preservice training to meet the needs of people from diverse cultural backgrounds. *Asha, 35*, 29–32.

Chappell, A. L. (1992) Towards a sociological critique of the normalization principle. *Disability, Handicap and Society, 7*(1), 35–51

Cowen, E. L., Wyman, P. A., Work, C., and Iker, M.R. (1995). A preventive intervention for enhancing resilience among highly stressed urban children. *Journal of Primary Prevention, 15*(3), 247–260.

STIMULUS CONFIGURATIONS

Bernard, R. M. (1990). Effects of processing instructions on the usefulness of a graphic organizer and structural cuing in text. *Instructional Science, 19*(3), 207–217.

Broadbent, D. E. (1992). Listening to one of two synchronous messages. *Journal of Experimental Psychology General, 121*(2), 125–127.

Cantor, J., and Engle, R. W. (1989). The influence of concurrent load on mouthed and vocalized modality effects, *Memory and Cognition, 17*(6), 701–711.

Cave, K. R., Pinker, S., Giorgi, L., Thomas, C. E., et al. (1994).The representation of location in visual images, *Cognitive Psychology, 26*(1), 1–32.

Cooper, B. A., Letts, L., and Rigby, P. (1993). Exploring the use of color cueing on an assistive device in the home: Six case studies. *Physical and Occupational Therapy in Geriatrics, 11*(4), 47–59.

Cuvo, A .J., and Klatt, K. P. (1992). Effects of community-based, videotaped, and flash card instruction of community-referenced sight words on students with mental retardation. *Journal of Applied Behavior Analysis, 25*(2), 499–512.

Dee Lucas, D., and Larkin, J. H. (1991). Equations in scientific proofs: Effects on comprehension. *American Educational Research Journal, 28*(3), 661–682.

Dunston, P. J. (1992). A critique of graphic organizer research. *Reading Research and Instruction, 31*(2), 57–65.

Frensch, P. A., and Miner, C. S. (1994). Effects of presentation rate and individual differences in short-term memory capacity on an indirect measure of serial learning. *Memory and Cognition, 22*(1), 95–110.

Frensch, P. A., Buchner, A., and Lin, J. (1994). Implicit learning of unique and ambiguous serial transitions in the presence and absence of a distractor task. *Journal of Experimental Psychology Learning, Memory, and Cognition, 20*(3), 567–584.

Gillstrom, A., and Ronnberg, J. (1994). Prediction accuracy of text recall: Ease, effort and familiarity. *Scandinavian Journal of Psychology, 35*(4), 367–385.

Glenberg, A. M., and Langston, W. E. (1992). Comprehension of illustrated text: Pictures help to build mental models. *Journal of Memory and Language, 31*(2), 129–151.

Goolkasian, P., Van Wallendael, L. R., and Terry, W. S. (1991). Recognition memory for easy and difficult text. *Journal of General Psychology, 118*(4), 375–393.

Greenfield, P. M., deWinstanley, P., Kilpatrick, H., and Kaye, D. (1994). Action video games and informal education: Effects on strategies for dividing visual attention. Special Issue: Effects of interactive entertainment technologies on development. *Journal of Applied Developmental Psychology, 15*(1), 105–123.

Hegarty, M., and Just, M. A. (1993). Constructing mental models of machines from text and diagrams. *Journal of Memory and Language, 32*(6), 717–742.

Jubis, R. M. (1990). Coding effects on performance in a process control task with uniparameter and multiparameter displays. *Human Factors, 32*(3), 287–297.

Kulhavy, R. W., Stock, W. A., and Kealy, W. A. (1993).How geographic mapsincrease recall of instructional text. *Educational Technology Research and Development, 41*(4) 47–62.

Livesay, J. R., and Porter, T. (1994). EMG and cardiovascular responses to emotionally provocative photographs and text. Special Issue *Perceptual and Motor Skills, 79*(1, Pt. 2), 579–594.

Locher, P. J., and Wagemans, J. (1993). Effects of element type and spatial grouping on symmetry detection. *Perception, 22*(5), 565–587.

Macrae, C. N., and Shepherd, J. W. (1991). Categorical effects on attributional inferences: A response-time analysis. *British Journal of Social Psychology, 30*(3) 235–245.

Meng, K., and Patty, D. (1991). Field dependence and contextual organizers. *Journal of Educational Research, 84*(3), 183–189.

Miller, H. R., and Davis, S. F. (1993).Recall of boxed material in textbooks. *Bulletin of the Psychonomic Society, 31*(1), 31–32.

Miyaji, N. T. (1993). The power of compassion: Truth-telling among American doctors in the care of dying patients. *Social Science and Medicine, 36*(3), 249–264.

O'Brien, E. J., and Albrecht, J. E. (1991). The role of context in accessing antecedents in text. *Journal of Experimental Psychology Learning, Memory, and Cognition, 17*(1), 94–102.

Riccio, D. C., Ackil, J. K., and Burch-Vernon, A. (1992) Forgetting of stimulus attributes: Methodological implications for assessing associative phenomena. *Psychological Bulletin; 112*(3), 433–445.

Roberts, M. J., Wood, D. J., and Gilmore, D. J. (1994). The sentence-picture verification task: Methodological and theoretical difficulties. *British Journal of Psychology, 85*(3), 413–432.

Short, K. G. (1992). Intertextuality: Searching for patterns that connect. *National Reading Conference Yearbook, 41*, 187–197.

Skotnikova, I. G. (1990). Psychophysical characteristics of visual discrimination and the cognitive style. *Soviet Journal of Psychology, 11*(1), 40–53.

Spiegel, G. F., and Barnfield, J. P. (1994). The effects of a combination of text structure awareness and graphic postorganizers on recall and retention of science knowledge. Special Issue: The reading-science learning-writing connection. *Journal of Research Science Teaching, 31*(9) 913–932.

Ward, L. M. (1994). Supramodal and modality-specific mechanisms for stimulus-driven shifts of auditory and visual attention. Special Issue: Shifts of visual attention. *Canadian Journal of Experimental Psychology, 48*(2) 242–259.

STRATEGIES

Alderman, D. L., Evans, F. R., and Wilder, G. (1981). The validity of written simulation exercises for assessing clinical skills in legal education. *Educational and Psychological Measurement, 41*(4), 1115–1126.

Alexander, J. M., and Schwanenflugel, P. (1994). Strategy regulation: the role of intelligence, metacognitive attributions, and knowledge base. *Developmental Psychology, 30*(5), 709–723.

Anderson, A.H., Clark, A,. and Mullin, J. (1994). Interactive communication between children: Learning how to make language work in dialogue. *Journal of Child Language, 21*(2), 439–463.

Bivens, J. A., and Berk, L. E. (1990). A longitudinal study of the development of elementary school children's private speech. *Merrill Palmer Quarterly, 36*(4), 443–463.

Blakemore, B., Shindler, S., and Conte, R. (1993). A problem solving training program for parents of children with attention deficit hyperactivity disorder. *Canadian Journal of School Psychology, 9*(1, Special Issue), 66–85.

Bleile, K. M. (1995). *Manual of articulation and phonological disorders.* San Diego, CA: Singular Publishing Group.

Bock, M. A. (1994). Acquisition, maintenance, and generalization of a categorization strategy by children with autism. *Journal of Autism and Developmental Disorders, 24*(1), 39–51.

Borkowski, J. G., and Buchel, F. P. (1981). Learning and memory strategies in the mentally retarded. In M. Pressley and J. R. Levin (Eds.), *Cognitive strategy research: psychological foundation.* (pp. 103–128). New York: Springer-Verlag.

Brackney, B. E., and Karabenick, S. A. (1995). Psychopathology and academic performance: The role of motivation and learning strategies. *Journal of Counseling Psychology, 42*(4), 456–465.

Brammer, L. M. (1992). Coping with life transitions. Special Section: counseling and health concerns. *International Journal for the Advancement of Counseling, 15*(4), 239–253.

Brammer, L. (1990, Fall). Teaching personal problem solving to adults. Special Issue: Problem solving and cognitive therapy. *Journal of Cognitive Psychotherapy.* pp. 267–279.

Butler, D. L. (1995). Promoting strategic learning by postsecondary students with learning disabilities. *Journal of Learning Disabilities, 28*(3) 170–190.

Chandler, M. C., and Mason, W. H. (1995). Solution-focused therapy: An alternative approach to addictions nursing. *Perspectives in Psychiatric Care, 31*(1), 8–13.

Chapey, R. (Ed.). (1986). *Language intervention strategies in adult aphasia.* Baltimore, MD: Williams and Wilkins.

Chen, L. C. (1990). The effects of attributional feedback and strategy training on achievement behaviors with mathematical learning disabled students. *Bulletin of Educational Psychology, 23*, 143–158.

Chi, M. T., de Leeuw, N., Chie, M. H., and LaVancher, C. (1994). Eliciting self-explanations improves understanding. *Cognitive Science, 18*(3) 439–477.

Cooke, R. A., and Szumal, J. L. (1994). The impact of group interaction styles on problem-solving effectiveness. *Journal of Applied Behavioral Science, 30*(4) 415–437.

Culatta, R., and Goldberg, S. A. (1995). *Stuttering therapy: An integrated approach to theory and practice.* Boston: Allyn and Bacon.

Daly, D. A. (1984). Treatment of the young chronic stutterer: Managing stuttering. In R. F. Curlee and W. H. Perkins (Eds.), *Nature and treatment of stuttering: New directions.* San Diego: College-Hill Press.

Daly, D. A. (1988). *The freedom of fluency: A therapy program for the chronic stutterer,* Moline, IL: LinguiSystems.

Davis-Dorsey, J., Ross, S. M., and Morrison, G. R. (1991). The role of rewording and context personalization in the solving of mathematical word problems. *Journal of Educational Psychology. 83*(1) 61–68.

Deacon, D., and Campbell, K. B. (1991). Decision-making following closed-head injury: Can response speed be retrained? *Journal of Clinical and Experimental Neuropsychology, 13*(5) 639–651.

Dee, S. M., Dansereau, D. F., Peel, J. L., Boatler, J. G., et al. (1991). Using conceptual matrices, knowledge maps, and scripted cooperation to improve personal management strategies. *Journal of Drug Education, 21*(3) 211–230.

Dee Lucas, D., and Larkin, J. H. (1991). Equations in scientific proofs: Effects on comprehension. *American Educational Research Journal, 28*(3), 661–682.

Delclos, V. R., and Harrington, C. (1991). Effects of strategy monitoring and proactive instruction on children's problem-solving performance. *Journal of Educational Psychology, 83*(1), 35–42.

Duchan, J. F., Hewitt, L. E., and Sonnenmeier, R.M. (1994). *Pragmatics: From theory to practice.* Englewood Cliffs, NY: Prentice-Hall.

Duffy, G. G., and Roehler, L. R. (1989). Why strategy instruction is so difficult and what we need to do about it. In C. B. McCormick, G. Miller, and M. Pressley (Eds.), *Cognitive strategy research: From basic research to educational applications.* City; Publisher.

Dugas, M. J., Letarte, H., Rheaume, J., Freeston, M. H., et al. (1995). Worry and problem solving: Evidence of a specific relationship. *Cognitive Therapy and Research, 19*(1), 109–120.

Dunston, P. J. (1992). A critique of graphic organizer research. *Reading Research and Instruction, 31*(2), 57–65.

Dworkin, J. P. (1991). *Motor speech disorders: A treatment guide.* Boston: Mosby Year Book.

Eldredge, N., and Carrigan, J. (1992). Where do my kindred dwell? Using art and storytelling to understand the transition of young Indian men who are deaf. *Arts in Psychotherapy, 19*(1), 29–38.

Fabiani, M., Buckley, J., Gratton, G., Coles, M. G., et al. (1989). The training of complex task performance. Special Issue: The Learning Strategies program: An examination of the strategies in skill acquisition. *Acta Psychologica, 71*(1–3), 259–299.

Fatout, M. F. (1995). Using limits and structures for empowerment of children in groups. *Social Work with Groups, 17*(4), 55–69.

Feltz, D. L., and Landers, D. M. (1983). The effects of mental practice on motor skill learning and performance: A meta-analysis. *Journal of Sport Psychology, 5*(1), 25–57.

Foxx, R. M., Kyle, M. S., Faw, G. D., and Bittle, R. G. (1989). Teaching a problem solving strategy to inpatient adolescents: Social validation, maintenance, and generalization. *Child and Family Behavior Therapy, 11*(3–4), 71–88.

Frank, B. M., and Keene, D. (1993). The effect of learners' field independence, cognitive strategy instruction, and inherent word-list organization on free-recall memory and strategy use. *Journal of Experimental Education, 62*(1), 14–25.

Frederiksen, J. R., and White, B. Y. (1989). An approach to training based upon principled task decomposition. Special Issue: The Learning Strategies program: An examination of the strategies in skill acquisition. *Acta Psychologica, 71*(1–3), 89–146.

Gambrell, L. B., and Jawitz, P. B. (1993). Mental imagery, text illustrations, and childrens story comprehension and recall. *Reading Research Quarterly, 28*(3), 264–276.

Garner, R. (1990). When children and adults do not use learning strategies: Toward a theory of settings. Special Issue: Toward a unified approach to learning as a multisource phenomenon. *Review of Educational Research, 60*(4), 517–529.

Goldberg, S. A., and Culatta, R. (1996). *Five steps to fluency.* San Francisco: IntelliGroup Publishers.

Goldberg, S. A. (1981). *Behavioral cognitive stuttering therapy.* Tigard, OR: C. C. Publications.

Goldberg, S. A. (1993). *Clinical intervention: A philosophy and methodology for clinical practice.* New York: Merrill/Macmillan.

Gopher, D., Weil, M., and Siegel, D. (1989). Practice under changing priorities: An approach to the training of complex skills. Special Issue: The Learning Strategies program: An examination of the strategies in skill acquisition. *Acta Psychologica, 7*(1–3), 147–177.

Gorrell, J. , Tricou, C., and Graham, A. (1991). Children's short- and long-term retention of science concepts via self-generated examples. *Journal of Research in Childhood Education, 5*(2), 100–108.

Greene, B. A., and Royer, J. M. (1994). A developmental review of response time data that support a cognitive components model of reading. Special Issue: Cognitive approaches to reading diagnostics. *Educational Psychology Review, 6*(2), 141–172.

Greenfield, P. M., deWinstanley, P., Kilpatrick, H., and Kaye, D. (1994). Action video game-sand informal education: Effects on strategies for dividing visual attention. Special Issue: Effects of interactive entertainment technologies on development. *Journal of Applied Developmental Psychology, 15*(1), 105–123.

Harlow, R. E., and Cantor, N. (1994). Personality as problem solving: A framework for the analysis of change in daily-life behavior. Special Issue: Cognitive science and psychotherapy. *Journal of Psychotherapy Integration, 4*(4), 355–385.

Heather, N., Kissoon-Singh, J., and Fenton, G. W. (1990). Assisted natural recovery from alcohol problems: Effects of a self-help manual with and without supplementary telephone contact. *British Journal of Addiction. 85*(9), 1177–1185.

Heinze-Fry, J. A., and Novak, J. D. (1990). Concept mapping brings long-term movement toward meaningful learning. *Science Education, 74*(4), 461–472.

Hird, J. S., Landers, D. M., Thomas, J. R., and Horan, J. J. (1991). Physical practice is superior to mental practice in enhancing cognitive and motor task performance. *Journal of Sports Exercise Psychology, 13*, 281–293.

Hodson, B., and Paden, E. (1991). *Targeting intelligible speech*. Austin, TX: Pro-Ed.

Hunt, P., Goetz, L., Alwell, M., and Sailor, W. (1986). Teaching generalized communication responses through an interrupted behavior chain strategy. *Journal of the Association for Persons with Severe Handicaps, 11*, 196–204.

Hynd, C. R., McWhorter, J., YeVette, P., Virginia, L., and Suttles, C. W. (1994). The role of instructional variables in conceptual change in high school physics topics. Special Issue: The reading-science learning-writing connection. *Journal of Research in Science Teaching, 31*(9), 933–946.

Jayanthi, M., and Friend, M. (1992). Interpersonal problem solving: A selective literature review to guide practice. *Journal of Educational and Psychological Consultation, 3*(1), 39–53.

Johnson, K., and Korn, E. R. (1980). Hypnosis and imagery in the rehabilitation of a brain-injured patient. *Journal of Mental imagery, 4*(2), 35–39.

Johnson, M., and Nelson, T. M. (1978). Game playing with juvenile delinquents. *Simulation and Games, 9*(4), 461–475.

Katz, N. (1990). Problem solving and time: Functions of learning style and teaching methods. *Occupational Therapy Journal of Research, 10*(4), 221–236.

Kiewra, K. A., Mayer, R. E., Christensen, M., Kim, S. I., et al. (1991). Effects of repetition on recall and note-taking: Strategies for learning from lectures. *Journal of Educational Psychology 83*(1) 120–123.

Kohl, F. L., and Beckman, P. J. (1990). The effects of directed play on the frequency and length of reciprocal interactions with preschoolers having moderate handicaps. *Education and Training in Mental Retardation, 25*(3), 258–266.

Krascum, R. M. (1993). Feature-based versus exemplar-based strategies in preschoolers' category learning. *Journal of Experimental Child Psychology, 56*(1) 1–48.

Kruger, L. (1988). Programmatic change strategies at the building level. In J. L. Graden, J. E. Zins, and M. J. Curtis (Eds.), *Alternative educational delivery systems: Enhancing instructional options for all students* (pp. 491–512). Washington, DC: National Association of School Psychologists.

Lamar, P., and Siegler, R. S. (1995). Four aspects of strategic change: Contributions to children's learning of multiplication. *Journal of Experimental Psychology General, 124*(1), 83–97.

Lange, G., and Pierce, S. H. (1992). Memory-strategy learning and maintenance in preschool children. *Developmental Psychology, 28*(3) 453–462.

Lange, G., Griffith, S. B., and Nida, R. E. (1990). Form characteristics of category-retrieval relationships in children and adults. *Journal of General Psychology, 117*(1), 5–14.

Lawton, J. T. (1991). Effects of verbal rule instruction on young children's learning. *Journal of Structural Learning, 11*(1), 1–11.

Lenz, B. K., Ellis, E. S., and Scanlon, D. (1996). *Teaching learning strategies to adolescents and adults with learning disabilities*. Austin, TX: Pro-Ed.

Lifter, K., Sulzer-Azaroff, B., Anderson, S. R., and Cowdery, G.E. (1993). Teaching play activities to preschool children with disabilities: The importance of developmental considerations. *Journal of Early Intervention, 17*(2), 139–159

Lonka, K., Lindblom, Y., and Maury, S. (1994). The effect of study strategies on learning from text. *Learning and Instruction, 4*(3), 253–271.

Loranger, A. L. (1994). The study strategies of successful and unsuccessful high school students. *Journal of Reading Behavior, 26*(4), 347–360.

Lyytinen, P., Rasku-Puttonen, H., Poikkeus, A. M., Laakso, M. L., et. al. (1994). Mother-child teaching strategies and learning disabilities. *Journal of Learning Disabilities, 27*(3), 186–192.

Macario, J. F. (1991). Young children's use of color in classification: Foods and canonically colored objects. *Cognitive Development, 6*(1), 17–46.

Mayer, R. E. (1988). Learning strategies: An overview. In C. E. Weinstein, E. T. Goetz, and P. A. Alexander (Eds.), In learning and study strategies (pp. 11–22). New York: Academic Press.

Holland, A., and Ferber, M. (1993). *Aphasia treatment: World perspective.* San Diego: Singular Publishing Group.

Rzoska, K. M., and Ward, C. (1991). The effects of cooperative and competitive learning methods on the mathematics achievement, attitudes toward school, self-concepts, and friendship choices of Maori, Pakeha and Samoan children. *New Zealand Journal of Psychology, 20*(1) 17–24.

Mayer, R. E. (1983). *Thinking, problem solving, cognition.* New York: W. H. Freeman.

Rueter, M. A., and Conger, R. D. (1995). Interaction style, problem-solving behavior, and family problem-solving effectiveness. *Child Development. 66*(1) 98–115.

McDougall, G. J. (1995). Memory self-efficacy and strategy use in successful elders. *Educational Gerontology, 21*(4), 357–373.

McKeachie, W. J. (1988). The need for study strategy training. In C. E. Weinstein, E. T. Goetz and P. A. Alexander (Eds.) *In learning and study strategies* (pp. 3–9). New York: Academic Press.

McWilliams, R., Nietupski, J., and Hamre-Nietupski, S. (1990). Teaching complex activities to students with moderate handicaps through the forward chaining of shorter total cycle response sequences. *Education and Training in Mental Retardation, 25*(3), 292–298.

Melot, A. M. and Corroyer, D. (1992). Organization of metacognitive knowledge: A condition for strategy use in memorization. *European Journal of Psychology of Education, 7*(1), 23–38.

Meloth, M. S., and Deering, P. D. (1994). Task talk and task awareness under different cooperative learning conditions. *American Educational Research Journal, 31*(1), 138–165.

Meltzer, L. J., Solomon, B., Fenton, T., and Levine, M. D. (1989). A developmental study of problem-solving strategies in children with and without learning difficulties. *Journal of Applied Developmental Psychology, 10*(2), 171–193.

Mishra, R. C. (1988). Learning strategies among children in the modern and traditional schools. *Indian Psychologist, 5*(1), 17–24.

Nelson, J. R., Smith, D. J., and Dodd, J. M. (1992). The effects of teaching a summary skills strategy to students identified as learning disabled on their comprehension of science text. *Education and Treatment of Children, 15*(3) 228–243.

Norman, G. R., and Schmidt, H. G. (1992). The psychological basis of problem-based learning: A review of the evidence. *Academic Medicine, 67*(9), 557–565.

Overholser, J. C. (1991). The use of guided imagery in psychotherapy: Modules for use with passive relaxation training. *Journal of Contemporary Psychotherapy, 21*(3), 159–172.

Paivio, A. (1971). Imagery and verbal processes. New York: Holt, Rinehart and Winston.

Parsons, J. E., and Durst, D. (1992). Learning contracts: Misunderstood and underutilized. *Clinical Supervisor, 10*(1) 145–156.

Peterson, S. E. (1992). The cognitive functions of underlining as a study technique. *Reading Research and Instruction. 31*(2) 49–56.

Pfiffner, L. J., Jouriles, E. N., Brown, M. M., Etscheidt, M.A., et al. (1990). Effects of problem-solving therapy on outcomes of parent training for single-parent families. *Child and Family Behavior Therapy, 12*(1), 1–11.

Pinkard, C. M. (1990). Mental imagery methods in rehabilitative services. *Journal of Applied Rehabilitation Counseling, 21*(1), 20–24.

Rabinowitz, M. (1991). Semantic and strategic processing: Independent roles in determining memory performance. *American Journal of Psychology, 104*(3) 427–437.

Rekrut, M. D. (1994). Teaching to learn: Strategy utilization through peer tutoring. *High School Journal, 77*(4) 304–314.

Rettig, K. D. (1993). Problem-solving and decision-making as central processes of family life: An ecological framework for family relations and family resource management. *Marriage and Family Review, 18*(304), 187–222.

Reynolds, R. E., Shepard, C., Lapan, R., Kreek, C., et al. (1990). Differences in the use of selective attention by more successful and less successful tenth-grade readers. *Journal of Educational Psychology, 82*(4), 749–759.

Richardson, A. (1969). *Mental imagery.* New York: Springer Pub. Co.

Rollin, W. J. (1987). *The psychology of communication disorders in individuals and their families.* Englewood Cliffs, NJ: Prentice-Hall

Rosenbek, J. C. , LaPointe, L. L. and Wertz, R. T. (1989). *Aphasia: A clinical approach.* Austin, TX: Pro-Ed.

Sachse, R. (1993). The effects of intervention phrasing on therapist-client communication. *Psychotherapy Research, 3*(4), 260–277.

Schunk, D. H., and Rice, J. M. (1993). Strategy fading and progress feedback: Effects on self-efficacy and comprehension among students receiving remedial reading services. *Journal of Special Education, 27*(3), 257–276.

Seifert, T. L. (1994). Enhancing memory for main ideas using elaborative interrogation. *Contemporary Educational Psychology, 19*(3), 360–366.

Shames, G. H. and Florance, C. L. (1980). *Stutter-free speech: A goal for Therapy.* Columbus, OH: Charles E. Merrill.

Shine, R. E. (1980) Systematic fluency training for children. Tigard, OR: C. C. Publications.

Siegler, R. S. (1991). Strategy choice and strategy discovery. *Learning and Instruction, 1*(1), 89–102.

Simpson, M. L., Olejnik, S., Tam, A. Y. W., and Supattathum, S. (1994). Elaborative verbal rehearsals and college students' cognitive performance. *Journal Educational Psychology, 86*(2), 267–278.

Sinatra, C. (1990). Five diverse secondary schools where learning style instruction works. *Journal of Reading, Writing, and Learning Disabilities International, 6*(3), 323–334.

Singer, R. N., Flora, L. A., and Abourezk, T. L. (1989). The effect of a five-step cognitive learning strategy on the acquisition of a complex motor task. *Journal of Applied Sport Psychology, 1*(2), 98–108.

Skaggs, L. P., Rocklin, T. R., Dansereau, D. F., Hall, R. H., et al. (1990). Dyadic learning of

technical material: Individual differences, social interaction, and recall. *Contemporary Educational Psychology, 15*(1), 47–63.

Snapp, J. C., and Glover, J. A. (1990). Advance organizers and study questions. *Journal of Educational Research, 83*(5), 266–271.

Sommer, R. (1978). *The mind's eye: Imagery in everyday life.* New York: Delacorte Press.

Starnes, W. R., and Loeb, R. C. (1993). Locus of control differences in memory recall strategies when confronted with noise. *Journal of General Psychology, 120*(4), 463–471.

Thames, D. G., and Reeves, C. K. (1994). Poor readers' attitudes: Effects of using interests and trade books in an integrated language arts approach. Special Issue: Assessment and intervention in reading/literacy education: Research and practice. *Reading Research and Instruction, 33*(4), 293–307.

Thompson, L. A. (1994). Dimensional strategies dominate perceptual classification. *Child Development, 65*(6), 1627–1645

Turner, L. A., Dofny, E. M., and Dutka, S. (1994). Effect of strategy and attribution training on strategy maintenance and transfer. *American Journal on Mental Retardation, 98*(4), 445–454.

Umbach, B., Darch, C., and Halpin, G. (1989). Teaching reading to low performing first-graders in rural schools: A comparison of two instructional approaches. *Journal of Instructional Psychology, 16*(3), 112–121.

Valle, J. D. (1990). The development of a learning styles program in an affluent, suburban New York elementary school. *Journal of Reading, Writing, and Learning Disabilities International, 6*(3), 315–322.

Vealey, R. S. (1986). Imagery training for performance enhancement. In J. M. William (Ed.), *Applied sport psychology* (pp. 209–234). San Francisco: Mayfield Publications.

Vitz, P. (1992). Narrative and counseling I.: From analysis of the past to stories about it. *Journal of Psychology and Theology, 20*(91), 11–19.

Waters, H. S., and Andreassen, C. (1983) Children's use of memory strategies under instruction. In M. Pressley and J.R. Levin (Eds.), *Cognitive strategy research: psychological foundations* (pp. 3–24). New York: Springer-Verlag.

Watson, K. L., and Lawson, M. J. (1995). Improving access to knowledge: The effect of strategy training for question answering in high school geography. *British Journal of Educational Psychology, 65*(1), 97–111.

Webster, R. L. (1974). *The precision fluency shaping program: Speech reconstruction for stutterers.* Roanoke, VA: Communications Development Corporation, Ltd.

Webster, R. L. (1974). A behavioral analysis of stuttering: Treatment and theory. In K. S. Calhoun, H. E. Adams, and H. E. Mitchel (Eds.), Innovative treatment methods in Psychopathology. New York: John Wiley.

Webster, R. (1980). Evolution of a target-based therapy for stuttering. *Journal of Fluency Disorders, 5,* 303–320.

Wertz, R. T., LaPointe, L. L., and Rosenbek, J. C. (1991). *Apaxia of speech in adults.* San Diego, CA: Singular Publishing Group.

Wilkinson, P., and Mynors-Wallis, L. (1994). Problem-solving therapy in the treatment of unexplained physical symptoms in primary care: A preliminary study. *Journal of Psychosomatic Research, 38*(6), 591–598.

Willoughby, T., Wood, E., and Khan, M (1994). Isolating variables that impact on or detract from the effectiveness of elaboration strategies. *Journal of Educational Psychology, 86*(2), 279–289.

Willoughby, T. and Wood, E., (1994). Elaborative interrogation examined at encoding and retrieval. *Learning and Instruction, 4*(2), 139–149.

Wilson, B. A., Baddeley, A., Evans, J., and Shiel, A. (1994). Errorless learning in the rehabilitation of memory impaired people. *Neuropsychological Rehabilitation, 4*(3), 307–326.

Wood, E., Willoughby, T., Kaspar, V., and Idle, T. (1994). Enhancing adolescents' recall of factual content: The impact of provided versus self-generated elaborations. *Alberta Journal of Educational Research, 40*(1), 57–65.

Wood, E., Needham, D. R., Williams, J., and Roberts, R. (1994). Evaluating the quality and impact of mediators for learning when using associative memory strategies. *Applied Cognitive Psychology, 8*(7), 679–692.

Wood, E., Miller, G., Symons, S., Canough, T., et al. (1993). Effects of elaborative interrogation on young learners' recall of facts. Special Issue: Strategies instruction. *Elementary School Journal, 94*(2), 245–254.

Wood, D., Bruner, J. S., and Ross, G. (1976). The role of tutoring in problem-solving. *Journal of Child Psychology and Psychiatry, 17*, 89–100.

TREATMENT EFFICACY

Baer, D. M. (1990). The critical issue in treatment efficacy is knowing why treatment was applied: A student's response to Roger Ingham. In *Treatment Efficacy Research in Communication Disorders.* Rockville, MD: American Speech-Language-Hearing Association.

Dowd, E. T., and Hingst, A. G. (1983). Matching therapists' predicates: An in vivo test of effectiveness. *Perceptual and Motor Skills, 57*(1), 207–210

Dowling, S., and Bliss, L. S. (1984). Cognitive complexity, rhetorical sensitivity: Contributing factors in clinical skill? *Journal of Communication Disorders, 17*(1) 9–17.

Finch, J., Mattson, D., and Moore, J. (1993). Selecting a theory of counseling: Personal and professional congruency for counseling students. Special Issue: Counselor educators' theories of counseling. *TCA Journal., 21*(1), 97–102.

Forsythe, G. B., McGaghie, W. C., and Friedman, C. P. (1985). Factor structure of the Resident Evaluation Form. *Educational and Psychological Measurement, 45*(2), 259–264.

Fortune, A. E., Pearling, B., and Rochelle, C. D. (1991). Criteria for terminating treatment. *Families in Society, 72*(6) 366–370.

Frosh, S. (1991). The semantics of therapeutic change. *Journal of Family Therapy, 13*(2), 171–186.

Gallagher, J. S., and Hargie, O. D. (1992). The relationship between counselor interpersonal skills and the core conditions of client-centered counseling. *Counseling Psychology Quarterly, 5*(1), 3–16.

Ginsburg, A. D. (1985) Comparison of training evaluation with tests of clinical ability in medical students. *Journal of Medical Education, 60*(1), 29–36.

Goodwin, R. E., and Bolton, D. P. (1991). Decision making in cognitive rehabilitation: A clinical model. *Cognitive Rehabilitation, 9*(4), 12–19.

Haynes, W. O. and Oratio, A. R. (1978). A study of clients' perceptions of therapeutic effectiveness. *Journal of Speech and Hearing Disorders, 43*(1), 21–33.

Kahn, W. A. (1992). To be fully there: Psychological presence at work. *Human Relations, 45*(4), 321–349.

Kahn, D. L., and Steeves, R. H. (1988). Caring and practice: Construction of the nurse's world. *Scholarly Inquiry for Nursing Practice, 2*(3), 201–216.

Kanfer, F. (1968). Issues and ethics in behavior manipulation. In H. N. Sloane, Jr., and B. D. MacAulay (Eds.), *Operant procedures in remedial speech and language training* (pp. 411–423). New York: Houghton Mifflin,

Kirshbaum, H. (1991). Disability and humiliation. Special Issue: The humiliation dynamic: Viewing the task of prevention from a new perspective: I. *Journal of Primary Prevention, 12*(2), 169–181.

Kleckner, T., Frank, L., Bland, C., Amendt, J. H., et al. (1992). The myth of the unfeeling strategic therapist. *Journal of Marital and Family Therapy, 18*(1) 41–51.

Klein, H. B., and Moses, N. (1994). *Intervention planning for children with communication disorders.* Englewood Cliffs: Prentice-Hall.

McCollum, E. E. (1994). "Which set of problems do you want to deal with?" *Journal of Family Psychotherapy, 5*(4), 75–77.

McGovern, M. A., and Davidson, J. (1983). Student perceptions of performance. British *Journal of Disorders of Communication, 18*(3), 181–185

Meredith, G. M. (1985). Two rating indicators of excellence in teaching in lecture-format courses. *Psychological Reports, 56*(1), 52–54

Mozdzierz, G. J., and Greenblatt, R.L. (1992). Clinical paradox and experimental decision making. *Individual Psychology Journal of Adlerian Theory, Research and Practice, 48*(3), 302–312.

Murphy, A.T. (1982). The clinical process and the speech-language pathologist. In G. H. Shames and E. H. Wiig, *Human communication disorders* (pp. 453–474). Columbus, OH: Charles E. Merrill.

Oliver, J. M., Lightfoot, S. L., Searight, H. R., and Katz, B. (1990). Consistency in individual and family theoretical orientation from assessment to therapy: Its impact on the effectiveness of therapy. *American Journal of Family Therapy, 18*(3), 236–245.

Oratio, A. R., and Hood, S. B. (1977). Certain select variables as predictors of goal achievement in speech therapy. *Journal of Communication Disorders, 10*(4), 331–342.

Oz, S. (1995). A modified balance-sheet procedure for decision making in therapy: Cost-cost comparisons. *Professional Psychology Research and Practice, 21*(3), 78–81.

Ozechowski, T. J. (1994). The integration of emotion in solution-focused therapy: Comment. *Journal of Marital and Family Therapy, 20*(2), 205–206.

O'Donohue, W., Fisher, J. E., Plaud, J. J., and Link W. (1989). What is a good treatment decision? The client's perspective. *Professional Psychology Research and Practice, 20*(6), 404–407.

Pollock, D. C., Shanley, D. F., and Byrne, P. N. (1985). Psychiatric interviewing and clinical skills. *Canadian Journal of Psychiatry, 30*(1) 64–68.

Potter, W. J. and Emanuel, R. (1990). Students preferences for communication styles and their relationship to achievement. *Communication Education, 39*(3), 234–249.

Rennie, D. L. (1994). Clients' deference in psychotherapy. Special Section: Qualitative research in counseling process and outcome. *Journal of Counseling Psychology, 41*(4), 427-437.

Rosenberg, C. M., Gerrein, J. R., Manohar, V. and Liftik, J. (1976). Evaluation of training of alcoholism counselors. *Journal of Studies on Alcohol, 37*(9) 1236–1246

Safran, J. D. (1989). Insight and action in psychotherapy. Journal of Integrative and Eclectic Psychotherapy, 8(3), 233–239.

Sagie, A., Elizur, D., and Koslowsky, M. (1990). Effect of participation in strategic and tactical decisions on acceptance of planned change. *Journal of Social Psychology, 130*(4), 459–465.

Shaffer, P., Murillo, N., and Michael, W. B. (1978). The factorial validity of a scale for evaluation of counselors in a university counseling and testing center. *Educational and Psychological Measurement, 38*(4), 1085–1096.

Shames, G. H. and Rubin, H. (1986). The roles of the client and the clinician during therapy. In G. H. Shames and H. Rubin (Eds.), *Stuttering, then and now* (pp. 61–270). Columbus, OH: Charles E. Merrill.

Silove, D., Parker, G., and Manicavasagar, V. (1990). Perceptions of general and specific therapist behaviors. Journal of Nervous and Mental Disease. 178 (5) 292-299.

Stolk, Y., and Perlesz, A. J. (1990). Do better trainees make worse family therapists? A follow up study of client families. *Family Process, 29*(1), 45–58.

Strickland, T. L., Jenkins, J. O., Myers, H. F. and Adams, H. E .(1988). Diagnostic judgments as a function of client and therapist race. *Journal of Psychopathology and Behavioral Assessment, 10*(2), 141–151.

Strupp, H. H., and Hadley, S. W. (1979). Specific vs. nonspecific factors in psychotherapy: A controlled study of outcome. *Archives of General Psychiatry, 36*(10), 1125–1136.

Trinchero, R. L. (1974). The longitudinal measurement of teacher effectiveness: Gains in overall class performance versus changes in pupil aptitude-performance relationships. *California Journal of Educational Research,. 25*(3), 121–127.

Vourlekis, B. S., Bembry, J., Hall, G., and Rosenblum, P. (1992). Evaluating the interrater reliability of process recordings. *Research on Social Work Practice, 2*(2), 198–206.

Wiseman, H., and Rice, L. N. (1989). Sequential analyses of therapist-client interaction during change events: A task-focused approach. *Journal of Consulting and Clinical Psychology, 57*(2), 281–286.

A P P E N D I X   B

Multicultural/Bilingual Resource Materials

ASIAN AMERICAN/PACIFIC ISLANDERS

Language

Cheng, L. R. (1991). *Assessing Asian language performance: Guidelines for evaluating limited-english-proficient students*. Oceanside, CA: Academic Communication Associates.

Mattes, L. J. (1995). *Bilingual vocabulary assessment measure: Chinese*. Oceanside, CA: Academic Communication Associates.

Miscellaneous

Trueba, H. T., Cheng, L. L., and Ima, K. (1993). *Myth or reality: Adaptive strategies of Asian Americans in California*. Washington, DC: The Falmer Press

Trueba, H. T., Jacobs, L., and Kirton, E. (1990). *Cultural conflict and adaptation: The case of the Hmong children in American Society*. Washington, DC: The Falmer Press

AFRICAN AMERICAN

Articulation and Phonology

Iglesias, A., and Anderson, H. B. (1993). Dialectal variations. In J. Bernthall and N. Bankson (Eds.), *Articulation and phonological disorders* (pp. 147–161). Englewood Cliffs, NJ: Prentice-Hall.

Stuttering

Leith, W., and Mims. (1975). cultural influences in the development and treatment of stuttering: A preliminary report on the black stutterer. *Journal of Speech and Hearing Research, 40,* 459–466.

Miscellaneous

Dillard, J. L. (1972). *Black English: Its history and usage in the United States*. New York: Random House.

Dillard, J. M. (1968). *Multicultural counseling*. Chicago: Nelson-Hall.

Nuru, N. (1993). Multicultural aspects of deafness. In D. Battle (Ed.), *Communication disorders in multicultural populations* (pp. 287–302). Boston: Andover Medical Publishers.

HISPANIC

Articulation and Phonology

Canfield, D. L. (1981). *Spanish pronunciation in the Americas*. Chicago: University of Chicago Press.

Carrow, E. (1974). *Austin Spanish articulation test*. Austin, TX: Learning Concepts.

Hodson, B. W. (1986). *The assessment of phonological processes—Spanish.* San Diego, CA: Los Amigos.

Lindamood, C., and Lindamood, P. (1971). *Lindamood Auditory Conceptualization Test* (LAC). Chicago: Riverside Publishing Company.

Mattes, L. J. (1995). *Spanish Articulation Measures.* Distributed by Speech Bin

Mattes, L. J., and Santiago, G. (1994). *Teaching Spanish speech sounds: Drills for articulation therapy.* Oceanside, CA: Aca-demic Communication Associates

Toronto, A. S. (1977). *Southwestern Spanish Articulation Test (SSAT).* Austin, TX: Academic Tests. Inc.

Language

Benton, A. Sivan, A. B., and Hamsher, K. (1994). *Multilingual Aphasia Examination (MAE)* (3rd ed.). San Antonio, TX: The Psychological Corporation.

Burt, M. K., and Dulay, H. C. (1978). *Bilingual Syntax Measure and I and II (BSM I, BSM II).* San Antonio, TX: The Psychological Corporation

Carrow-Woolfolk, E. (1985). *Test for Auditory Comprehension of Language, Revised—English/Spanish (TACL-R).* Allen, TX: DLM Teaching Resources.

Casas, C., and Portillo, P. (1989). *Language Learning Everywhere We Go.* Oceanside, CA: Academic Communication Associates.

Critchlow, D. C. (1974). *Dos Amigos Verbal Language Scales (Dos Amigos).* East Aurora, NY: United Educational Services.

Dunn, L. M., Padilla, E. R., Lugo, D. E., and Dunn, L. M. (1987). *Test de Vocabulario en Imagenes Peabody.* Cedar Pines, MN: American guidance Service.

Hannah, E. P., and Gardner, J. O. (1985). *Hannah-Garder Test of Verbal and Nonverbal Language Functioning-English/Spanish.* Northridge, CA: Linguia Press.

Hresko, W. P., Reid, D. K., and Hammill, D. D. (1982). *A Standardized Test of the Spanish Spoken Language for Children Ages 3 to 7 Years (Prueba del Desarrollo Inicial del Lenguaje).* Austin, TX: Pro-Ed.

James, P. (1984). *James Language Dominance-English/Spanish.* Austin, TX: Learning Concepts.

Mattes, L. J. (1995). *Spanish Language Assessment Procedures.* Oceanside, CA: Academic Communication Associates.

Nugent, T. M., Shipley, K. G., and Provencio, D. O. (1989). *Spanish Test for Assessing Morphological Production (STAMP).* Oceanside, CA: Academic Communication Associates.

Payan, R. (1984). Language assessment for Bilingual Exceptional Children. In L. M. Baca and H. T. Cervantes (Eds.), *The bilingual interface.* St. Louis, MO: Times Mirror/Mosley.

Rosenberg, L. R. (1984) *Cuban-Spanish Edition of the Sequenced Inventory of Communication Development (SICD-R).* New York: Slosson Educational Publications.

Toronto, A. (1973). *Screening Test of Spanish Grammar (STSG).* Evanston, IL: Northwestern University Press.

Toronto, A. (1977). *Toronto Tests of Receptive Vocabulary (Spanish/English).* Austin, TX: National Education Laboratory.

Toronto, A. S., Leverman, D., Hanna, C., Rosenzweig, P., and Maldonado, A. (1978). *Del Rio Language Screening Test.* Austin, TX: National Educational Laboratory Publishers.

Woodcock, R. W. (1981). *Woodcock Language Proficiency Battery–Spanish (WLPB-S)* Allen, TX: DLM Teaching Resources.

Woodcock, R. W., and Munoz-Sandoval, A. (1993). *Woodcock-Munoz Language Survey, English and Spanish Forms.* Chicago: Riverside Publishing Company.

Zimmerman, I. L., Steiner, V. G., and Pond, R. E. (1992). *Preschool Language Scale—3, Spanish Edition (PLS-3 Spanish).* San Antonio, TX: The Psychological Corporation.

Psychological/Educational

Bruininks, R. H., Woodcock, R. W., Weatherman, R. F., and Hill, R. K. (1984). *Scales of Independent Behavior (SIB).* Chicago: Riverside Publishing Company.

Isser, A. V., and Kirk, W. (1991). *Prueba Illinois de Habilidades Pscolinguisticas (Spanish adaptation of ITPA).* San Antonio, TX: The Psychological Corporation.

Riverside Performance Assessment Series (R-PAS). Chicago: Riverside Publishing Company.

Wechsler, D. (1992). *Escala de Inteligencia Wechsler para Ninos—Revisada.* San Antonio, TX: Psychological Corporation.

Woodcock, R. W. (1982). *Woodcock Spanish Psycho-Educational Battery. (Bateria Woodcock Psico-Educativa en Espanol).* Chicago: Riverside Publishing Company.

Miscellaneous

Bruininks, R. H., Hill, R. K. Weatherman, R. F., and Woodcock, R. W. (1986). *Inventory for Client and Agency Planning (ICAP).* Chicago: Riverside Publishing Company.

Hamayan, E. V., and Damico, J. S. (Eds) (1991). *Limiting Bias in the Assessment of the Bilingual Child.* Austin, TX: Pro-Ed.

Kayser, H. (1993). Hispanic cultures. In D. Battle (Ed.), *communication disorders in multicultural populations* (pp. 114–157). Boston, MA: Andover Medical Publishers.

Langdon, H. W., and Cheng, L. L. (Eds.). (1992). *Hispanic children and adults with communication disorders: Assessment and intervention.* Gaithersburg, MD: Aspen Publishers.

Mattes, L. J., and Omark, D. R. (1991). *Speech and language assessment for he bilingual handicapped.* Austin, TX: Pro-Ed.

Ramos, M., and Ciccia, G. G. (1995). *Speech and language handouts, Spanish version.* Austin, TX: Pro-Ed.

Valdez, C. G. (1985). *Bilingual health and developmental history questionnaire.* Oceanside, CA: Academic Communication Associates.

MISCELLANEOUS

Adler, S. (1993). *Multicultural communication skills in the classroom.* Boston: Allyn & Bacon.

Battle, D. E. (1993). *Communication disorders in multicultural populations.* Stoneham, MA: Andover Medical Publishers.

Bilingual children with communicative disorders: Referral guidelines. Oceanside, CA: Academic Communication Associates.

Bryer, J. (1993). *Rap n 'Rock.* Oceanside, CA: Academic Communication Associates

Bryer, J. (1994). *Rap 'n Rock 2.* Oceanside, CA: Academic Communication Associates

Cole, L., and Snope, T. (1981). Resource guide to multicultural tests and materials. *Asha, 23,* 639–649.

Deal, V. R., and Rodriguez, V. L. (1987). *Resource guide to multicultural tests and materials in communicative disorders.* Rockville, MD: ASHA.

Deal, V. R., and Yan, M. A. (1985). Resource Guide to multicultural tests and materials, Supplement II. *Asha, 27,* 43–49.

Mattes, L. J., and Omark, D. R. (1991). *Speech and language assessment for the bilingual handicapped.* Oceanside, CA: Academic Communication Associates.

Roberts, P. and Roberts, C. (1993). *Celebrating cultural diversity through music.* Oceanside, CA: Academic Communication Associates

Roseberry-McKibbin, C. (1993). *Bilingual classroom communication profile: An observational screening tool.* Oceanside, CA: Academic Communication Associates.

Roseberry-McKibbin, C. (1994). *Multicultural students with special language needs: Practical strategies for assessment and intervention.* Oceanside, CA: Academic Communication Associates

Sue, D. W., and Sue, D. (1990). *Counseling the culturally different: Theory and practice.* New York: John Wiley.

Taylor, O. (Ed.). (1986). *Nature of communication disorders in culturally and linguistically diverse populations.* San Diego, CA: College-Hill Press.

Weakland, M. (1992). *Rap it Up!* Oceanside, CA: Academic Communication Associates.

Westby, E. C. (1994). Multicultural issues. In B. Tomblin, H. L. Morris, and D. C. Spriestersbach (Eds)., *Diagnosis in speech-language pathology* (pp. 29–50). San Diego, CA: Singular Publishing Group.

Bibliography

Aberbach, D. (1995, August). Charisma and attachment theory: A cross disciplinary interpretation. *International Journal of Psycho Analysis, 76*(4), 845–855.

Afflerbach, P. and Walker, B. (1992). Main idea instruction: An analysis of three basal reader series. *Reading Research and Instruction, 32*(1), 11–28.

Agbayani-Stewart, P. (1994). Filipino American culture and family: Guidelines for practitioners. *Families in Society, 75*(7), 429–438.

Ager, A. (1987). Minimal intervention: a strategy for generalized behavior change with mentally handicapped individuals. *Behavioral Psychotherapy, 15*(1), 16–30.

Albano, M., Cox, B., York, J., and York, R. (1981). Educational teams for students with severe and multiple handicaps. In R. York, W.K. Schofield, D.J. Donder, D.L. Ryndak, and B. Reguly (Eds.), *Organizing and implementing services for students with severe and multiple handicaps,* (pp. 23–24). Springfield: Illinois State Board of Education.

Albertini, J.A., Smith, J.M., and Metz, D.E. (1983). Small group versus individual speech therapy with hearing-impaired young adults. *Volta-Review, 85,* 83–89.

Alderman, D. L., Evans, F.R., and Wilder, G. (1981, Winter). The validity of written simulation exercises for assessing clinical skills in legal education. *Educational and Psychological Measurement, 41*(4), 1115–1126.

Alexander, J. F., and Newberry, A.M. (1988). The interview process in functional family therapy. *Family Therapy Collections, 24,* 33–48.

Alexander, J.M., and Schwanenflugel, P. (1994). Strategy regulation: the role of intelligence, metacognitive attributions, and knowledge base. *Developmental Psychology, 30*(5), 709–723.

Alston, R. and Mngadi, S. (1992). The interaction between disability status and the African American experience: Implications for rehabilitation counseling. *Journal of Applied Rehabilitation Counseling. 23*(2), 12–16.

Anderson, A.H., Clark, A., and Mullin, J. (1994, June). Interactive communication between children: Learning how to make language work in dialogue. *Journal of Child Language, 21*(2), 439–463.

Andrews, J. A., and Andrews, M. (1990). *Family based treatment in communicative disorders—a systemic approach.* Sandwich, IL: Janelle Publications.

Andrews, M.L. (1995). *Manual of Voice Treatment.* San Diego, CA: Singular Publishing Group.

Archer, J. (1994). Achievement goals as a measure of motivation in university students. *Contemporary Educational Psychology, 19*(4) 430–446.

Aronson, A.E. (1990). *Clinical Voice Disorders.* New York: Thieme.

Astrom, J., Thorell, L.H., and D'Elia, G. (1993). Attitudes towards and observations of nonverbal communication in a psychotherapeutic greeting situation: III. An interview study of outpatients. *Psychological Reports, 73*(1), 151–168

Ausubel, D.P. (1968). *Educational psychology: A cognitive view.* New York: Holt, Rinehart, and Winston.

Baer, D.M. (1990). The critical issue in treatment efficacy is knowing why treatment was applied: A student's response to Roger Ingham. In *Treatment Efficacy Research in Communication Disorders.* Rockville, MD: American Speech-Language-Hearing Association.

Balajthy, E. and Weisberg, R. (1990). Transfer effects of prior knowledge and use of graphic organizers on college developmental readers' summarization and comprehension of expository text. *National Reading Conference Yearbook, 39,* 339–345.

Bales, R.F. (1950). *Interaction process analysis.* Cambridge, England: Addison-Wesley.

Balluerka, N. (1995). The influence of instructions, outlines, and illustrations on the comprehension and recall of scientific texts. *Contemporary Educational Psychology, 20*(3), 369–375.

Bandura, A. (1969). *Principles of behavior modification.* New York: Holt, Rinehart, and Winston.

Baptiste, D.A. (1990). Therapeutic strategies with Black-Hispanic families: Identify problems of a neglected minority. *Journal of Family Psychotherapy, 1*(3), 15–38.

Barbara, D.A. (1954). *Stuttering: a psychodynamic approach to its understanding and treatment.* New York: Julian Press.

Barfield, J. (1976). Biological influences on sex differences in behavior. In M.S. Teitelbaum (Ed.), *Sex differences: social and biological perspectives* (pp. 62–121). Garden City, NY: Anchor Press.

Barksdale-Ladd, M.A., and Thomas, K.F. (1993). Eight teachers' reported pedagogical dependency on basal readers. *Elementary School Journal, 94*(1), 49–72.

Barnes, D., and Keenan, M. (1993). Concurrent activities and instructed human fixed-interval performance. *Journal of the Experimental Analysis of Behavior, 59*(3), 501–520.

Barnes, H.N., O'Neill, S.F., Aronson, M.D., and Delbanco, T.L. (1984). Early detection and outpatient management of alcoholism: a curriculum for medical residents. *Journal of Medical Education, 59*(11, Pt. 1), 904–906

Baroff, G.S. (1976). On the use of aversive techniques in controlling self-injurious behavior. *American Psychologist, 31*(8), 616.

Baum, B.E., and Gray, J. (1992). Expert modeling, self-observation using videotape, and acquisition of basic therapy skills. *Professional Psychology Research and Practice, 23*(3), 220–225.

Baxter, J.C., Winters, E.P., and Hammer, R.E. (1968). Gestural behavior during a brief interview as a function of cognitive variables. *Journal of Personality and Social Psychology, 8,* 303–307.

Beck, A.T. (1976). *Cognitive therapy and the emotional disorders.* New York: International Universities Press.

Beckwith, J.B.(1994). Prejudice, reverse prejudice, and positive attitude towards differences among people with intellectual disabilities. *Psychological Reports, 74*(3, Pt. 1), 938.

Belfiore, P.J., and Browder, D.M. (1992). The effects of self-monitoring on teacher's data-based decisions and on the performance of adults with severe mental retardation. *Education and Training in Mental Retardation, 27*(1), 60–67.

Berg, I.K., and Jaya, A. (1993, January). Different and same: family therapy with Asian American families. *Journal of Marital and Family Therapy, 19*(1), 31–38.

Berg, I.K., and Miller, S.P. (1992). Working with Asian American clients: one person at a time. Special issue: Multicultural practice. *Families in Society, 73*(6), 356–363.

Berg, J.H., and Wright-Buckley, C. (1988, October). Effects of racial similarity and interviewer intimacy in a peer counseling analogue. *Journal of Counseling Psychology, 35*(4), 377–384.

Berger, M.M. (1978). *Videotape techniques in psychiatric training and treatment.* New York: Brunner/Mazel.

Bergin, J.J. (1989). Building group cohesiveness through cooperation activities. Special Issue: Preventive and developmental counseling. *Elementary School Guidance and Counseling, 24*(1), 90–94.

Berlo, D.K. (1960). *The process of communication.* New York: Holt, Rinehart, and Winston.

Bernard, R.M. (1990). Effects of processing instructions on the usefulness of a graphic organizer and structural cuing in text. *Instructional Science, 19*(3), 207–217.

Berne, E. (1966). *Principles of group treatment.* New York: Oxford University Press.

Bernthal, J.E., and Bankson, N.W. (1981). *Articulation disorders.* Englewood Cliffs, NJ: Prentice-Hall, Inc.

Berry, D. C. (1991). The role of action in implicit learning. *Quarterly Journal of Experimental Psychology Human Experimental Psychology, 43A*(4), 881–906.

Best, D. L. (1993). Inducing children to generate mnemonic organizational strategies: an examination of long-term retention and materials. *Developmental Psychology, 29*(2), 324–336.

Beukelman, D.R., and Yorkston, K.M. (1991). *Communication disorders following traumatic brain injury.* Austin, TX: Pro-Ed.

Bielaczyc, K., Pirolli, P. L., and Brown, A. L. (1995). Training in self-explanation and self-regulation strategies: Investigating the effects of knowledge acquisition activities on problem solving. *Cognition and Instruction, 13*(2), 221–252.

Biggs, J. B. (1988). Assessing student approaches to learning. *Australian Psychologist, 23*(2), 197–206.

Billings, B. P. (1994). The importance of involvement in counseling. *Journal of Reality Therapy, 13*(2), 26–30.

Bivens, J.A., and Berk, L.E. (1990). A longitudinal study of the development of elementary school children's private speech. *Merrill Palmer Quarterly, 36*(4), 443–463.

Blair, C. (1992). Objective: recruitment-student perspective. *ASHA, 34,* 43–44.

Blakemore, B., Shindler, S., and Conte, R. (1993, Spring). A problem solving training program for parents of children with attention deficit hyperactivity disorder. [Special issue.] *Canadian Journal of School Psychology, 9*(1), 66–85.

Blanck, P.D., Rosenthal, R., Vannicelli, M., and Lee, T.D. (1986). Therapists' tone of voice: Descriptive, psychometric, interactional, and competence analyses. *Journal of Social and Clinical Psychology, 4*(2), 154–178.

Bleile, K.M. (1995). *Manual of articulation and phonological disorders.* San Diego, CA: Singular Publishing Group.

Bock, M.A. (1994). Acquisition, maintenance, and generalization of a categorization strat-egy by children with autism. *Journal of Autism and Developmental Disorders, 24*(1), 39–51.

Bolton, B., Bonge, D., and Marr, J. (1979). Ratings of instruction, examination performance, and subsequent enrollment in psychology courses. *Teaching of Psychology, 6*(2), 82–85.

Boone, D.R. (1983). *Voice and voice therapy.* Englewood Cliffs, NJ: Prentice-Hall.

Borkowski, J.G., and Buchel, F.P. (1981). Learning and memory strategies in the mentally retarded. In M. Pressley and J.R. Levin (Eds.), *Cognitive strategy research: Psychological foundations,* (pp. 103–128). New York: Springer-Verlag,

Borus, J.F., et al. (1979). Psychotherapy in the goldfish bowl. *Archives of General Psychiatry, 36*(2), 187–190.

Bowman, V.E. and DeLucia, J.L. (1993). Preparation for group therapy: The effects of preparer and modality on group process and individual functioning. *Journal for Specialists in Group Work, 18*(2), 67–79.

Boyd-Franklin, N. (1989). Five key factors in the treatment of Black families. *Journal of Psychotherapy and the Family, 6*(1–2), 53–69.

Boyd-Franklin, N., and Shenouda, N.T. (1990). A multisystems approach to the treatment of a Black, inner-city family with a schizophrenic mother. *American Journal of Orthopsychiatry, 60*(2), 186–195.

Brackney, B. E. and Karabenick, S.A. (1995). Psychopathology and academic performance: The role of motivation and learning strategies. *Journal of Counseling Psychology, 42*(4), 456–465.

Brammer, L. (1990, Fall). Teaching personal problem solving to adults: problem solving and cognitive therapy. [Special issue.] *Journal of Cognitive Psychotherapy,* 267–279.

Brammer, L.M. (1992). Coping with life transitions: Counseling and health concerns. *International Journal for the Advancement of Counseling, 15*(4), 239–253.

Brennan, S.E. and Williams, M. (1995). The feeling of another's knowing: prosody and filled pauses as cues to listeners about the metacognitive states of speakers. *Journal of Memory and Language, 34*(3), 383–398.

Bricker, W.A., and Campbell, P. (1980). Interdisciplinary assessment and programming for multihandicapped students. In W. Sailor, B. Wilcox, and L. Brown (Eds.), *Methods of instruction for severely handicapped students* (pp. 3–45). Baltimore: Paul H. Brookes.

Broadbent, D.E. (1992). Listening to one of two synchronous messages. *Journal of Experimental Psychology General, 121*(2), 125–127.

Brondolo, E., Baruch, C., Conway, E., and Marsh, L. (1994). Aggression among inner-city minority youth: a biopsychosocial model for school-based evaluation and treatment. Special Issue: Multicultural views on domestic violence. *Journal of Social Distress and the Homeless, 3*(1), 53–80.

Brooke, M., Uomoto, J.M., Mclean, A. Jr., and Fraser, R.T. (1991). *Rehabilitation of persons with traumatic brain injury: A continuum of care*. Austin, TX: Pro-Ed.

Brown, A.K., Brown, J.L., and Poulson, C.L. (1995). Generalization of children's identity matching-to-sample performances to novel stimuli. *Psychological Record, 45*(1), 29–43.

Brown, A.L., Smiley, S.S., and Lawton, S.C. (1978). The effects of experience on the selection of suitable retrieval cues for studying text. *Child Development, 49*, 829–835.

Brutten, E.J., and Shoemaker, D.J. (1967). *The modification of stuttering*. Englewood Cliffs, NJ: Prentice-Hall.

Bryngelson, B. (1935). Sidedness as an etiological factor in stuttering. *Journal of Genetics and Psychology, 47*, 204–217.

Buenting, Julie A. (1992). Health life-styles of lesbian and heterosexual women: Lesbian health: What are the issues? [Special issue.] *Health Care for Women International, 13*(2), 165–171.

Bull, P. E. (1987). *Posture and gesture*. New York: Pergamon Press.

Butler, D., and Geis, F. L. (1990, January). Nonverbal affect responses to male and female leaders: implications for leadership evaluations. *Journal of Personality and Social Psychology, 58*(1), 48–59,

Butler, D.L. (1995). Promoting strategic learning by postsecondary students with learning disabilities. *Journal of Learning Disabilities, 28*(3), 170–190.

Calas, M. B. (1993). Deconstructing charismatic leadership: Re-reading Weber from the darker side. *Charismatic leadership: Neo Weberian perspectives*. [Special issue.] *P. Quarterly, 4*(3–4), 305–328.

Cameron, C. (1994). Women survivors confronting their abusers: Issues, decisions, and outcomes. *Journal of Child Sexual Abuse, 3*(1), 7–35.

Campbell, L.R., Brennan, D.G., and Steckol, K.F. (1992). Preservice training to meet the needs of people from diverse cultural backgrounds. *Asha, 35*, 29–32.

Cantor, J., and Engle, R.W. (1989, November). The influence of concurrent load on mouthed and vocalized modality effects, *Memory and Cognition, 17*(6), 701–711.

Capelli, C., Nakagawa, N., and Madden, C. M. (1990, December). How children understand sarcasm: The role of context and intonation. *Child Development, 61*(6), 1824–1841.

Carter, R.T,. and Helms, J.E. (1992, October) The counseling process as defined by relationship types: A test of Helms's interactional model: Gender and relationships. [Special issue.] *Journal of Multicultural Counseling and Development, 20*(4), 181–201.

Carver, R.P., and Leibert, R.E. (1995, January–March). The effect of reading library books at different levels of difficulty upon gain in reading ability. *Reading Research Quarterly, 30*(1), 26–48.

Cave, K. R., Pinker, S., Giorgi, L., Thomas, C.E., et al. (1994, February).The representation of location in visual images, *Cognitive Psychology, 26*(1), 1–32.

Chan, F., Hedl, J. J., Parker, H. J., Lam, C. S., et al. (1988). Differential attitudes of Chinese students toward people with disabilities: A cross-cultural perspective. *International Journal of Social Psychiatry, 34*(4) 267–273.

Chan, F., Lam, C. S., Wong, D., Leung, P., et al. (1988). Counseling Chinese Americans with disabilities. [Special issue.] *Journal of Applied Rehabilitation Counseling, 19*(4), 21–25.

Chan, L. K. S. (1994). Relationship of motivation, strategic learning, and reading achievement in Grades 5, 7, and 9. *Journal of Experimental Education, 62*(4), 319–339.

Chan-ho, M.W. (1988). From classroom to clinic: Promoting the transfer of knowledge and clinical skills: A personal view. *Bulletin of the Hong Kong Psychological Society*, July-January (19–20), 78-86.

Chandler, M. C., and Mason, Walter H. (1995). Solution-focused therapy: An alternative approach to addictions nursing. *Perspectives in Psychiatric Care, 31*(1), 8–13.

Chang, P. (1994). Effects of interviewer questions and response type on compliance: An analogue study. *Journal of Counseling Psychology, 41*(1), 74–82.

Chapey, R. (Ed.). (1986). *Language intervention strategies in adult aphasia.* Baltimore, MD: Williams and Wilkins.

Chappell, A.L. (1992). Towards a sociological critique of the normalization principle. *Disability, Handicap, and Society, 7*(1), 35–51.

Chen, L. C. (1990). The effects of attributional feedback and strategy training on achievement behaviors with mathematical learning disabled students. *Bulletin of Educational Psychology, 23*, 143–158.

Cheng, A.H.H. (1973). Rapport in initial counseling interview and its impact on effectiveness. *Acta Psychologica Taiwanica, 15*, 31–40.

Cheng, L.L. (1992). Objective: Recruitment—Asians and Pacific Islanders. *Asha, 34*, 41–42.

Cheng, L.R.I. (1987). Cross cultural and linguistic considerations in working with Asian populations. *Asha, 29*, 33–37.

Chevron, E.S., Rounsaville, B.J., Rothblum, E.D., and Weissman, M.M (1983). Selecting psychotherapists to participate in psychotherapy outcome studies: Relationship between psychotherapist characteristics and assessment of clinical skills. *Journal of Nervous and Mental Disease, 171*(6), 348–353.

Chi, M.T., de Leeuw, N., Chie, M.H., and LaVancher, C. (1994). Eliciting self-explanations improves understanding. *Cognitive Science, 18*(3), 439–477.

Chideya, F. (1995). *Don't believe the hype: Fighting cultural misinformation about African Americans.* New York: Penguin Books.

Chomsky, N. (1972). *Language and mind.* New York: Harcourt Brace Jovanovich.

Christenson, S.L., and Cleary, M. (1990). Consultation and the parent-educator partnership: A perspective. *Journal of Educational and Psychological Consultation, 1*(3) 219–241.

Clutton-Brock, T.H. and Parker, G.A. (1995). Sexual coercion in animal societies. *Animal Behaviour, 49*(5), 1345–1365.

Cohn, E.S. (1989). Fieldwork education: Shaping a foundation for clinical reasoning. *American Journal of Occupational Therapy, 43*(4), 240–244.

Cole, L. (1989). E pluribus pluribus: Multicultural imperatives for the 1990s and beyond. *Asha, 31*, 65–70.

Cole, L. (1992). We're Serious. *Asha, 32*, 38–39.

Cole, L., and Deal, V.R. (Eds.). (In Press). *Communication disorders in multicultural populations.* Rockville, MD: American Speech-Language-Hearing Association.

Compton, C. (1990). *A guide to 85 tests for special education.* Belmont, CA: Fearon Education.

Cooke, R.A., and Szumal, J. L. (1994). The impact of group interaction styles on problem-solving effectiveness. *Journal of Applied Behavioral Science, 30*(4) 415–437.

Cooper, B.A., Letts, L., and Rigby, P. (1993). Exploring the use of color cueing on an assistive device in the home: Six casestudies. *Physical and Occupational Therapy in Geriatrics, 11*(4), 47–59.

Corey, G. (1990). *Theory and practice of group counseling* (3rd ed.). Pacific Grove, CA: Brooks/Cole.

Cornett, B.S., and Chabon, S.S. (1988). *The clinical practice of speech-language pathology.* Columbus, OH: Merrill.

Costello, J. (1982). Techniques of therapy based on operant conditioning. In W. Perkins (Ed.), *General Principles of Therapy.* New York: Thieme-Stratton.

Costello, J., and Ingham, R.J. (1984). Stuttering as an operant disorder. In R. Curlee and W. Perkins (Eds.), *Nature and treatment of stuttering.* San Diego. CA: College-Hill Press.

Costello, J.M. (1980). Operant conditioning and the treatment of stuttering. *Seminars in Speech, Language, and Hearing, 1*, 311–325.

Coufal, K.L. (1993). Collaborative consultation for speech-language pathologists. *Topics in Language Disorders, 14*(1), 1–14.

Cowen, E.L., Wyman, P.A., Work, C., and Iker, M.R. (1995). A preventive intervention for enhancing resilience among highly stressed urban children. *Journal of Primary Prevention, 15*(3), 247–260.

Crais, E. (1991). Moving from "parent involvement" to family-centered services. American *Journal of Speech-Language Pathology, 1*, 5–8.

Cramer, P. and Skidd, J. E. (1992). Correlates of self-worth in preschoolers: The role of gender-stereotyped styles of behavior. *Sex Roles, 26*(9–10), 369–390.

Crary, M.A. (1993). *Developmental motor speech disorders.* San Diego, CA: Singular Publishing Group.

Crowder, R.G. (1976). *Principles of learning and memory.* Hillsdale, NJ: Lawrence Erlbaum.

Culatta, R., and Goldberg, S.A. (1995). *Stuttering therapy: An integrated approach to theory and practice.* Boston: Allyn and Bacon.

Culatta, R. and Rubin, H. (1973). A program for the initial stages of fluency therapy. *Journal of Speech and Hearing Research, 16,* 556–567.

Cuvo, A.J., and Klatt, K.P. (1992). Effects of community-based, videotaped, and flash card instruction of community-referenced sight words on students with mental retardation. *Journal of Applied Behavior Analysis, 25*(2), 499–512.

Daly, D.A. (1984). Treatment of the young chronic stutterer: Managing stuttering. In R.F. Curlee and W.H. Perkins (Eds.), *Nature and treatment of stuttering: New directions.* San Diego: College-Hill Press.

Daly, D.A. (1988). *The freedom of fluency: A therapy program for the chronic stutterer.* Moline, IL: LinguiSystems.

Darou, W.G. (1987). Counseling and the northern native. *Canadian Journal of Counseling, 21*(1), 33–41.

Darrow, A.A., and Johnson, C.M. (1994). Junior and senior high school music student's attitudes toward individuals with a disability. *Journal of Music Therapy, 31*(4), 266–279.

Das, A.K., and Littrell, J.M. (1989). Multicultural education for counseling: A reply to Lloyd. *Counselor Education and Supervision, 29*(1), 7–15.

Davis, D.L., and Boster, L.H. (1992). Cognitive-behavioral-expressive interventions with aggressive and resistant youths. North American out-of-home care conference: Out-of-home care: Challenging the new realities (1991, St. Louis, MO). *Child Welfare, 71*(6), 557–573.

Davis, I.P. (1938). The speech aspects of reading readiness. Newer practices in reading in the elementary school. 17th yearbook of the department of elementary school principals, *NEA, 17*(7), 282–289.

Davis, L.E., and Gelsomino, J. (1994). An assessment of practitioner cross-racial treatment experiences. *Social Work, 39*(1), 116–123.

Davis-Dorsey, J., Ross, S. M., and Morrison, G. R. (1991). The role of rewording and context personalization in the solving of mathematical word problems. *Journal of Educational Psychology, 83*(1) 61–68.

de Luca, R.V. and Holborn, S.W. (1992). Effects of a variable-ratio reinforcement schedule with changing criteria on exercise in obese and nonobese boys. *Journal of Applied Behavior Analysis, 25*(3), 671–679.

Deacon, D., and Campbell, K.B. (1991). Decision-making following closed-head injury: Can response speed be retrained? *Journal of Clinical and Experimental Neuropsychology, 13*(5), 639–651.

Dee, S. M., Dansereau, D. F., Peel, J. L., Boatler, J. G., et al. (1991). Using conceptual matrices, knowledge maps, and scripted cooperation to improve personal management strategies. *Journal of Drug Education, 21*(3) 211–230.

Dee Lucas, D., and Larkin, J.H. (1991). Equations in scientific proofs: Effects on comprehension. *American Educational Research Journal, 28*(3), 661–682.

Delclos, V.R., and Harrington, C. (1991). Effects of strategy monitoring and proactive instruction on children's problem-solving performance. *Journal of Educational Psychology, 83*(1), 35–42.

Delgado, M., and Humm-Delgado, D. (1984). Hispanics and group work: A review of the literature. *Social Work Groups, 7*(3), 85–96.

Denis, M. (1974). Religious education among North American Indian peoples. *Religious Education, 69* (3), 343–354.

Dent, V., and Seligman, S. (1993). The dynamic functions of the act of reading. *International Journal of Psycho Analysis, 74*(6), 1253–1267.

Deutsch, M. (1949). An experimental study of the effects of cooperation and competition upon group process. *Human Relations, 2,* 199–231.

Devereaux, D. (1991). The issue of race and the client-therapist assignment. *Issues in Mental Health Nursing, 12*(3), 283–290,

Dickinson, A.M. (1989). The detrimental effects of extrinsic reinforcement on "intrinsic motivation." *Behavior Analyst, 12*(1), 1–15.

Diedrich, W., and Bangert, J. (1980). *Articulation learning*. San Diego, CA: College-Hill Press.

Dinkmeyer, D.C., Dinkmeyer, D.C., Jr., and Sperry. L. (1987). *Adlerian counseling and psychotherapy* (2nd ed.). Columbus, OH: Merrill.

Donahue-Kilburg, G. (1992). *Family-centered early intervention for communication disorders*. Gaithersburg, MD: Aspen Publishers.

Dooley, J.G. (1996). *Albert Renger-Patzsch: The magic of material things*. Malibu, CA. The J. Paul Getty Museum.

Dorpat, T.L. (1993). Clinical education: 1: Response. *Journal of Clinical Psychoanalysis, 2*(3), 318–320.

Dortch, H. L. and Trombly, C. A. (1990). The effects of education on hand use with industrial workers in repetitive jobs. *American Journal of Occupational Therapy, 44*(9), 777–782.

Dowd, E.T., and Hingst, A.G. (1983). Matching therapists' predicates: An in vivo test of effectiveness. *Perceptual and Motor Skills, 57*(1), 207–210.

Dowling, S. (1986). Supervisory training: Impetus for clinical supervision. *Clinical Supervisor, 4*(4), 27–34.

Dowling, S., and Bliss, L.S. (1984). Cognitive complexity, rhetorical sensitivity: Contributing factors in clinical skill? *Journal of Communication Disorders, 17*(1) 9–17.

Dresser, N. (1996). *Multicultural manners*. New York: John Wiley and Sons.

Dreyfus, H.L., and Dreyfus, S.E. (1986). *Mind over machine*. New York: The Free Press.

DuBray, W.H. (1985). American Indian values: Critical factor in casework. *Social Casework, 66*(1), 30–37.

Duchan, J.F. (1984). Language assessment: The pragmatics revolution. In R.C. Naremore (Ed.), *Language science* (pp. 147–180). San Diego, CA.: College-Hill Press.

Duchan, J.F., Hewitt, L.E., and Sonnenmeier, R.M. (1994). *Pragmatics: From theory to practice*. Englewood Cliffs, NJ: Prentice-Hall.

Duffy, G.G., and Roehler, L.R. (1989). Why strategy instruction is so difficult and what we need to do about it. In C.B. McCormick, G. Miller, and M. Pressley (Eds.), *Cognitive strategy research: From basic research to educational applications*. City: Publisher?

Dugas, M.J., Letarte, H., Rheaume, J., Freeston, M.H., et al. (1995). Worry and problem solving: Evidence of a specific relationship. *Cognitive Therapy and Research, 19*(1), 109–120.

Dunlap, G., and Plienis, A. J. (1991). The influence of task size on the unsupervised task performance of students with developmental disabilities. *Education and Treatment of Children, 14*(2), 85–95.

Dunn, L. (1965). *Peabody picture vocabulary test*. Circle Pines, MN: American Guidance Service.

Dunn, L., and Dunn, L. (1981). *Peabody Picture Vocabulary Test—revised*. Circle Pines, MN: American Guidance Service.

Dunn, R. (1990). Cross-cultural differences in learning styles of elementary-age students from four ethnic backgrounds. *Journal of Multicultural Counseling and Development, 18*(2), 68–93.

Dunn, R., and Griggs, S.A. (1990). Research on the learning style characteristics of selected racial and ethnic groups. *Journal of Reading, Writing, and Learning Disabilities International, 6*(3), 261–280.

Dunston, P.J. (1992). A critique of graphic organizer research. *Reading Research and Instruction, 31*(2), 57–65.

Durdic, S. (1983). Odnos izmedu terapeuta I pacijenta u bihejvior psihoterapiji [The therapist-patient relationship in behavioral psychotherapy]. *Psihijatrija Danas, 15*(2–3), 265–269.

Durlak, J.A. (1979). Comparative effectiveness of paraprofessional and professional helpers. *Psychological Bulletin, 86*(1), 80–92.

Durvasula, R.S., and Mylvaganam, G.A. (1994) Mental health of Asian Indians: Relevant issues and community implications: Asian-American mental health. [Special issue.] *Journal of Community Psychology, 22*(2), 97–108.

Dworkin, J.P. (1991). *Motor speech disorders: A treatment guide*. Boston: Mosby Year-Book.

Edwards, E.D., and Edwards, M.E. (1984). Group work practice with American Indians. *Social Work with Groups, 7*(3), 7–21.

Egan, V. (1993). Can specific inspection time strategies be inferred by their latency? *Irish Journal of Psychology, 14*(2), 253–269.

Eisenberg, A.M., and Smith, R.R., Jr. (1971). *Nonverbal communication*. New York: Bobbs-Merrill.

Eisendrath, S. J. (1989). Factitious physical disorders: Treatment without confrontation. 34th Annual Meeting of the Academy of Psychometric Medicine (1987, Las Vegas, NV). *Psychosomatics, 30*(4), 383–387.

Ekman, P. (1964). Body position, facial expression, and verbal behavior during interviews. *Journal of Abnormal and Social Psychology, 68*(3), 295–301.

Ekman, P. (1985). *Telling lies.* New York: Norton.

Ekman, P., and Friesen, W. (1968). Nonverbal behavior in psychotherapy research. *Research in Psychotherapy, 3,* 179–215.

Ekman, P., and Friesen, W. (1971). *Emotion in the human face.* New York: Bobbs-Merrill.

Ekman, P., and Friesen, W. (1974). Detecting deception from the body or face. *Journal of Personality and Social Psychology, 29,* 288–298.

Elbert, M. (1989). Generalization in the treatment of phonological disorders. In L.V. McReynolds and J.E. Spradlin (Eds.), *Generalization strategies in the teatment of communication disorders* (pp. 31–43). Philadelphia: B.C. Decker.

Eldredge, N., and Carrigan, J. (1992). Where do my kindred dwell? Using art and storytelling to understand the transition of young Indian men who are deaf. *Arts in Psychotherapy, 19*(1), 29–38.

Ellinwood, C. (1989). The young child in person-centered family therapy. Person-centered ability, affective states, and psychological distress. [Special issue.] *Journal of Counseling Psychology, 42*(1), 105–115.

Elliott, R.T., Sherwin, E., Harkins, S.W., and Marmarosh, C. (1995). Self-appraised problem-solving ability, affective states, and psychological distress. [Special issue.] *Journal of Counseling Psychology, 42*(1), 105–115.

Ellis, A. (1962). *Reason and emotion in psychotherapy.* New York: Lyle Stuart.

Esten, G., and Willmott, L. (1993). Double bind messages: The effects of attitude towards disability on therapy. Special Issue: Women with disabilities: Found voices. *Women and Therapy 14*(3–4), 29–41.

Exum, H.A., and Lau, E. (1988). Counseling style preference of Chinese college students. *Journal of Multicultural Counseling and Development, 16*(2), 84–92.

Fabiani, M., Buckley, J., Gratton, G., Coles, M.G., et al. (1989). The training of complex task performance: The Learning Strategies program: An examination of the strategies in skill acquisition. [Special issue.] *Acta Psychologica, 71*(1–3), 259–299.

Fairbanks, G. (1954). A theory of the speech organism as a servosystem. *Journal of Speech and Hearing Disorders, 19,* 133–139.

Farver, J.A., and Howes, C. (1988). Cross-cultural differences in social interaction: A comparison of American and Indonesian children. *Journal of Cross-Cultural Psychology, 19*(2), 203–215.

Fatout, M. F. (1995). Using limits and structures for empowerment of children in groups. *Social Work with Groups, 17*(4), 55–69.

Feldman, P. (1994). The use of therapeutic questions to restructure dysfunctional triangles in marital therapy: A psychodynamic family therapy approach. *Journal of Family Psychotherapy, 5*(3), 55–67.

Feltz, D.L. and Landers, D.M. (1983). The effects of mental practice on motor skill learning and performance: A meta-analysis. *Journal of Sport Psychology, 5*(1), 25–57.

Ferraro, K.F. (1993). Are Black older adults health-pessimistic? *Journal of Health and Social Behavior, 34*(3), 201–214.

Ferster, C.B. (1957). Withdrawal of positive reinforcement as punishment. *Science, 126,* 509.

Feyereisen, P., and de Lannoy, J. (1991). *Gestures and speech: Psychological investigations.* New York: Cambridge Press.

Fiene, J.I., and Taylor, P.A. (1991). Serving rural families of developmentally disabled children: A case management model. *Social Work, 36*(4), 323–327.

Finch, J., Mattson, D., and Moore, J. (1993). Selecting a theory of counseling: Personal and professional congruency for counseling students. Special Issue: Counselor educators' theories of counseling. *TCA Journal, 21*(1), 97–102.

Fine, M.J., and Gardner, A. (1994). Collaborative consultation with families of children with special needs: Why bother? *Journal of Educational and Psychological Consultation, 5*(4), 283–308.

Fishman, J.A., and Luders, E. (19??). What has the sociology of language to say to the teacher? In C.B. Cazden, V.P. John, and D. Hymes (Eds.), *The functions of language.* New York: Teachers College Press.

Flaskerud, J.H. (1986). The effects of culture-compatible intervention on the utilization of mental health services by minority clients. *Community Mental Health Journal, 22*(2), 127–141.

Flora, S. R. (1990). Undermining intrinsic interest from the standpoint of a behaviorist. *Psychological Record, 40*(3), 323–346.

Florsheim, M. J., and Herr, J.J. (1990). Family counseling with elders. Special Issue: Counseling and therapy for elders. *Generations, 14*(1), 40–42.

Flower, R.M. (1984). *Delivery of speech-language pathology and audiology services.* Baltimore, MD: Williams and Wilkins.

Forlin, C., and Cole, P. (1994). Attributions of the social acceptance and integration of children with mild intellectual disability. *Australia and New Zealand Journal of Developmental Disabilities, 19*(1), 11–23

Forsythe, G.B., McGaghie, W.C., and Friedman, C.P. (1985). Factor structure of the Resident Evaluation Form. *Educational and Psychological Measurement, 45*(2), 259–264.

Fortune, A. E., Pearling, B., and Rochelle, C. D. (1991). Criteria for terminating treatment. *Families in Society, 72*(6) 366–370.

Fox, L. (1989). Stimulus generalization of skills and persons with profound mental handicaps. *Education and Training in Mental Retardation, 24*(3), 219–229.

Foxx, R. M., Kyle, M. S., Faw, G. D., and Bittle, R.G. (1989). Teaching a problem solving strategy to inpatient adolescents: Social validation, maintenance, and generalization. *Child and Family Behavior Therapy, 11*(3–4), 71–88.

Frank, B.M. and Keene, D. (1993). The effect of learners' field independence, cognitive strategy instruction, and inherent word-list organization on free-recall memory and strategy use. *Journal of Experimental Education, 62*(1), 14–25.

Frank, J.D. (1961). *Persuasion and healing.* Baltimore: Johns Hopkins Press.

Frankel, S.A., and Frankel, E.B. (1970). Nonverbal behavior in a selected group of Negro and white males. *Psychosomatics, 11*(2), 127–132.

Frankish, C. (1995). Intonation and auditory grouping in immediate serial recall: Donald Broadbent and applied cognitive psychology. [Special issue.] *Applied Cognitive Psychology, 9*, S5–S22.

Franklin, A.J. (1992). Therapy with African American men: Multicultural practice. [Special issue.] *Families in Society, 73*(6), 350–355.

Frazier, N., and Sadker, M. (1973). *Sexism in school and society.* New York: Harper and Row.

Frederiksen, J.R., and White, B.Y. (1989). An approach to training based upon principled task decomposition: The Learning Strategies program: An examination of the strategies in skill acquisition. [Special issue.] *Acta Psychologica, 71*(1–3), 89–146.

Freed, A.O. (1992). Discussion: Minority elderly. *Journal of Geriatric Psychiatry, 25*(1), 105–111.

French, D.C., and Stright, A.L.(1991). Emergent leadership in children's small groups. *Small Group Research, 22*(2), 187–199.

Frensch, P.A., Buchner, A., and Lin, J. (1994). Implicit learning of unique and ambiguous serial transitions in the presence and absence of a distractor task. *Journal of Experimental Psychology Learning, Memory, and Cognition, 20*(3), 567–584.

Frensch, P. A., and Miner, C. S. (1994). Effects of presentation rate and individual differences in short-term memory capacity on an indirect measure of serial learning. *Memory and Cognition, 22*(1), 95–110.

Freud, S. (1933). *A general introduction to psychoanalysis.* New York: Norton.

Friedlander, R. (1993). BHSM comes to the Flathead Indian Reservation. *Asha, 35*, 29–30.

Friedman, W. J. (1991). The benefits of suffering and the costs of well-being: Secondary gains and losses. *Medical Hypnoanalysis Journal, 6*(3), 111–116.

Fromm-Reichmann, F. (1963). Psychiatric aspects of anxiety. In M.R. Stein, A.J. Vidich, and D.M. White (Eds.), *Identity and anxiety* (pp. 129–144). New York: The Free Press.

Frosh, S. (1991). The semantics of therapeutic change. *Journal of Family Therapy, 13*(2), 171–186.

Gagné, R.M. (1970). *The conditions of learning.* New York: Holt, Rinehart, and Winston.

Gagné, R.M., Briggs, L.J., and Wager, W.W. (1988). *Principles of instructional design.* New York: Holt, Rinehart, and Winston.

Galea, L.A., and Kimura, D. (1993). Sex differences in route-learning. *Personality and Individual Differences, 14*(1), 53–65.

Gallagher, J.S., and Hargie, O.D. (1992). The relationship between counselor interpersonal skills and the core conditions of client-centered counseling. *Counseling Psychology Quarterly, 5*(1), 3–16.

Gallant, J.P., Thyer, B.A., and Bailey, J.S. (1991). Using bug-in-the-ear feedback in clinical supervision: Preliminary evaluations. *Research on Social Work Practice, 1*(2), 175–187.

Gambrell, L. B., and Jawitz, P. B. (1993). Mental imagery, text illustrations, and children's story comprehension and recall. *Reading Research Quarterly, 28*(3), 264–276.

Gardner, R.A. (1982). *Psychotherapeutic approaches to the resistant child.* New York: Aronson.

Garner, R. (1990). When children and adults do not use learning strategies: Toward a theory of settings: Toward a unified approach to learning as a multisource phenomenon. [Special issue.] *Review of Educational Research, 60*(4), 517–529.

Garza, R. T., Lipton, J. P., and Isonio, S. A. (1989). Group ethnic composition, leader ethnicity, and task performance: An application of social identity theory. *Genetic, Social, and General Psychology Monographs, 115*(3), 295–314.

Gelinas-Chebat, C., and Chebat, J. C. (1992). Effects of two voice characteristics on the attitudes toward advertising messages. *Journal of Social Psychology, 132*(4), 447–459.

George, R.L., and Dustin D. (1988). *Group counseling: Theory and practice.* Englewood Cliffs, NJ: Prentice-Hall.

Georgia, Robert T. (1994). Preparing to counsel clients of different religious backgrounds: A phenomenological approach. *Counseling and Values, 38*(2), 143–151.

Gesuelle-Hart, S., Kaplan, L.W., and Kikoski, C. (1990). Assessing the family in context: Working with the urban poor. [Special issue.] *Journal of Strategic and Systemic Therapies, 9*(3), 1–13.

Giangreco, M. (1989). Making related service decisions for students with severe handicaps in public schools: Roles, criteria, and authority. *Dissertation Abstracts International, 50,* 1624A. (University Microfilms No. DA8919516)

Gierut, J.E.M., and Dinnsen, D. (1987). A functional analysis of phonological knowledge and generalization learning in misarticulating children. *Journal of Speech and Hearing Research, 30*(4), 462–479.

Giles, S., and Dryden, W. (1991). Fears about seeking therapeutic help: The effect of sex on subjects, sex of professional, and title of professional. *British Journal of Guidance and Counseling, 19*(1) 81–92.

Gillan, D. J., and Lewis, R. (1994). A componential model of human interaction with graphs: I. Linear regression modeling. *Human Factors, 36*(3), 419-440.

Gillstrom, A., and Ronnberg, J. (1994). Prediction accuracy of text recall: Ease, effort, and familiarity. *Scandinavian Journal of Psychology, 35*(4), 367–385.

Gim, R.H. , Atkinson, D.R., and Whiteley, S. (1990). Asian-American acculturation, severity of concerns, and willingness to see a counselor. *Journal of Counseling Psychology, 37*(3), 281–285.

Ginsburg, A. D. (1985) Comparison of training evaluation with tests of clinical ability in medical students. *Journal of Medical Education, 60*(1), 29–36.

Gladding, S.T. (1991). *Group work: A counseling specialty.* New York: Merrill.

Glenberg, A.M., and Langston, W.E. (1992). Comprehension of illustrated text: Pictures help to build mental models. *Journal of Memory and Language, 31*(2), 129–151.

Goldberg, S.A. (1981). *Behavioral cognitive stuttering therapy.* Tigard, OR: C. C. Publications.

Goldberg, S.A. (1990, November). *Identification of clinical skills and their relationship to clinical training.* Presentation at the American Speech-Language-Hearing Association Annual Convention. Seattle, WA.

Goldberg, S.A. (1993). *Clinical intervention: A philosophy and methodology for clinical practice.* New York: Merrill/Macmillan.

Goldberg, S.A,. and Culatta, R. (1996). *Five steps to fluency.* San Francisco: IntelliGroup Publishers.

Goldstein, G.S. (1974). Behavior modification: Some cultural factors. *Psychological Record, 24*(1), 89–91.

Goldstein, M. D., Hopkins, J. R., and Strube, M. J. (1994). The eye of the beholder: A classroom demonstration of observer bias. *Teaching of Psychology, 21*(3), 154–157.

Golffing, F. (1956). *Nietzsche: The birth of tragedy and the genealogy of morals* (Trans.). Garden City, NY: Doubleday .

Gollnick, D., and Chinn, P. (1990). *Multicultural education in a pluralistic society* (3rd ed.). New York: Merrill/Macmillian.

Goodare, H. (1994). Counseling people with cancer: Questions and possibilities. *Advances, 10*(2), 4–17.

Goodenough, W. (1987). Multi-culturalism as the normal human experience. In E.M. Effy and W.L. Partridge (Eds.), *Applied anthropology in America* (2nd ed.). New York: Columbia University Press.

Goodwin, R.E., and Bolton, D.P. (1991). Decision making in cognitive rehabilitation: A clinical model. *Cognitive Rehabilitation, 9*(4), 12–19.

Goolkasian, P., Van Wallendael, L.R., and Terry, W.S. (1991). Recognition memory for easy and difficult text. *Journal of General Psychology, 118*(4), 375–393.

Gopher, D., Weil, M., and Siegel, D. (1989). Practice under changing priorities: An approach to the training of complex skills: The Learning Strategies program: An examination of the strategies in skill acquisition. [Special issue.] *Acta Psychologica, 71*(1–3), 147–177.

Gorrell, J., Tricou, C., and Graham, A. (1991). Children's short- and long-term retention of science concepts via self-generated examples. *Journal of Research in Childhood Education, 5*(2), 100–108.

Gotlib, I.H. (1982). Self-reinforcement and depression in interpersonal interaction: The role of performance level. *Journal of Abnormal Psychology, 91*, 3–13.

Grant, E.C. (1968). An ethological description of non-verbal behavior during interview. *British Journal of Medical Psychology, 4*(2), 177–184.

Greene, Barbara A., and Royer, J. M. (1994). A developmental review of response time data that support a cognitive components model of reading: Cognitive approaches to reading diagnostics. [Special issue.] *Educational Psychology Review, 6*(2), 141–172.

Greenfield, P. M., deWinstanley, P., Kilpatrick, H., and Kaye, D. (1994). Action video games and informal education: Effects on strategies for dividing visual attention: Effects of inter-active entertainment technologies on development. [Special issue.] *Journal of Applied Developmental Psychology, 15*(1), 105–123.

Gregory, K., Wells, K.B., and Leake, B. (1987). Medical students' expectations for encounters with minority and nonminority patients. *Journal of the National Medical Association, 79*(4), 403–408.

Griener, T. (1992, May). Objective recruitment—public schools. *Asha, 34*, 40–41.

Griffith, E.E. (1986, January). Blacks and American psychiatry. *Hospital and Community Psychiatry, 37*(1), 5.

Gross, D. (1990) Communication and the elderly. *Physical and Occupational Therapy in Geriatrics, 9*(1), 49–64.

Gross, P.R. (1994). A pilot study of the contribution of empathy to burnout in Salvation Army officers. *Work and Stress, 8*(1) 68–74.

Hagen, D., and Behrman, M. (1984). Using computers with mildly and moderately handicapped children. In M. Behrmann (Ed.), *Handbook of microcomputers in special education* (pp. 79–101). San Diego: College-Hill Press.

Hains, A.A., and Fouad, N.A. (1994). The best laid plans...: Assessment in an inner-city high school: Multicultural assessment. [Special issue] *Measurement and Evaluation in Counseling and Development, 27*(2), 116–124.

Hall, E.T. (1959). *The silent language*. Garden City, NY: Doubleday.

Hall, L.E., and Tucker, C.M. (1985) Relationships between ethnicity, conceptions of mental illness, and attitudes associated with seeking psychological help. *Psychological Reports, 57*(3, Pt. 1), 907–916.

Hall, T., and Lloyd, C. (1990). Non-verbal communication in a health care setting. *British Journal of Occupational Therapy, 53*(9) 383–386.

Halpern, R. (1990). Poverty and early childhood parenting: Toward a framework for intervention. *American Journal of Orthopsychiatry, 60*(1), 6–18.

Halpert, J.A. (1990). The dimensionality of charisma. *Journal of Business and Psychology, 4*(4), 399-410.

Hanser, S.B. and Furman, C.E. (1980). The effect of videotape-based feedback vs. field-based feedback on the development of applied clinical skills. *Journal of Music Therapy, 17*(3) 103–112.

Hanson, M.J., and Lovett, D. (1992). Personnel preparation for early interventionists: A cross-disciplinary survey. *Journal of Early Intervention, 16*(2), 123–135.

Hare, A.P. (1994). Types of roles in small groups: A bit of history and a current perspective. *Small Group Research, 25*(3), 433–448.

Harel, Z. (1986). Older Americans act related homebound aged: What difference does racial background make?: Ethnicity and gerontological social work. *Journal of Gerontological Social Work.* [Special issue.] *9*(4), 133–143.

Haring, T.G., and Lovinger, L. (1989). Promoting social interaction through teaching generalized play initiation responses to preschool children with autism. *Journal of the Association for Persons with Severe Handicaps, 14*(1), 58–67.

Harlow, R. E., and Cantor, N. (1994). Personality as problem solving: A framework for the analysis of change in daily-life behavior: Cognitive science and psychotherapy. [Special issue.] *Journal of Psychotherapy Integration, 4*(4), 355–385

Harre, R. (1988). The social context of self-deception. In B.P. McLaughlin and A.O. Rorty (Eds.), *Perspectives on self-deception* (pp. 364–379). Berkeley, CA: University of California Press.

Hartley, L.L. (1995). *Cognitive-communicative abilities following brain injury.* San Diego, CA: Singular Publishing Group.

Hatfield, E., Hsee, C. K. , Costello, J., Weisman, M. S., et al. (1995). The impact of vocal feedback on emotional experience and expression. *Journal of Social Behavior and Personality, 10*(2), 293–312.

Hawkins, K.W. (1995). Effects of gender and communication content of leadership emergence in small task-oriented groups. *Small Group Research, 26*(2), 234–249.

Haynes, N.M., and Gebreyesus, S. (1992). Cooperative learning: A case for African-American students. *School Psychology Review, 21*(4), 577–585.

Haynes, W.O., and Oratio, A.R. (1978). A study of clients' perceptions of therapeutic effectiveness. *Journal of Speech and Hearing Disorders, 43*(1), 21–33.

Heather, N., Kissoon-Singh, J., and Fenton, G.W. (1990). Assisted natural recovery from alcohol problems: Effects of a self-help manual with and without supplementary telephone contact. *British Journal of Addiction, 85*(9), 1177–1185.

Hector, M.A., and Fray, J.S. (1987). The counseling process, client expectations, and cultural influences: A review. *International Journal for the Advancement of Counselling, 10*(4), 237–247.

Hegarty, M., and Just, M.A. (1993). Constructing mental models of machines from text and diagrams. *Journal of Memory and Language, 32*(6), 717–742.

Hegde, M.N., and Davis, D. (1995). *Clinical methods and practicum in speech-language pathology* (2nd ed.). San Diego, CA: Singular Publishing Group.

Heinze-Fry, J.A., and Novak, J.D. (1990). Concept mapping brings long-term movement toward meaningful learning. *Science Education, 74*(4), 461–472.

Heller, T., Markwardt, R., Rowitz, L., and Farber, B. (1994). Adaptation of Hispanic families to a member with mental retardation. *American Journal on Mental Retardation, 99*(3), 289–300

Hempel, C.G. (1995). *Aspects of scientific explanation.* New York: The Free Press.

Henriksen, E.M. (1991). A peer helping program for the middle school. *Canadian Journal of Counselling, 25*(1), 12–18.

Herbert, J.T., and Cheatham, H.E. (1988). Africentricity and the Black disability experience: A theoretical orientation for rehabilitation counselors. *Journal of Applied Rehabilitation Counseling, 19*(4, Special Issue), 50–54.

Hermans, H. J., Fiddelaers, R., de-Groot, R., and Nauta, J. F. (1990). Self-confrontation as a method for assessment and intervention in counseling. *Journal of Counseling and Development, 69*(2), 156–162.

Herring, R. D. (1992). Seeking a new paradigm: Counseling Native Americans. *Journal of Multicultural Counseling and Development, 20*(1), 35–43

Hersen, M., and Van Hasselt, V. B. (1992). Behavioral assessment and treatment of anxiety in the elderly. *Clinical Psychology Review, 12*(6), 619–640.

Hewes, G.W. (1957). World distribution of certain postural habits. *American Anthropologist, 57*, 231-244.

Higgins, E., and Warner, R. (1975). Counseling blacks. *Personnel and Guidance Journal, 53*, 383-386.

Hill, C.E., and Stephany, A. (1990). Relation of nonverbal behavior to client reactions. *Journal of Counseling Psychology, 37*(1), 22–26.

Hill, J., and Carper, M. (1985). Group therapeutic approaches with the head injured. *Cognitive Rehabilitation, 3*, 18–29.

Hines, P.M., Garcia-Preto, N., McGoldrick, M., Almeida, R., et al. (1992). Intergenerational relationships across cultures: Multicultural practice. [Special issue.] *Families in Society, 73*(6), 323–338.

Hird, J.S., Landers, D.M., Thomas, J.R., and Horan, J.J. (1991). Physical practice is superior to mental practice in enhancing cognitive and motor task performance. *Journal of Sports Exercise Psychology, 13*, 281–293.

Hirschberg, J., and Ward, G. (1992). The influence of pitch range, duration, amplitude, and spectral features on the interpretation of the rise-fall-rise intonation contour in English. *Journal of Phonetics, 20*(2), 241–251.

Hittner, A., and Bornstein, H. (1990). Group counseling with older adults: Coping with late-onset hearing impairment: Techniques for counseling older persons. [Special issue.] *Journal of Mental Health Counseling, 12*(3), 332–341.

Hodge, R., and Kress, G. (1988). *Social semiotics*. Cambridge: Policy Press.

Hodson, B., and Paden, E. (1991). *Targeting intelligible speech*. Austin, TX: Pro-Ed.

Hoffman, L.W. (1988). Cross-cultural differences in childrearing goals. *New Directions for Child Development, 40*, 99–122.

Holland, A., and Ferber, M. (1993). *Aphasia treatment: World perspective*. San Diego, CA: Singular Publishing Group.

Holland, A.L. (1967). Some applications of behavioral principles to clinical speech problems. *Journal of Speech and Hearing Disorders, 32*, 11–18.

Holland, A.L. and Matthews, J. (1963). Application of teaching machine concepts to speech pathology and audiology. *Asha, 5*.

Hollander, M., and Kazaoka, K. (1988). Behavior therapy groups. In S. Long (Ed.), *Six group therapies* (pp. 257–326). New York: Plenum.

Hollingshead, A.B. (1958). Factors associated with prevalence of mental illness. In E.E. Maccoby, T.M. Newcomb, and E. L. Harley (Eds.), *Readings in social psychology* (pp. 425–436). New York: Holt, Rinehart, and Winston.

Hunt, P., Goetz, L., Alwell, M., and Sailor, W. (1986). Teaching generalized communication responses through an interrupted behavior chain strategy. *Journal of the Association for Persons with Severe Handicaps, 11*, 196–204.

Hunt, P.L. (1987). Black clients: Implications for supervision of trainees. *Psychotherapy, 24*(1), 114–119.

Huxley, R., and Ingram, E. (Eds.). (1971). *Language acquisition: Models and methods*. New York: Academic Press.

Hyde, R., and Weinberg, D. (1991). The process of the MPD therapist and the use of the study group. *Dissociation Progress in the Dissociative Disorders, 4*(2), 105–108.

Hynan, M.T. (1981). On the advantages of assuming that the techniques of psychotherapy are ineffective. *Psychotherapy Theory, Research and Practice, 18*(1), 11–13.

Hynd, C.R., McWhorter, J., YeVette, P., Virginia, L., and Suttles, C.W. (1994). The role of instructional variables in conceptual change in high school physics topics: The reading-science learning-writing connection. [Special issue.] *Journal of Research in Science Teaching, 31*(9), 933–946.

Ingham, R.J. (1984). *Stuttering and behavior therapy: Current status and experimental foundations*. San Diego, CA: College-Hill Press.

Jackson, E. (1985). Peer rated therapeutic talent and affective sensitivity: A multiple regression approach. *Psychology: A Quarterly Journal of Human Behavior, 22* (3-4), 28–35.

Janowsky, D.S., Kraft, A., Clopton, P., and Huey, L. (1984). Relationships of mood and interpersonal perceptions. *Comprehensive Psychiatry, 25*(6), 546–551.

Jayanthi, M., and Friend, M. (1992). Interpersonal problem solving: A selective literature review to guide practice. *Journal of Educational and Psychological Consultation, 3*(1), 39–53.

Jochums, B.L. (1989). Behavioral versus insight-oriented marital therapy: Labels can be misleading. Counseling and curriculum opportunities in the training of disadvantaged adults. *College Student Journal, 23*(3), 243–250.

Johnson, D.W., and Johnson, R.T. (1989). *Cooperation and competition: Theory and research.* Edina, MN: Interaction Book Company.

Johnson, K., and Korn, E.R. (1980). Hypnosis and imagery in the rehabilitation of a brain-injured patient. *Journal of Mental Imagery, 4*(2), 35–39.

Johnson, M., and Nelson, T.M. (1978). Game playing with juvenile delinquents. *Simulation and Games, 9*(4), 461–475.

Johnson, W. (1934). The influence of stuttering on the attitudes and adaptations of the stutterer. *Journal of Social Psychology, 5,* 410–420.

Jones, N.S. (1990). Black/White issues in psychotherapy: A framework for clinical practice. *Journal of Social Behavior and Personality, 5*(5), 305–322.

Jubis, R.M. (1990). Coding effects on performance in a process control task with uniparameter and multiparameter displays. *Human Factors, 32*(3), 287–297.

Kahn, D.L., and Steeves, R.H. (1988). Caring and practice: Construction of the nurse's world. *Scholarly Inquiry for Nursing Practice, 2*(3), 201–216.

Kahn, W.A. (1992). To be fully there: Psychological presence at work. *Human Relations, 45*(4), 321–349.

Kalunger, G., and Kalunger, M.F. (1986). *Human development: The span of life* (3rd ed.). Columbus, OH: Merrill/Macmillan.

Kalyanpur, M., and Rao, S.S. (1991). Empowering low-income Black families of handicapped children. *American Journal of Orthopsychiatry, 61*(4), 523–532.

Kanfer, F. (1968). Issues and ethics in behavior manipulation. In H.N. Sloane, Jr., and B.D. Mac Aulay (Eds.), *Operant procedures in remedial speech and language training* (pp. 411–423). New York: Houghton Mifflin.

Karge, B.D., McClure, M., and Patton, P.L. (1995). The success of collaboration resource programs for students with disabilities in Grades 6 through 8. *Remedial and Special Education, 16*(2), 79–89.

Kashner, T. M., Rodell, D. E., Ogden, S. R., Guggenheim, F. G., et al. (1992). Outcomes and costs of two VA inpatient treatment programs for older alcoholic patients. *Hospital and Community Psychiatry, 43*(10), 985–989.

Katz, N. (1990). Problem solving and time: Functions of learning style and teaching methods. *Occupational Therapy Journal of Research, 10*(4), 221–236.

Katz, P. (1981). Psychotherapy with native adolescents. *Canadian Journal of Psychiatry, 26*(7), 455–459.

Kausler, D. (1974). *Psychology of verbal learning and memory.* New York: Academic Press.

Kayser, H. (Ed.). (1995). *Bilingual speech-language pathology: An Hispanic focus.* San Diego, CA: Singular Publishing Group.

Keany, K.C., and Glueckauf, R. L. (1993). Disability and value change: An overview and reanalysis of acceptance of loss theory. *Rehabilitation Psychology, 38*(3), 199–210

Kember, D., and Gow, L. (1990). Cultural specificity of approaches to study. *British Journal of Educational Psychology, 60*(3), 356–363.

Kendall, P.C. (1984). Cognitive processes and procedures in behavior therapy. *Annual Review of Behavior Therapy Theory and Practice, 9,* 132–179.

Kern, C.W., and Watts, R.E. (1993). Adlerian counseling. *TCA Journal, 21*(1), 85–95.

Kernis, M.H., Brockner, J., and Frankel, B. S. (1989). Self-esteem and reactions to failure: The mediating role of overgeneralization. *Journal of Personality and Social Psychology, 57*(4), 707–714.

Kiewra, K.A., Mayer, R.E., Christensen, M., Kim, S.I., et al. (1991). Effects of repetition on recall and note-taking: Strategies for learning from lectures. *Journal of Educational Psychology, 83*(1), 120–123.

King, A. (1994). Autonomy and question asking: The role of personal control in guided student-generated questioning: Individual differences in question asking and strategic listening processes. [Special issue.] *Learning and Individual Differences, 6*(2), 163–185.

Kinnunen, R., and Vauras, M. (1995). Comprehension monitoring and the level of comprehension in high- and low-achieving primary school children's reading. *Learning and Instruction, 5*(2), 143-165.

Kinseth, L.M. (1989). Nonverbal training for psychotherapy: Overcoming barriers to clinical work with client nonverbal behavior. *Clinical Supervisor, 7*(1), 5–25.

Kinzie, J.D., Leung, P., Bui, A., Ben, R., et al. (1988). Group therapy with Southeast Asian refugees. *Community Mental Health Journal, 24*(2), 157–166.

Kirshbaum, H. (1991). Disability and humiliation: The humiliation dynamic: Viewing the task of prevention from a new perspective: I. [Special issue.] *Journal of Primary Prevention, 12*(2), 169–181.

Kivlighan, D. M., Mullison, D.D., Flohr, D. F., Proudman, S., et al. (1992). The interpersonal structure of "good" versus "bad" group counseling sessions:A multiple-case study. *Psychotherapy, 29*(3), 500–508.

Kleckner, T., Frank, L., Bland, C., Amendt, J. H., et al. (1992). The myth of the unfeeling strategic therapist. *Journal of Marital and Family Therapy, 18*(1), 41–51.

Klein, H.B., and Moses, N. (1994). *Intervention planning for children with communication disorders.* Englewood Cliffs, NJ: Prentice-Hall.

Klein, J.D., and Freitag, E. (1991). Effects of using an instructional game on motivation and performance. *Journal of Educational Research, 84*(5), 303–308.

Klitzke, M.J., and Lombardo, T.W. (1991). A "bug-in-the-eye" can be better than a "bug-in-the-ear": A teleprompter technique for on-line therapy skills training, *Behavior Modification, 15*(1), 113–117.

Knafl, K., Breitmayer, B., Gallo, A., and Zoeller, L. (1992). Parents' views of health care providers: An exploration of the components of a positive working relationship. *Children's Health Care, 21*(2) 90–95.

Kohl, F.L., and Beckman, P.J. (1990). The effects of directed play on the frequency and length of reciprocal interactions with preschoolers having moderate handicaps. *Education and Training in Mental Retardation, 25*(3), 258–266.

Koocher, G.P. (1976). Civil liberties and aversive conditioning for children. *American Psychologist, 31*(1), 94–95.

Kottman, T. (1990) Counseling middle school students: Techniques that work. *Elementary School Guidance and Counseling, 25*(2), 138–145

Krascum, R.M. (1993). Feature-based versus exemplar-based strategies in preschoolers' category learning. *Journal of Experimental Child Psychology, 56*(1) 1–48.

Kratz, N.A., and Marshall, L. L. (1988). First impressions: Analog experiment on counselor behavior and gender. *Representative Research in Social Psychology, 18*(1), 41–50.

Krishnamurti, J. (1970). *Think on these things.* New York: Harper and Row.

Kruger, L. (1988). Programmatic change strategies at the building level. In J.L. Graden, J.E. Zins, and M.J. Curtis (Eds.), *Alternative educational delivery systems: Enhancing instructional options for all students* (pp. 491–512). Washington, DC: National Association of School Psychologists.

Kulhavy, R.W., Stock, W.A., and Kealy, W.A. (1993). How geographic maps increase recall of instructional text. *Educational Technology Research and Development, 41*(4), 47–62.

Kupfer, D.J., Maser, J.D., Blehar, M.C., and Miller, R. (1987). Behavioral assessment in depression. In J.D. Maser (Ed.), *Depression and Expressive Behavior* (pp. 1–15). Hillsdale, NJ: Lawrence Erlbaum.

Kyrios, M., Prior, M., Oberklaid, R., Demetriou, A., La Trobe, U., and Bundoora, V. (1989). Cross-cultural studies of temperament: Temperament in Greek infants. *International Journal of Psychology, 24*(5), 585–603.

Lafleur, L.J. (1960). *Descartes: Discourse on method and meditations* (Trans.). New York: Bobbs-Merrill.

LaFromboise, T.D. (1992). An interpersonal analysis of affinity, clarification, and helpful responses with American Indians. *Professional Psychology Research and Practice, 23*(4), 281–286.

Lahey, M. (1988). *Language disorders and language development.* New York: MacMillan.

Lamar, P., and Siegler, R.S. (1995). Four aspects of strategic change: Contributions to children's learning of multiplication. *Journal of Experimental Psychology General, 124*(1), 83–97.

Lambert, M.C., Weisz, J.R., and Knight, F. (1989). Over- and undercontrolled clinic referral problems of Jamaican and American children and adolescents: The culture general and the culture specific. *Journal of Consulting and Clinical Psychology, 57*(4), 467–472.

Lange, G., Griffith, S.B., and Nida, R.E. (1990) Form characteristics of category-retrieval relationships in children and adults. *Journal of General Psychology, 117*(1), 5–14.

Lange, G., and Pierce, S.H. (1992). Memory-strategy learning and maintenance in preschool children. *Developmental Psychology, 28*(3), 453–462.

Larson, G.W., and Summers, P.A. (1976). Response patterns of preschool-age children to the Northwestern Syntax Screening Test. *Journal of Speech and Hearing Disorders, 41*, 486–497.

Law, M., and Dunn, W. (1993). Perspectives on understanding and changing the environments of children with disabilities. *Physical and Occupational Therapy in Pediatrics, 13*(3), 1–17.

Lawton, J.T. (1991). Effects of verbal rule instruction on young children's learning. *Journal of Structural Learning, 11*(1), 1–11.

Leader, E. (1991). Why adolescent group therapy? *Journal of Child and Adolescent Group Therapy, 1*(2), 81–93.

LeCroy, C.W. (1986). An analysis of the effects of gender on outcome in group treatment with young adolescents. *Journal of Youth and Adolescence, 15*, 497–508.

Lee, D.Y., and Hallberg, E.T. (1982). Nonverbal behaviors of "good" and "poor" counselors. *Journal of Counseling Psychology, 29*(4), 414–417.

Lee, T.M.C., and Rodda, M. (1994). Modification of attitudes toward people with disabilities. *Canadian Journal of Rehabilitation, 7*(4), 229–238.

Lenz, B.K., Ellis, E.S., and Scanlon, D. (1996). *Teaching learning strategies to adolescents and adults with learning disabilities.* Austin, TX: Pro-Ed.

Levy, J.E. (1988). The effects of labeling on health behavior and treatment programs among North American Indians. [Monograph.] *American Indian and Alaska Native Mental Health Research, 1,* 211–231.

Levy, L.H. (1983). Evaluation of students in clinical psychology programs: A program evaluation perspective. *Professional Psychology Research and Practice, 14*(4), 497–503

Lieberman, M.A. (1990). Understanding how groups work: A study of homogeneous peer group failures. *International Journal of Group Psychotherapy, 40*(1), 31–52

Lifter, K., Sulzer-Azaroff, B., Anderson, S.R., and Cowdery, G.E. (1993). Teaching play activities to preschool children with disabilities: The importance of developmental considerations. *Journal of Early Intervention, 17*(2), 139–159.

Lindstrom, B., and Kohler, L. (1991). Youth, disability, and quality of life. *Pediatrician, 18*(2), 121–128.

Little Soldier, L. (1985). To soar with the eagles: Enculturation and acculturation of Indian children. *Childhood Education, 61*(3), 185–191.

Livesay, J. R., and Porter, T. (1994). EMG and cardiovascular responses to emotionally provocative photographs and text. [Special issue.] *Perceptual and Motor Skills, 79*(1, Pt. 2), 579–594.

Lloyd, J.W. , Bateman, D.F., Landrum, Y.J., and Hallahan, D.P. (1989). Self-recording of attention versus productivity. *Journal of Applied Behavior Analysis, 22*(3), 315–323.

Locher, P. J., and Wagemans, J. (1993). Effects of element type and spatial grouping on symmetry detection. *Perception, 22*(5), 565–587.

Lockhart, B. (1981). Historic distrust and the counseling of American Indians and Alaskan Natives. *White Cloud Journal, 2*(3), 31-34.

Long, S. (1988). The six group therapies compared. In S. Long (Ed.), *Six group therapies* (pp. 327–338). New York: Plenum.

Lonka, K., Lindblom, Y., and Maury, S. (1994). The effect of study strategies on learning from text. *Learning and Instruction, 4*(3), 253–271.

Loranger, A.L. (1994). The study strategies of successful and unsuccessful high school students. *Journal of Reading Behavior, 26*(4), 347–360.

Loschen, E.L. (1993). Using the objective structured clinical examination in a psychiatry residency. *Academic Psychiatry, 17*(2), 95–104.

Lovaas, O.I. (1966). A program for the establishment of speech in psychotic children. In J.K. Wing (Ed.), *Early childhood autism.* New York: Pergamon.

Lovaas, O.I., Freitag, G., Gold, V.J., and Kassorla, I.C. (1965). Experimental studies in childhood schizophrenia: Analysis of self-destructive behavior. *Journal of Experimental Child Psychology, 2*, 67–84.

Lowenstein, L. F. (1991). The relationship of psychiatric disorder and conduct disorders with substance abuse. *Journal of Psychoactive Drugs, 23*(3), 283–287.

Lowith, K. (1964). *From Hegel to Nietzsche.* New York: Holt, Rineholt, and Winston.

Lowman, J. (1990). Failure of laboratory evaluation of CAI to generalize to classroom settings: The SuperShrink interview simulation. *Behavior Research Methods, Instruments, and Computers, 22*(5), 429–432.

Lund, N.J., and Duchan, J.F. (1988). *Assessing children's language in naturalistic contexts.* Englewood Cliffs, NJ.: Prentice-Hall.

Lundberg, M. A., Fox, P. W., and Punccohar, J. (1994). Highly confident but wrong: Gender differences and similarities in confidence judgments. *Journal of Educational Psychology, 86*(1), 114–121.

Lyon, S., and Lyon, G. (1980). Team functioning and staff development: A role release approach to providing integrated educational services for severely handicapped students. *Journal of the Association for the Severely Handicapped, 5*(3), 250–263.

Lyytinen, P., Rasku-Puttonen, H., Poikkeus, A.M., Laakso, M.L., et al. (1994). Mother-child teaching strategies and learning disabilities. *Journal of Learning Disabilities, 27*(3), 186–192.

Macario, J.F. (1991). Young children's use of color in classification: Foods and canonically colored objects. *Cognitive Development, 6*(1), 17–46.

Maccoby, E.E. (1990). Gender and relationships: A developmental account. American Psychological Association: Distinguished Scientific Contributions Award Address (1989, New Orleans, LA). *American Psychologist, 45*(4), 513–520.

Macrae, C.N., and Shepherd, J.W. (1991). Categorical effects on attributional inferences: A response-time analysis. *British Journal of Social Psychology, 30*(3) 235–245.

Madonna, J.M., and Caswell, P. (1991).The utilization of flexible techniques in group therapy with delinquent adolescent boys. *Journal of Child and Adolescent Group Therapy, 1*(2), 147–157.

Malgady, R.G., Rogler, L.H., and Costantino, G. (1990). Culturally sensitive psychotherapy for Puerto Rican children and adolescents: A program of treatment outcome research. *Journal of Consulting and Clinical Psychology, 58*(6), 704–712.

Manolis, M.B., and Milich, R. (1993). Gender differences in social persistence. *Journal of Social and Clinical Psychology, 12*(4), 385–405.

Marek, L.I., Sandifer, D.M., Beach, A., Coward, R.L., et al. (1994). Supervision without the problem: A model of solution-focused supervision. *Journal of Family Psychotherapy, 5*(2), 57–64

Markowitz, J.C. (1994). Religiosity and psychopathology. *Journal of Clinical Psychiatry, 55*(9), 414–415.

Marshall, C.A., Martin, W.W., Thomason, T.C., and Johnson, J.J. (1991). Multiculturalism and rehabilitation counselor training: Recommendations for providing culturally appropriate counseling services to American Indians with disabilities: Multiculturalism as a fourth force in counseling. [Special issue.] *Journal of Counseling and Development, 70*(1), 225–234.

Marshall, R.C., Neuburger, S.I., and Phillips, D. S. (1994). Verbal self-correction and improvement in treated aphasic clients. *Aphasiology, 8*(6), 535–547.

Martinez, M.E. (1992). Interest enhancements to science experiments: Interactions with student gender. *Journal of Research in Science Teaching, 29*(2), 167–177.

Matthews, G.A., and Harley, T.A. (1993). Effects of extroversion and self-report arousal on semantic priming: A connectionist approach. *Journal of Personality and Social Psychology, 65*(4), 735–756.

Mayadas, N.S., and Duehn, W.D. (1977). The effects of training formats and interpersonal discriminations in education for clinical social work practice. *Journal of Social Service Research, 1*(2), 147–161.

Mayer, R.E. (1983). *Thinking, problem solving, cognition.* New York: W.H. Freeman.

Mayer, R.E. (1987). Instructional variables that influence cognitive processes during reading. In B.K. Britton and S.M. Glynn (Eds.), *Historical foundations of educational psychology* (pp. 327–347). New York: Plenum Press.

Mayer, R.E. (1988). Learning strategies: An overview. In C.E. Weinstein, E.T. Goetz, and P.A. Alexander (Eds.), *Learning and study strategies* (pp. 11–22). New York: Academic Press.

McCarthey, S. J., Hoffman, J.V., Christian, C., and Corman, L., et al. (1994). Engaging the new basal readers. *Reading Research and Instruction, 33*(3), 233–256.

McCarty, T.L., Wallace, S., Lynch, R.H., and Benally, A. (1991). Classroom inquiry and Navajo learning styles: A call for reassessment. *Anthropology and Education Quarterly, 22*(1), 42–59.

McClean, A.P. (1995). Contrast and reallocation of extraneous reinforcers as a function of component duration and baseline rate of reinforcement. *Journal of the Experimental Analysis of Behavior, 36*(2), 203–224.

McCollum, E.E. (1994). "Which set of problems do you want to deal with?" *Journal of Family Psychotherapy, 5*(4), 75–77.

McDougall, G. J. (1995). Memory self-efficacy and strategy use in successful elders. *Educational Gerontology, 21*(4), 357–373.

McGovern, M.A., and Davidson, J. (1983). Student perceptions of performance. *British Journal of Disorders of Communication, 18*(3), 181–185.

McKeachie, W.J. (1988). The need for study strategy training. In C.E. Weinstein, E.T. Goetz, and P.A. Alexander (Eds.), *Learning and study strategies* (pp. 3–9). New York: Academic Press.

McKinley, V. (1987). Group therapy as a treatment modality of special value for Hispanic patients. *International Journal of Group Psychotherapy, 37*(2), 255–268.

McKirnan, D.J., and Hamayan, E.V. (1984). Speech norms and attitudes toward outgroup members: A test of a model in a bicultural context. *Journal of Language and Social Psychology, 3,* 21-38.

McMillon, H.G. (1994). Developing problem solving and interpersonal communication skills through intentionally structured groups. *Journal for Specialists in Group Work, 19*(1), 43–47.

McMullen, L.M., and Pasloski, D.D. (1992). Effects of communication apprehension, familiarity of partner, and topic on selected "women's language" features. Annual Convention of the Canadian Psychological Association (1990, Ottawa, Canada). *Journal of Psycholinguistic Research, 21*(1), 17–30.

McNair, L.D. (1992). African American women in therapy: An afrocentric and feminist synthesis: Finding voice: Writing by new authors. [Special issue.] *Women and Therapy, 12*(1–2), 5-19.

McQuaide, S. (1989). Working with Southeast Asian refugees. *Clinical Social Work Journal, 17*(2), 165–176.

McShane, D. (1987). Mental health and North American Indian/native communities: Cultural transactions, education, and regulation. *American Journal of Community Psychology, 15*(1), 95–116.

McWilliams, R., Nietupski, J., and Hamre-Nietupski, S. (1990). Teaching complex activities to students with moderate handicaps through the forward chaining of shorter total cycle response sequences. *Education and Training in Mental Retardation, 25*(3), 292–298.

Mead, M. (1930). Adolescence in primitive and modern society. In V.F. Calverton and S.D. Schmalhausen (Eds.), *The new generation.* New York: Macauley.

Meadow, D. (1988). Preparation of individuals for participation in a treatment group: Development and empirical testing of a model. *International Journal of Group Psychotherapy, 38*(3), 367–385.

Meadows, J.L. (1991). Multicultural communication. *Physical and Occupational Therapy in Pediatrics, 11*(4) 31-42.

Meichenbaum, D. (1977). *Cognitive-behavior modification.* New York: Plenum Press.

Melot, A.M., and Corroyer, D. (1992). Organization of metacognitive knowledge: A condition for strategy use in memorization. *European Journal of Psychology of Education, 7*(1), 23–38.

Meloth, M.S., and Deering, P.D. (1994). Task talk and task awareness under different cooperative learning conditions. *American Educational Research Journal, 31*(1), 138–165.

Meltzer, L.J., Solomon, B., Fenton, T., and Levine, M.D. (1989). A developmental study of problem-solving strategies in children with and without learning difficulties. *Journal of Applied Developmental Psychology, 10*(2), 171–193.

Meng, K., and Patty, D. (1991). Field dependence and contextual organizers. *Journal of Educational Research, 84*(3), 183–189.

Meredith, G.M. (1985). Two rating indicators of excellence in teaching in lecture-format courses. *Psychological Reports, 56*(1), 52–54.

Meyer, S. L., Murphy, C. M., Cascardi, M., and Birns, B. (1991). Gender and relationships: Beyond the peer group. *American Psychologist, 46*(5), 537.

Miles, M. (1992). Concepts of mental retardation in Pakistan: Toward cross-cultural and historical perspectives. *Disability, Handicap, and Society, 7*(3), 235–255.

Miller, A.D., Hall, S.W., and Heard, W.L. (1995). Effects of sequential 1-minute time trials with and without inter-trial feedback and self-correlation on general and special education students' fluency with math facts. *Journal of Behavioral Education, 5*(3), 319-345.

Miller, D.L., and Kelley, M.L. (1992). Treatment acceptability: The effects of parent gender, marital adjustment, and child behavior. *Child and Family Behavior Therapy, 14*(1), 11–23.

Miller, E.S. (1979). *Introduction to cultural anthropology.* Englewood Cliffs, NJ: Prentice-Hall.

Miller, H.R., and Davis, S. F. (1993).Recall of boxed material in textbooks. *Bulletin of the Psychonomic Society, 31*(1), 31–32.

Miller, S.D. (1993). Increasing the adjustment success of the disabled African American. *Journal of Health and Social Policy, 5*(2), 87–104.

Mills, A. (1991). Art therapy on a residential treatment team for troubled children. *Journal of Child and Youth Care, 6*(4), 49–59

Mir, M.A., Evans, R.W., Marshall, R. J., Newcombe, R.G., et al. (1989). The use of video recordings of medical postgraduates in improving clinical skills. *Medical Education, 23*(3), 276–281.

Mishra, R.C. (1988). Learning strategies among children in the modern and traditional schools. *Indian Psychologist, 5*(1), 17–24.

Miyaji, N. T. (1993). The power of compassion: Truth-telling among American doctors in the care of dying patients. *Social Science and Medicine, 36*(3), 249–264.

Molyneaux, D., and Lane, V.W. (1982). *Effective interviewing.* Boston: Allyn and Bacon.

Molyneaux, D. and Lane, V.W. (1992). *Dynamics of communication development.* Englewood Cliffs, NJ: Prentice-Hall.

Montagu, A. (1972). Statement on race: An annotated elaboration and exposition of the four statements on race issues by the United Nations Educational, Scientific, and Cultural Organization. New York: Oxford University Press.

Montes, J., and Erickson, J.G. (1990). Bilingual stuttering: Exploring a diagnostic dilemma. *Ethnotes, 1*, 14–15.

Moran, M.R. (1992). Effects of sexual orientation similarity and counselor experience level on gay men's and lesbians' perceptions of counselors. *Journal of Counseling Psychology, 39*(2), 247–251.

Morgenstern, J. (1956). Socioeconomic factors in stuttering. *Journal of Speech and Hearing Disorders, 21*, 25–33.

Morran, D. K., Stockton, R., and Bond, L. (1991). Delivery of positive and corrective feedback in counseling groups. *Journal of Counseling Psychology, 38*(4), 410–414.

Morris, G.B. (1991). Perceptions of leadership traits: Comparison of adolescent and adult school leaders. *Psychological Reports, 69*(3, Pt. 1), 723–727.

Morrow, D., Worthington, E.L., and McCullough, M.E. (1993). Observers' perceptions of a counselor's treatment of a religious issue. *Journal of Counseling and Development, 71*(4), 452–456.

Morse, J.M., Anderson, G., Bottorff, J.L., Yonge, O., et al. (1992). Exploring empathy: A conceptual fit for nursing practice? *IMAGE Journal of Nursing Scholarship, 24*(4) 273–280.

Mozdzierz, G.J., and Greenblatt, R.L. (1992). Clinical paradox and experimental decision making. *Individual Psychology Journal of Adlerian Theory, Research and Practice, 48*(3), 302–312.

Murphy, A.T. (1982). The clinical process and the speech-language pathologist. In G.H. Shames and E.H. Wiig (Eds.), *Human communication disorders* (pp. 453–474). Columbus, OH: Charles E.Merrill.

Murphy, L.O., and Ross, S.M. (1990). Protagonist gender as a design variable in adapting mathematics story problems to learner interests. *Educational Technology Research and Development, 38*(3), 27–37.

Myrick, R.D. (1987). *Developmental guidance and counseling: A practical approach.* Minneapolis, MN: Educational Media Corporation.

Myrick, R. D., Highland, W.H., and Sabella, R. A. (1995). Peer helpers and perceived effectiveness. *Elementary School Guidance and Counseling, 29*(4), 278–288.

Nagel, E. (1961). *The structure of science.* New York: Harcourt, Brace, and World.

Nangle, D.W., Carr-Nagle, R.E., and Hansen, D.J. (1994). Enhancing generalization of a contingency-management intervention through the use of family problem-solving training: Evaluation with a severely conduct-disordered adolescent. *Child and Family Behavior Therapy, 16*(2), 65–76.

Naremore, R.C. (Ed.). (1984). *Language science.* San Diego, CA.: College-Hill Press.

Naremore, R.C., Densmore, A.E., and Harman, D.R. (1995). *Language intervention with school-aged children.* San Diego, CA: Singular Publishing Group.

Neimeyer, R.A., and Feixas, G. (1990). The role of homework and skill acquisition in the outcome of group cognitive therapy for depression. *Behavior Therapy, 21*(3), 281–292.

Nelson, J. R., Smith, D. J., and Dodd, J. M. (1992). The effects of teaching a summary skills strategy to students identified as learning disabled on their comprehension of science text. *Education and Treatment of Children, 15*(3), 228–243.

Neufeldt, S. A. (1994). Use of a manual to train supervisors. *Counselor Education and Supervision, 33*(4) 327–336.

Newbern, V.B. (1992). Failure to thrive: A growing concern in the elderly. *Journal of Gerontological Nursing, 18*(8), 21–25.

Nikelly, A.G., and Majors, R.G. (1986). Techniques for counseling Black students. *Techniques, 2*(1), 48–54.

Norman, G.R., and Schmidt, H.G. (1992). The psychological basis of problem-based learning: A review of the evidence. *Academic Medicine, 67*(9), 557–565.

Norris, D. (1994). A quantitative multiple-levels model of reading aloud: Modeling visual word recognition. [Special issue.] *Journal of Experimental Psychology Human Perception and Performance, 20*(6), 1212–1232.

Nosek, M.A., Fuhrer, M. J., and Hughes, S. O. (1991). Perceived counselor credibility by persons with physical disability: Influence of counselor disability status, professional status, and the counseling content. *Rehabilitation Psychology, 36*(3), 153–161.

O'Brien, E. J., and Albrecht, J. E. (1991). The role of context in accessing antecedents in text. *Journal of Experimental Psychology Learning, Memory, and Cognition, 17*(1), 94–102.

O'Donohue, W., Fisher, J.E., Plaud, J.J., and Link W. (1989). What is a good treatment decision? The client's perspective. *Professional Psychology Research and Practice, 20*(6), 404–407.

O'Sullivan, M.J., Peterson, P.D., Cox, G.B., and Kirkeby, J. (1989). Ethnic populations: Community mental health services ten years later. *American Journal of Community Psychology, 17*(1), 17-30.

Oakhill, J. (1993). Children's difficulties in reading comprehension: European educational psychology. [Special issue.] *Educational Psychology Review, 5* (3), 223–237.

Oliver, J.M., Lightfoot, S.L., Searight, H.R., and Katz, B. (1990). Consistency in individual and family theoretical orientation from assessment to therapy: Its impact on the effectiveness of therapy. *American Journal of Family Therapy, 18*(3), 236–245.

Oratio, A.R., and Hood, S.B. (1977). Certain select variables as predictors of goal achievement in speech therapy. *Journal of Communication Disorders, 10*(4), 331–342.

Orleans, C.S., Houpt, J.L., and Larson, D.B. (1980). Interpersonal factors in the psychiatry clerkship: New findings. *American Journal of Psychiatry, 137*(9), 1101–1103.

Overholser, J. C. (1991). The use of guided imagery in psychotherapy: Modules for use with passive relaxation training. *Journal of Contemporary Psychotherapy, 21*(3), 159–172.

Oz, S. (1995). A modified balance-sheet procedure for decision making in therapy: Cost-cost comparisons. *Professional Psychology Research and Practice, 21*(3), 78–81.

Ozechowski, T.J. (1994). The integration of emotion in solution-focused therapy: Comment. *Journal of Marital and Family Therapy, 20*(2), 205–206.

Pachalska, M.K. (1982). Presentation of the state of social dependence of patients afflicted with aphasia. *American Journal of Social Psychiatry, 2,* 51–53.

Paden, E.P. (1970). *A history of the American Speech and Hearing Association, 1925–1958.* Washington, DC.: American Speech and Hearing Association.

Paivio, A. (1971). *Imagery and verbal processes.* New York: Holt, Rinehart, and Winston.

Parsons, J.E., and Durst, D. (1992). Learning contracts: Misunderstood and underutilized. *Clinical Supervisor, 10*(1), 145–156.

Patterson, C.H. (1990). Involuntary clients: A person-centered view. *Person Centered Review, 5*(3), 316–320.

Patterson, L.E., Rak, C.F., Chermonte, J., and Roper, W. (1992). Automaticity as a factor in counselor skills acquisition. *Canadian Journal of Counseling, 26*(3), 189–200.

Pearson, J.B. (1993). The process of change in cognitive therapy: Schema change or acquisition of compensatory skills? *Cognitive Therapy and Research, 17*(2), 123–137.

Perigoe, C., and Ling, D. (1986). Generalization of speech skills in hearing-impaired children. *Volta Review, 8*(7) 351–366.

Perls, F.S. (1965). *Three approaches to psychotherapy, I: Frederick Perls.* Psychological Films, Inc.

Perls, F.S. (1969). *Ego, hunger, and aggression.* New York: Random House.

Perls, F.S., Hefferline, R.E., and Goodman, P. (1951). *Gestalt therapy.* New York: Dell Publishing.

Peters, T.J., and Guitar, B. (1991). *Stuttering: An integrated approach to its nature and treatment.* Baltimore, MD: Williams and Wilkins.

Peterson, S. E. (1992). The cognitive functions of underlining as a study technique. *Reading Research and Instruction, 31*(2), 49–56.

Pfiffner, L. J., Jouriles, E. N., Brown, M. M., Etscheidt, M.A., et al. (1990). Effects of problem-solving therapy on outcomes of parent training for single-parent families. *Child and Family Behavior Therapy, 12*(1), 1–11.

Piaget, J. (1954). *The construction of reality in the child.* New York: Basic Books.

Piaget, J. (1963). *The origins of intelligence in children.* New York: The Norton Library.

Piaget, J. (1972). *Psychology of the child.* New York: Basic Books.

Piercy, F., and Sprenkle, D. (1986). *Family therapy source book.* New York: Guilford.

Pinkard, C.M. (1990). Mental imagery methods in rehabilitative services. *Journal of Applied Rehabilitation Counseling, 21*(1), 20–24.

Pletts, M. (1981). Principles and practice of clinical teaching—a need for structure. *British Journal of Disorders of Communication, 16*(2), 129–134.

Polcin, D. L. (1991). Prescriptive group leadership. *Journal for Specialists in Group Work, 16*(1), 8–15.

Pollock, D.C., Shanley, D.F., and Byrne, P. N. (1985). Psychiatric interviewing and clinical skills. *Canadian Journal of Psychiatry, 30*(1) 64–68.

Ponzo, Z. (1991). Critical factors in group work: Clients' perceptions. *Journal for Specialists in Group Work, 16*(1), 16–23.

Poole, E. (1934). Genetic development of articulation of consonant sounds in speech. *Elementary English Review, 11*, 159–161.

Poston, W. C., Craine, M., and Atkinson, D.R. (1991). Counselor dissimilarity confrontation, client cultural mistrust, and willingness to self-disclose. *Journal of Multicultural Counseling and Development, 19*(2), 65–73.

Potter, W.J., and Emanuel, R. (1990). Students' preferences for communication styles and their relationship to achievement. *Communication Education, 39*(3), 234–249.

Powell, T.W., Gospel, M.D., and Williams, A.L. (1991). Attitudes toward the clinical supervisory model: Results from in-service training. *Clinical Supervisor, 9*(2), 53–62.

Prelock, P.A. (1995). Rethinking collaboration: A speech-language pathology perspective. *Journal of Educational and Psychological Consultation, 6*(1), 95–99.

Presley, D.B. (1992). Three approaches to religious issues in counseling. *Journal of Psychology and Theology, 20*(1), 39–46.

Rabinowitz, M. (1991). Semantic and strategic processing: Independent roles in determining memory performance. *American Journal of Psychology, 104*(3), 427–437.

Rainforth, B., York, J., Macdonald, C., and Dunn, R. (1992). Collaborative Assessment. In Rainforth, B., York, J., and Macdonald C. (Eds.), *Collaborative teams for students with severe disabilities.* Baltimore: Paul H. Brookes.

Ramirez, M., and Castaneda, A. (1974). *Cultural democracy, bicognitive development, and education.* New York: Academic Press.

Ramsay, J.E., and Oatley, K. (1992). Designing minimal computer manuals from scratch: Computers and writing: Issues and implementations. [Special issue.] *Instructional Science, 21*(1–3), 85–98.

Ratner, H.H., and Hill, L. (1991). The development of children's action memory: When do actions speak louder than words? *Psychological Research Psychologische Forschung, 53*(3), 195–202.

Redfern, S., Dancey, C.P., and Dryden, W. (1993). Empathy: Its effect on how counselors are perceived. *British Journal of Guidance and Counseling, 21*(3), 300–309.

Rekrut, M.D. (1994). Teaching to learn: Strategy utilization through peer tutoring. *High School Journal, 77*(4), 304–314.

Rennie, D.L. (1994). Clients' deference in psychotherapy: Qualitative research in counseling process and outcome. [Special section.] *Journal of Counseling Psychology, 41*(4), 427–437.

Resendiz, P.S., and Fox, R.A. (1985). Reflection-impulsivity in Mexican children: Cross-cultural relationships. *Journal of General Psychology, 112*(3), 285–290.

Resnick, L., and Ford, W. (1981). *The psychology of mathematics for instruction.* Hillsdale, NJ: Erlbaum.

Rettig, K.D. (1993). Problem-solving and decision-making as central processes of family life: An ecological framework for family relations and family resource management. *Marriage and Family Review, 18*(304), 187–222.

Reynolds, R.E., Shepard, C., Lapan, R., Kreek, C., et al. (1990). Differences in the use of selective attention by more successful and less successful tenth-grade readers. *Journal of Educational Psychology, 82*(4), 749–759.

Riccio, D. C., Ackil, J. K., and Burch-Vernon, A. (1992). Forgetting of stimulus attributes: Methodological implications for assessing associative phenomena. *Psychological Bulletin, 112*(3), 433–445.

Richardson, A. (1969). *Mental Imagery.* New York: Springer..

Roberts, M. J., Wood, D. J., and Gilmore, D. J. (1994). The sentence-picture verification task: Methodological and theoretical difficulties. *British Journal of Psychology, 85*(3), 413–432.

Roberts, S.D., and Bouchard, K.R. (1989). Establishing rapport in rehabilitative audiology. *Journal of the Academy of Rehabilitative Audiology, 22,* 67–73.

Robinson, D.D., Stockton, R., and Moran, D.K. (1990). Anticipated consequences of self-disclosure during early therapeutic group development. *Journal of Group Psychotherapy, Psychodrama, and Sociometry, 43*(1), 3–18.

Rogers, C.R. (1965). *Client-centered therapy.* New York: Houghton Mifflin.

Rogers, C.R. (1970). *On becoming a person.* Boston: Houghton Mifflin.

Rogers, W. A. and Fisk, A. D. (1990). A reconsideration of age-related reaction time slowing from a learning perspective: Age-related slowing is not just complexity-based: Fron-

tiers of learning and individual differences: Paradigms in transition. [Special issue.] *Learning and Individual Differences, 2*(2), 161–179.

Rollin, W.J. (1987). *The psychology of communication disorders in individuals and their families.* Englewood Cliffs, NJ: Prentice-Hall.

Rosenbek, J.C., LaPointe, L.L., and Wertz, R.T. (1989). *Aphasia: A clinical approach.* Austin, TX: Pro-Ed.

Rosenberg, C.M., Gerrein, J.R., Manohar, V., and Liftik, J. (1976). Evaluation of training of alcoholism counselors. *Journal of Studies on Alcohol, 37*(9), 1236–1246.

Rosenberg, P.P. (1984). Support groups: A special therapeutic entity. *Small Group Behavior, 15*(2), 173–186.

Rosenkrantz, A.L., and Holmes, G.R. (1974). A pilot study of clinical internship training at the William S. Hall Psychiatric Institute. *Journal of Clinical Psychology, 30*(3), 417–419.

Rossberg-Bempton, I., and Poole, G.D. (1993). The effects of open and closed postures on pleasant and unpleasant emotions: Research in the creative arts therapies. [Special issue.] *Arts in Psychotherapy, 20*(1), 75–82.

Rubin, H. (1986). Cognitive therapy. In G. Shames and H. Rubin (Eds.), *Stuttering then and now.* Columbus, OH: Merrill Publishing.

Rubin, H., and Culatta, R.A. (1971). A point of view about fluency. *Asha,* 13, 380–384.

Rubin, H., and Culatta, R.A. (1974). Stuttering as an after effect of normal developmental disfluency. *Clinical Pediatrics, 13,* 172–176.

Rubin, S.S., and Niemeier, D.L. (1992). Nonverbal affective communication as a factor in psychotherapy. *Psychotherapy, 29*(4) 596–602.

Rudd, R.E. and Comings, J.P. (1994). Learner developed materials: An empowering product: Community empowerment, participatory education, and health: II [Special issue.]. *Health Education Quarterly, 21*(3) 313–327.

Rueter, M.A., and Conger, R.D. (1995). Interaction style, problem-solving behavior, and family problem-solving effectiveness. *Child Development, 66*(1), 98–115.

Russell, B. (1961). Styles in ethics. In R. I. Egner and L.E. Denonn (Eds.), *The basic writings of Bertrand Russell* (p. 345). New York: Simon and Schuster.

Ryan, E.B., Hamilton, J.M., and See, S.K. (1994). Patronizing the old: How do younger and older adults respond to baby talk in the nursing home?: Intergenerational communication. [Special issue.] *International Journal of Aging and Human Development, 39*(1), 21–32.

Rzoska, K.M., and Ward, C. (1991). The effects of cooperative and competitive learning methods on the mathematics achievement, attitudes toward school, self-concepts, and friendship choices of Maori, Pakeha and Samoan children. *New Zealand Journal of Psychology, 20*(1), 17–24.

Sachse, R. (1993). The effects of intervention phrasing on therapist-client communication. *Psychotherapy Research, 3*(4), 260–277.

Sadker, M., Sadker, D., and Steindam, S. (1989). Gender equity and educational reform. *Educational Leadership, 46*(6), 44–47.

Safran, J.D. (1989). Insight and action in psychotherapy. *Journal of Integrative and Eclectic Psychotherapy, 8*(3), 233–239.

Sagen, C. (1977). *The Dragons of Eden*. New York: Ballantine Books.

Sagie, A., Elizur, D., and Koslowsky, M. (1990). Effect of participation in strategic and tactical decisions on acceptance of planned change. *Journal of Social Psychology, 130*(4), 459–465.

Sailor, W.S. (1991). Special education in the restructured school. *Remedial and Special Education, 12*(6), 8–22.

Salas, S.B., and Dickinson, D.J. (1990). The effect of feedback and three different types of corrections on student learning. *Journal of Human Behavior and Learning, 7*(2), 13–19.

Saleh, M.A. (1986). Cultural perspectives: Implications for counseling in the Arab world. *School Psychology International, 7*(2), 71–75.

Salerno, M., Farber, B. A., McCullough, L., Winston, A., et al. (1992). The effects of confrontation and clarification on patient affective and defensive responding. *Psychotherapy Research, 2*(3), 181–192.

Samuels, M., and Samuels, N. (1975). *Seeing through the mind's eye*. New York: Random House.

Sanchez-Iniguez, F. (1993). Estrategia para extraer el significado de un texto.[Strategy for extracting the meaning of a text]. *Revista de Psicologia de la Educacion, 13*, 63–75.

Sansone, C., and Morgan, C. (1992). Intrinsic motivation and education: Competence in context: Perspectives on intrinsic motivation. [Special issue.] *Motivation and Emotion, 16*(3), 249–270.

Sapir, E. (1921). *Language*. New York: Harcourt, Brace, and World, Inc.

Satir, V. (1967). Conjoint family therapy (rev. ed.). Palo Alto, CA: Science and Behavior Books.

Sayger, T.V., Szykula, S.A., and Laylander, J.A. (1991). Adolescent-focused family counseling: A comparison of behavioral and strategic approaches. *Journal of Family Psychotherapy, 2*(3), 57–80.

Sazar, L. and Kassinove, H. (1991). Effects of counselor's profanity and subject's religiosity on content acquisition of a counseling lecture and behavioral compliance. [Special issue.] *Psychological Reports, 69*(3, Pt. 2), 1059–1070.

Scheflen, A.E. (1967). On the structuring of human communication. *American Behavioral Scientist, 10*(8), 8–12.

Scheuerle, J. (1992). *Counseling in speech-language pathology and audiology*. Columbus, OH: Merrill.

Schultz, C.L., Kemm, M.A., Bruce, E.J., and Smyrnios, K.X. (1992). Caring for fathers and mothers of children with intellectual disability: A pilot study. *Australia and New Zealand Journal of Developmental Disabilities, 18*(1), 45–56.

Schunk, D. H., and Rice, J. M. (1993). Strategy fading and progress feedback: Effects on self-efficacy and comprehension among students receiving remedial reading services. *Journal of Special Education, 27*(3), 257–276.

Schutz, P.A. (1993). Additional influences on response certitude and feedback requests. *Contemporary Educational Psychology, 18*(4), 427–441.

Screen, R.M., and Anderson, N.B. (1994). *Multicultural perspectives in communication disorders*. San Diego, CA : Singular Publishing Group.

Seifert, T. L. (1994). Enhancing memory for main ideas using elaborative interrogation. *Contemporary Educational Psychology, 19*(3), 360–366.

Semmes, C.E. (1991). Developing trust: Patient-practitioner encounters in natural health care. *Journal of Contemporary Ethnography, 19*(4), 450–470.

Seymour, H.N., Ashton, N., and Wheeler, L. (1986). The effect of race on language elicitation. *Language, Speech, and Hearing Services in Schools, 17*(3), 146–151.

Seymour, C.M. (1992). Objective: Recruitment—mentoring fosters leadership. *Asha, 34,* 45–46.

Shaffer, P., Murillo, N., and Michael, W.B. (1978). The factorial validity of a scale for evaluation of counselors in a university counseling and testing center. *Educational and Psychological Measurement, 38*(4), 1085–1096.

Shames, G.H. (1989). Stuttering: An RFP for a cultural perspective. *Journal of Fluency Disorders, 14,* 67–77.

Shames, G.H., and Florance, C.L. (1980). *Stutter-free speech: A goal for therapy.* Columbus, OH: Charles E. Merrill.

Shames, G.H., and Rubin, H. (1986). The roles of the client and the clinician during therapy. In G.H. Shames and H. Rubin (Eds.), *Stuttering, then and now* (pp. 261–270). Columbus, OH: Charles E. Merrill.

Shames, G. H., and Sherrick, C.E., Jr. (1963). A discussion of nonfluency and stuttering as operant behavior. *Journal of Speech and Hearing Disorders, 28,* 13–18.

Shapiro, D.A., and Anderson, J.L. (1988). An analysis of commitments made by student clinicians in speech-language pathology and audiology. *Journal of Speech and Hearing Disorders, 53*(2), 202–210.

Shapiro, D.A., and Anderson, J.L. (1989). One measure of supervisory effectiveness in speech-language pathology and audiology. *Journal of Speech and Hearing Disorders, 54*(4), 549–557.

Sharf, R.S., and Lucas, M. (1993). An assessment of a computerized simulation of counseling skills. *Counselor Education and Supervision, 32*(4), 254–266.

Sheehan, J.G. (1978). Stuttering and recovery. In H.H. Gregory (Ed.), *Controversies about stuttering therapy.* Baltimore: University Park Press.

Shefelbine, J. L. (1990). Student factors related to variability in learning word meanings from context. *Journal of Reading Behavior, 22*(1), 71–97.

Sherer, M., and Rogers, R.W. (1980). Effects of therapists' nonverbal communication on rated skill and effectiveness. *Journal of Clinical Psychology, 36*(3), 696–700.

Shine, R.E. (1980). *Systematic fluency training for children.* Tigard, OR: C.C. Publications.

Shipley, K.G. (1992). *Interviewing and counseling in communicative disorders.* New York: Merrill.

Short, K. G. (1992). Intertextuality: Searching for patterns that connect. *National Reading Conference Yearbook, 41,* 187–197.

Siegel, S. M., Friedlander, M. L., and Heatherington, L. (1992). Nonverbal relational control in family communication. *Journal of Nonverbal Behavior, 16*(2), 117–139.

Siegler, R.S. (1991). Strategy choice and strategy discovery. *Learning and Instruction, 1*(1), 89–102.

Sigman, M., Heuman, K., Jansen, B., and Bwibo, D. (1989). Cognitive abilities of Kenyan children in relation to nutrition, family characteristics, and education. *Child Development, 60*(6), 1463–74.

Silove, D., Parker, G., and Manicavasagar, V. (1990). Perceptions of general and specific therapist behaviors. *Journal of Nervous and Mental Disease. 178*(5) 292–299.

Silverman, W.K., La Greca, A.M., and Wasserstein, S. (1995). What do children worry about? Worries and their relation to anxiety. *Child Development, 66*(3), 671–686

Simpson, M. L., Olejnik, S., Tam, A.Y.W., and Supattathum, S. (1994). Elaborative verbal rehearsals and college students' cognitive performance. *Journal Educational Psychology, 86*(2), 267–278.

Sinatra, C. (1990). Five diverse secondary schools where learning style instruction works. *Journal of Reading, Writing, and Learning Disabilities International, 6*(3), 323–334.

Singer, R. N., Flora, L. A., and Abourezk, T. L. (1989). The effect of a five-step cognitive learning strategy on the acquisition of a complex motor task. *Journal of Applied Sport Psychology, 1*(2), 98–108.

Skaggs, L.P., Rocklin, T.R., Dansereau, D.F., Hall, R.H., et al. (1990). Dyadic learning of technical material: Individual differences, social interaction, and recall. *Contemporary Educational Psychology, 15*(1), 47–63.

Skinner, B.F. (1948). *Walden two.* New York: MacMillian.

Skinner, B.F. (1953). *Science and human behavior.* New York: MacMillan.

Skinner, B.F. (1957). *Verbal behavior.* New York: Appletown-Century-Crofts.

Skotnikova, I.G. (1990). Psychophysical characteristics of visual discrimination and the cognitive style. *Soviet Journal of Psychology, 11*(1), 40–53.

Sloane, H.N. Jr., and Mac Aulay, B.D. (Eds.) (1968). *Operant procedures in remedial speech and language training.* New York: Houghton Mifflin Co.

Smart, J.F., and Smart, D.W. (1991). Acceptance of disability and the Mexican American culture. *Rehabilitation Counseling Bulletin, 34*(4), 357–367.

Smith, A.B., and Inder, P.M. (1993). Social interaction in same and cross gender preschool peer groups: A participant observation study. *Educational Psychology, 13*(1), 29–42.

Smith, D.C. (1994). A "last rights" group for people with AIDS. *Journal for Specialists in Group Work, 19*(1), 17–21.

Smith, J. A. (1993). Content learning: A third reason for using literature in teaching reading. *Reading Research and Instruction, 32*(3), 64–71.

Smith, S.E. (1994). Parent-initiated contracts: An intervention for school-related behaviors. *Elementary School Guidance and Counseling, 28*(3), 182–187.

Smith, V. L., and Clark, H. H. (1993). On the course of answering questions. *Journal of Memory and Language, 32*(1), 25–38.

Snapp, J.C., and Glover, J. A. (1990). Advance organizers and study questions. *Journal of Educational Research, 83*(5), 266-271.

Sommer, R. (1978). *The mind's eye: Imagery in everyday life.* New York: Delacorte Press.

Sommers-Flanagan, J., and Sommers-Flanagan, R. (1989). A categorization of pitfalls common to beginning interviews. *Journal of Training and Practice in Professional Psychology, 3*(1), 58–71.

Spaights, E. (1990). The therapeutic implications of working with the Black family. *Journal of Instructional Psychology, 17*(4), 183–189.

Spiegel, G. F., and Barnfield, J. P. (1994). The effects of a combination of text structure awareness and graphic postorganizers on recall and retention of science knowledge: The reading-science learning-writing connection. [Special issue.] *Journal of Research in Science Teaching, 31*(9), 913–932.

Spolsky, B. (1972). The language education of minority children. In B. Spolsky (Ed.), *The language education of minority children* (pp. 1–10). Rowley, MA: Newbury House,

Sriram, T.G., Chandrashekar, C.R., Isaac, M.K., and Srinivasa-Murthy, R. (1990). Development of case vignettes to assess the mental health training of primary care medical officers. *Acta Psychiatrica Scandinavica, 82*(2), 174–177.

Stackhouse, J., and Furnham, A. (1983). A student-centered approach to the evaluation of clinical skills. *British Journal of Disorders of Communication 18*(3), 171–179.

Starnes, W.R., and Loeb, R.C. (1993). Locus of control differences in memory recall strategies when confronted with noise. *Journal of General Psychology, 120*(4), 463–471.

Stevenson, H.C., and Renard, G. (1993). Trusting ole' wise owls: Therapeutic use of cultural strengths in African American families: 23rd Annual Mid-Winter Convention of Division 29 (Psychotherapy), 42 (Independent Practice), and 43 (Family Psychology) of the American Psychological Association (1992, Amelia Island Plantation, Florida). *Professional Psychology Research and Practice, 24*(4), 433–442.

Stewart, J.L. (1992). Native American populations. *Asha, 34,* 40–42.

Stillman, P.L., Regan, M.B., Swanson, D.B., and Case, S., et al. (1990). An assessment of the clinical skills of fourth-year students at four New England medical schools. *Academic Medicine, 65*(5), 320–326.

Stock, W. A., Winston, K. S., Behrens, J. T., and Harper-Marinick, M. (1989). The effects of performance expectation and question difficulty on text study time, response certitude, and correct responding. *Bulletin of the Psychonomic Society, 27*(6), 567–569.

Stockard, J., and Johnson, M.M. (1980). *Sex roles: Sex inequality and sex role development.* Englewood Cliffs, NJ: Prentice-Hall.

Stokes, T., and Baer, D. (1978). An implicit technology of generalization. *Journal of Applied Behavior Analyst, 11,* 285–303.

Stolk, Y., and Perlesz, A.J. (1990). Do better trainees make worse family therapists?: A follow up study of client families. *Family Process, 29*(1), 45–58.

Strickland, T.L., Jenkins, J.O., Myers, H.F., and Adams, H.E. (1988). Diagnostic judgments as a function of client and therapist race. *Journal of Psychopathology and Behavioral Assessment, 10*(2), 141–151.

Strupp, H.H., and Hadley, S.W. (1979). Specific vs. nonspecific factors in psychotherapy: A controlled study of outcome. *Archives of General Psychiatry, 36*(10), 1125–1136.

Sue, S., Fujino, D.C., Hu, L., Takeuchi, D.T., et al. (1991). Community mental health services for ethnic minority groups: A test of the cultural responsiveness hypothesis. *Journal of Consulting and Clinical Psychology, 59*(4), 533–540.

Sullivan, T. (1983). Native children in treatment: Clinical, social, and cultural issues. *Journal of Child Care, 1*(4), 75–94.

Suzuki, D.T. (1955). *Studies in Zen*. New York: Dell Publishing.

Swanson, D.B., and Stillman, P.L. (1990). Use of standardized patients for teaching and assessing clinical skills: Reflections on research in medical problem solving. [Special issue.] *Evaluation and the Health Professions, 13*(1), 79–103.

Sweller, J., and Chandler, P. (1994). Why some material is difficult to learn. *Cognition and Instruction, 12*(3), 185–233.

Sykes, D.K. (1987). An approach to working with Black youth in cross cultural therapy. *Clinical Social Work Journal, 15*(3), 260–270.

Szivos, S.E., and Griffiths, E. (1990). Group processes involved in coming to terms with a mentally retarded identity. *Mental Retardation, 28*(6) 333–341.

Tafoya, T. (1989). Circles and cedar: Native Americans and family therapy. *Journal of Psychotherapy and the Family, 6*(1–2), 71–98

Takeuchi, D.T., Mokuau, N., and Chun, C.A. (1992). Mental health services for Asian Americans and Pacific Islanders: Multicultural mental health and substance abuse services. [Special issue.] *Journal of Mental Health Administration, 19*(3), 237–245.

Tamura, T., and Lau, A. (1992). Connectedness versus separateness: Applicability of family therapy to Japanese families. *Family Process, 31*(4), 319–340.

Taylor, O. (1989). Old wine and new bottles: Some things change yet remain the same. *Asha, 31*(9), 72–73.

Taylor, O.L. (In press). In L. Cole and V.R. Deal (Eds.), *Communication Disorders in Multi-cultural Populations*. Rockville, MD: American Speech-Language-Hearing Association.

Teasdale, G., and Jennett, B. (1974). Assessment of coma and impaired consciousness. *Lancet, 2*, 81.

Tedeschi, G.J., and Willis, F.N. (1993). Attitudes toward counseling among Asian international and native Caucasian students. *Journal of College Student Psychotherapy 7*(4), 43–54.

Thames, D.G., and Reeves, C.K. (1994). Poor readers' attitudes: Effects of using interests and trade books in an integrated language arts approach: Assessment and intervention in reading/literacy education: Research and practice. [Special issue.] *Reading Research and Instruction, 33*(4), 293–307.

Thompson, B.M., Hearn, G.N. and Collins, M.J. (1992). Patient perceptions of health professional interpersonal skills. *Australian Psychologist, 27*(2), 91–95.

Thompson, L. A. (1994). Dimensional strategies dominate perceptual classification. *Child Development, 65*(6), 1627–1645.

Tickle-Degnen, L., and Rosenthal, R. (1990). The behavioral and cognitive response of brain-damaged patients to therapist instructional style. *Occupational Therapy Journal of Research, 10*(6), 345–359.

Tien, J.L., and Johnson, H.L. (1985). Black mental health client's preference for therapists: A new look at an old issue. *International Journal of Social Psychiatry, 31*(4), 258–266.

Todisco, M., and Salomone, P.R. (1991, October). Facilitating effective cross-cultural relationships: The White counselor and the Black client. *Journal of Multicultural Counseling and Development, 19*(4), 146–157.

Trinchero, R.L. (1974). The longitudinal measurement of teacher effectiveness: Gains in overall class performance versus changes in pupil aptitude-performance relationships. *California Journal of Educational Research, 25*(3), 121–127.

Turkel, S. (1972). *Working*. New York: Avon Books.

Turner, L.A., Dofny, E.M., and Dutka, S. (1994). Effect of strategy and attribution training on strategy maintenance and transfer. *American Journal on Mental Retardation, 98*(4), 445–454.

Tuters, E. (1988). The relevance of infant observation to clinical training and practice: An interpretation. *Infant Mental Health Journal, 9*(1), 93–104.

Tyler, J.D., and Clar, J.A. (1985). Promoting clinical expertise in academic faculty supervisors. *Professional Psychology Research and Practice, 16*(6), 902–904.

Uhlemann, M. R., Lee, D. Y., and Martin, J. (1993). Perceptions of counselors' intentions with high versus low quality counselor responses. *Canadian Journal of Counseling, 27*(2), 104–112.

Umbach, B., Darch, C., and Halpin, G. (1989). Teaching reading to low performing first-graders in rural schools: A comparison of two instructional approaches. *Journal of Instructional Psychology, 16*(3), 112–121.

Valle, J. D. (1990). The development of a learning styles program in an affluent, suburban New York elementary school. *Journal of Reading, Writing, and Learning Disabilities International, 6*(3), 315–322.

Van der Vleuten, C.P., and Swanson, D.B. (1990). Assessment of clinical skills with standardized patients: State of the art. *Teaching and Learning in Medicine, 2*(2), 58–76.

Van Galen, J. A. (1993). Caring in community: The limitations of compassion in facilitating diversity: Caring across educational boundaries: Redefinitions of caring within and by historically marginalized groups. [Special issue.] *Urban Review 25*(1), 5–24.

Van Riper, C. (1971). *The nature of stuttering.* Englewood Cliffs, NJ: Prentice-Hall.

Van Riper, C. (1973). *The management of stuttering.* Englewood Cliffs, NJ: Prentice-Hall

Van Riper, C. (1978). *Speech correction principles and methods.* Englewood Cliffs, NJ: Prentice-Hall.

Vandercook, T., and York, J. (1990). A team approach to program development and support. In W. Stainback and S. Stainback (Eds.), *Support networks for inclusive schooling: Interdependent integrated education* (pp. 95–122). Baltimore: Paul H. Brookes Publishing Co.

Vandereycken, W., Probst, M., and Van Bellinghen, M. (1992). Treating the distorted body experience of anorexia nervosa patients. 5th Congress of the International Association for Adolescent Health (1991, Montreux, Switzerland). *Journal of Adolescent Health, 13*(5), 403–405.

Vealey, R.S. (1986). Imagery training for performance enhancement. In J.M. William (Ed.), *Applied Sport Psychology,* (pp. 209–234). Los Angeles, CA: Mayfied Publications.

Ventres, W., and Gordon, P. (1990). Communication strategies in caring for the underserved. *Journal of Health Care for the Poor and Underserved, 3,* 305–314.

Vitz, P. (1992). Narrative and counseling, I: From analysis of the past to stories about it. *Journal of Psychology and Theology, 20*(91), 11–19.

Vitz, P.C. (1974). Learning numerical progressions. *Memory and Cognition, 2*(1-A), 121–126.

Volz, H.B., Klevans, D.R., Norton, S.J., and Putens, D.L. (1978). Interpersonal communication skills of speech-language pathology undergraduates: The effects of training. *Journal of Speech and Hearing Disorders, 43*(4), 524–541.

Vontress, C.E. (1974). Barriers in cross-cultural counseling. *Counseling and Values, 18*(3), 160–165.

Vourlekis, B.S., Bembry, J., Hall, G., and Rosenblum, P. (1992). Evaluating the interrater reliability of process recordings. *Research on Social Work Practice, 2*(2), 198–206.

Vrugt, A. (1990). Negative attitudes, nonverbal behavior, and self-fulfilling prophecy in simulated therapy interviews. *Journal of Nonverbal Behavior, 14*(2), 77–86.

Vu, N.V., Barrows, H.S., Marcy, M.L., and Verhulst, S.J., et al. (1992). Six years of comprehensive, clinical, performance-based assessment using standardized patients at the Southern Illinois University School of Medicine. *Academic Medicine, 67*(1), 42–50.

Wade, P., and Bernstein, B.L. (1991). Culture sensitivity training and counselor's race: Effects on Black female clients' perceptions and attrition. *Journal of Counseling Psychology, 38*(1), 9–15.

Walker, H.M. (1979). *The acting-out child.* Boston: Allyn and Bacon.

Walsh, M.E., and Buckley, M.A. (1994). Children's experiences of homelessness: Implications for school counselors. *Elementary School Guidance and Counseling, 29*(1), 9–15.

Ward, L. M. (1994). Supramodal and modality-specific mechanisms for stimulus-driven shifts of auditory and visual attention: Shifts of visual attention. [Special issue.] *Canadian Journal of Experimental Psychology, 48*(2), 242–259.

Waters, H.S., and Andreassen, C. (1983). Children's use of memory strategies under instruction. In M. Pressley and J.R. Levin (Eds.), *Cognitive strategy research: Psychological foundations* (pp. 3–24). New York: Springer-Verlag.

Watkins, C.E., and Terrell, F. (1988). Mistrust level and its effects on counseling expectations in Black client-White counselor relationships: An analogue study. *Journal of Counseling Psychology, 35*(2), 194–197.

Watkins, C.E., Terrell, F., Miller, F.S., and Terrell, S.L. (1989). Cultural mistrust and its effects on expectational variables in Black client-White counselor relationships. *Journal of Counseling Psychology, 36*(4), 447–450.

Watkins, D., and Ismail, M. (1994). Is the Asian learner a rote learner? A Malaysian perspective. *Contemporary Educational Psychology, 19*(4), 483–488.

Watson, K.L., and Lawson, M. J. (1995). Improving access to knowledge: The effect of strategy training for question answering in high school geography. *British Journal of Educational Psychology, 65*(1), 97–111.

Watts, A.W. (1957). *The way of Zen.* New York: New American Library.

Webster, R. (1980). Evolution of a target-based therapy for stuttering. *Journal of Fluency Disorders, 5*, 303–320.

Webster, R.L. (1974). A behavioral analysis of stuttering: Treatment and theory. In K.S. Calhoun, H.E. Adams, and H.E. Mitchel (Eds.), *Innovative treatment methods in psychopathology* (pp. 17–61). New York: John Wiley.

Webster, R.L. (1974). *The precision fluency shaping program: Speech reconstruction for stutterers.* Roanoke, VA: Communications Development Corporation, Ltd.

Webster-Stratton, C., and Herbert, M. (1993). What really happens in parent training? *Behavior Modification, 17*(4), 407-456.

Weeks, J.R., and Cuellar, J. B. (1983). Isolation of older persons: The influence of immigration and length of residence. *Research on Aging, 5*(3), 369–388.

Weisel, A., and Florian, V. (1990). Same- and cross-gender attitudes toward persons with physical disabilities. *Rehabilitation Psychology, 35*(4), 229–238.

Weiss, S.J. (1984). The effect of transition modules on new graduate adaptation. *Research in Nursing and Health, 7*(1), 51–59.

Wertz, R.T., LaPointe, L.L., and Rosenbek, J.C. (1991). *Apaxia of speech in adults.* San Diego, CA: Singular Publishing Group.

Wessler, R.L. (1986). Rational-emotive therapy in groups. In A. Ellis and R. Grieger (Eds.), *Handbook of rational-emotive therapy*, Vol. 2 (pp. 295–314). New York: Springer.

Westbrook, M.T., and Legge, V. (1993). Health practitioners' perceptions of family attitudes toward children with disabilities: A comparison of six communities in a multicultural society. *Rehabilitation Psychology, 38*(3), 177–185.

Westermeyer, J. (1987). Cultural factors in clinical assessment. *Journal of Consulting and Clinical Psychology, 55*(4), 471–478.

Wetzel, C.G., and Wright-Buckley, C. (1988). Reciprocity of self-disclosure: Breakdowns of trust in cross-racial dyads. *Basic and Applied Social Psychology, 9*(4), 277–288.

Wheeler, L., and Reis, H. T. (1991). Self-recording of everyday life events: Origins, types, and uses: Personality and daily experience. [Special issue.] *Journal of Personality, 59*(3), 339–354.

Whitaker, C.A., and Malone, T.P. (1953). *The roots of psychotherapy.* New York: McGraw-Hill.

Whitney, J.L., and Goldstein, H. (1989). Using self-monitoring to reduce disfluencies in speakers with mild aphasia. *Journal of Speech and Hearing Disorders, 54*(4), 576–586.

Wiener, M., Budney, S., Wood, L. and Russell, R.L. (1989). Nonverbal events in psychotherapy: Psychotherapy process research. [Special issue.] *Clinical Psychology Review, 9*(4), 487–504.

Wieselberg, H. (1992). Family therapy and ultra-orthodox Jewish families: A structural approach. *Journal of Family Therapy, 14*(3), 305–329.

Wilkinson, P., and Mynors-Wallis, L. (1994). Problem-solving therapy in the treatment of unexplained physical symptoms in primary care: A preliminary study. *Journal of Psychosomatic Research, 38*(6), 591–598.

Wilkinson, W. K., Parrish, J. M., and Wilson, F. E. (1994). Training parents to observe and record: A data-based outcome evaluation of a pilot curriculum. *Research in Developmental Disabilities, 15*(5), 343–354.

Williams, C., and Bybee, J. (1994). What do children feel guilty about? Developmental and gender differences. *Developmental Psychology, 30*(5), 617–623.

Willingham, D. B., Koroshetz, W. J., Treadwell, J. R., and Bennett, J. P. (1995). Comparison of Huntington's and Parkinson's disease patients' use of advanced information. *Neuropsychology, 9*(1), 39–46.

Willis, J.T. (1988). An effective counseling model for treating the Black family. *Family Therapy, 15*(2), 185–194.

Willoughby, T., and Wood, E. (1994). Elaborative interrogation examined at encoding and retrieval. *Learning and Instruction, 4*(2), 139–149.

Willoughby, T., Wood, E., and Khan, M. (1994). Isolating variables that impact on or detract from the effectiveness of elaboration strategies. *Journal of Educational Psychology, 86*(2), 279–289.

Wilson, B.A., Baddeley, A., Evans, J., and Shiel, A. (1994). Errorless learning in the rehabilitation of memory impaired people. *Neuropsychological Rehabilitation, 4*(3), 307–326.

Wilson, G.T. (1984). Clinical issues and strategies in the practice of behavior therapy. *Annual Review of Behavior Therapy Theory and Practice, 10,* 291–320.

Wilson, G.T. (1989). Behavior therapy. In R.J. Corsini and D. Wedding (Eds.), *Current psychotherapies,* (4th ed., pp. 241–282). Itasca, IL: Peacock.

Wilson, L.L., and Stith, S.M. (1991). Culturally sensitive therapy with Black clients. *Journal of Multicultural Counseling and Development, 19*(1) 32–43.

Winitz, H. (1969). *Articulatory acquisition and behavior.* Englewood Cliffs, NJ: Prentice-Hall.

Winner, E., and Leekam, S. (1991). Distinguishing irony from deception: Understanding the speaker's second-order intention: Perspectives on the child's theory of mind: II. [Special issue.] *British Journal of Developmental Psychology, 9*(2), 257–270.

Winnicott, D.W. (1971). *Playing and reality.* London: Tavistock.

Wiseman, H., and Rice, L.N. (1989). Sequential analyses of therapist-client interaction during change events: A task-focused approach.

Journal of Consulting and Clinical Psychology, 57(2), 281–286.

Wittmer, D.S., and Honig, A.S. (1991). Convergent or divergent? Teacher questions to three-year-old children in day care: Varieties of early child care research. [Special issue.] *Early Child Development and Care, 68,* 141–147.

Wolf, A. (1963). The psychoanalysis of groups. In M. Rosembaum and M. Berger (Eds.), *Group psychotherapy and group function.* New York: Hawthorn.

Wood, D., Bruner, J.S., and Ross, G. (1976). The role of tutoring in problem-solving. *Journal of Child Psychology and Psychiatry, 17,* 89–100.

Wood, E., Miller, G., Symons, S., Canough, T., et al. (1993). Effects of elaborative interrogation on young learners' recall of facts: Strategies instruction. [Special issue.] *Elementary School Journal, 94*(2), 245–254.

Wood, E., Needham, D.R., Williams, J., and Roberts, R. (1994). Evaluating the quality and impact of mediators for learning when using associative memory strategies. *Applied Cognitive Psychology, 8*(7), 679–692.

Wood, E., Willoughby, T., Kaspar, V., and Idle, T. (1994). Enhancing adolescents' recall of factual content: The impact of provided versus self-generated elaborations. *Alberta Journal of Educational Research, 40*(1), 57–65.

Woods, P. (1993). The charisma of the critical other: Enhancing the role of the teacher. *Teaching and Teacher Education, 9*(5–6), 545–557.

Yarczower, M., Kilbride, J.E., and Beck, A.T. (1991). Changes in nonverbal behavior of therapists and depressed patients during cognitive therapy. *Psychological Reports, 69*(3, Pt. 1), 915–919.

Yates, J. (1988). Demography as it affects special education. In A.A. Ortiz and B.A. Ramirez (Eds.), *Schools and the culturally diverse exceptional student: Promising practices and future directions.* Reston, VA: Council for Exceptional Children.

Yetman, N.R. (Ed.). (1985). *Majority and minority: The dynamics of race and ethnicity in American life* (4th ed.). Boston: Allyn and Bacon.

Zeskind, P.S. (1983). Cross-cultural differences in maternal perceptions of cries of low- and high-risk infants. *Child Development, 54*(5), 1119–1128.

Zabrucky, K., and Commander, N. (1993). Rereading to understand: The role of text coherence and reader proficiency. *Contemporary Educational Psychology, 18*(4), 442–452.

Zarbatany, L., Ghesquiere, K., and Mohr, K. (1992). A context perspective on early adolescents' friendship expectations. *Journal of Early Adolescence, 12*(1), 111–126.

Zimmerman, B.J. (1990). Self-regulating academic learning and achievement: The emergence of a social cognitive perspective. *Educational Psychology Review, 2*(2), 173–201.

Ziter, M.L. (1987). Culturally sensitive treatment of Black alcoholic families. *Social Work, 32*(2), 130–135.

Index